The Anatomy and Physiology Textbook for Midwives

Focusing on optimising the normal biological processes of reproduction and early life, and in line with the Nursing and Midwifery Council (NMC) Future Midwives Standards, this comprehensive textbook introduces the fundamental anatomy and physiology knowledge needed for midwifery practice.

This textbook follows the journey from preconception to the puerperium. Divided into six parts, it begins with foundational material before moving onto reproduction, embryology and fetal development. The central sections of the book consider maternal changes and adaptations during pregnancy, the intrapartum period, and the puerperium and transition from fetal to neonatal life. The book finishes with a section looking at lactation. Containing numerous full colour illustrations, each chapter includes 'Application to practice' boxes, 'challenge' sections and 'interrupters' to help you consolidate your learning. The text is accompanied by a downloadable interactive workbook to complete as you read.

Written in a clear and accessible style, *The Anatomy and Physiology Textbook for Midwives* is an essential read for preregistration midwifery students, studying at both BSc and MSc levels.

Jane Carpenter initially studied biology at BSc, MRes and DPhil level. She then completed her midwifery education. Jane is now Lead Midwife for Education at Oxford Brookes University, with a passion for midwifery education and midwifery research. She also maintains her lifelong love of biology, and more specifically, for all things anatomy and physiology in childbearing related.

Louise Hunter is a midwife and midwifery educator with a keen interest in inclusivity and lactation. A former Lead Midwife for Education, she is now an examiner for the NMC Test of Competence and a Breastfeeding Supporter for the Breastfeeding Network.

The Anatomy and Physiology Textbook for Midwives

Edited by Jane Carpenter and Louise Hunter

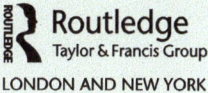
Routledge
Taylor & Francis Group

LONDON AND NEW YORK

Designed cover image: Image designed by Giada Giusmin

First published 2025
by Routledge
4 Park Square, Milton Park, Abingdon, Oxon OX14 4RN

and by Routledge
605 Third Avenue, New York, NY 10158

Routledge is an imprint of the Taylor & Francis Group, an informa business

British Library Cataloguing-in-Publication Data
A catalogue record for this book is available from the British Library

Library of Congress Cataloging-in-Publication Data
Names: Carpenter, Jane, 1971– editor. | Hunter, Louise, editor.
Title: The anatomy and physiology textbook for midwives /
edited by Jane Carpenter and Louise Hunter.
Description: Abingdon, Oxon ; New York, NY : Routledge, 2025. |
Includes bibliographical references and index.
Identifiers: LCCN 2024026151 (print) | LCCN 2024026152 (ebook) |
ISBN 9781032130859 (hardback) | ISBN 9781032130842 (paperback) |
ISBN 9781003227571 (ebook)
Subjects: MESH: Pregnancy–physiology | Reproductive Physiological Phenomena |
Labor, Obstetric–physiology
Classification: LCC RG525 .A64 2025 (print) | LCC RG525 (ebook) | NLM WQ 205 |
DDC 618.2–dc23/eng/20240625
LC record available at https://lccn.loc.gov/2024026151
LC ebook record available at https://lccn.loc.gov/2024026152

ISBN: 9781032130859 (hbk)
ISBN: 9781032130842 (pbk)
ISBN: 9781003227571 (ebk)

DOI: 10.4324/9781003227571

Typeset in Univers Lt
by Newgen Publishing UK

Access the Support Material: www.routledge.com/9781032130842

Contents

About the authors/ editors

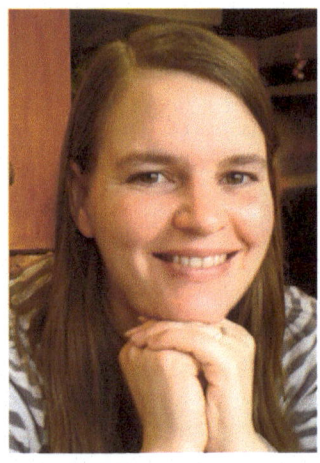

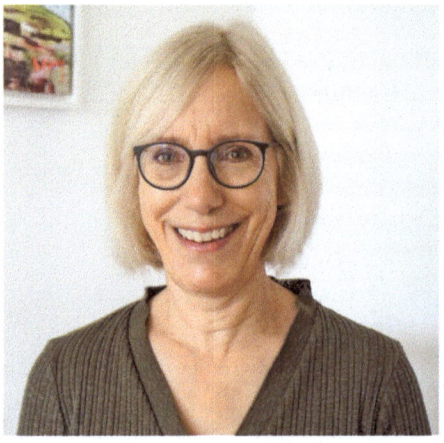

Jane Carpenter

Before becoming a midwife, Jane studied biology at BSc, MRes and DPhil level. She then completed her midwifery education. Jane is now Lead Midwife for Education at Oxford Brookes University, with a passion for midwifery education and midwifery research. She also maintains her lifelong love of biology, and more specifically, for all things anatomy and physiology in childbearing related.

Louise Hunter

Louise is a midwife and midwifery educator with a keen interest in inclusivity and lactation. A former Lead Midwife for Education, she is now an examiner for the NMC Test of Competence and a Breastfeeding Supporter for the Breastfeeding Network.

List of contributors

Key Contributors

Giada Giusmin, *Senior Lecturer, Oxford Brookes University*

Giada qualified as a midwife in Italy, before working in a range of midwifery settings in the UK. As a midwifery educator she has developed significant expertise in complex pregnancies and births and is currently undertaking a Professional Doctorate in Midwifery.

Ginny Mounce, *Senior Lecturer, Oxford Brookes University*

Ginny has practised midwifery in a number of clinical and research settings, developing considerable expertise in reproductive health; which has been invaluable in writing Section 2 of this book.

Contributors

Kirsten Baker, *Associate Lecturer, Oxford Brookes University*

Sarah Fleming, *Senior Lecturer, Oxford Brookes University*

Katherine Palles-Dimmock, *Lecturer, Oxford Brookes University*

Claire Smith, *Senior Lecturer, Oxford Brookes University*

Acknowledgements

We wish to acknowledge Liz Nightingale for helping us to articulate the birth process, Dr Ethel Burns for kindly allowing us to use her antenatal massage instructions, El Johnson from the Breastfeeding Network for reviewing Chapter 6.3, Stacey Zimmels for access to her artwork and Francesca Entwhistle from UNICEF Baby Friendly Initiative (BFI) for permission to use their graphics. We are also indebted to our publishers, and particularly Grace McInnes, who have been extraordinarily patient and have provided key guidance and support throughout.

The idea for this book evolved from the teaching of anatomy and physiology to many student midwife cohorts. We thank them all for their engagement, passion, dedication and encouragement. They have driven us to bring this book into existence. We would also like to thank all of our midwifery and health-care colleagues who have inspired and informed us over the years. This book would not have come to fruition without the love and support of our families, for which we are forever grateful.

How to use this book

The motivation for writing this book was simple; to create an anatomy and physiology textbook which is comprehensive yet easy to understand and that meets the educational needs of midwifery students, educators and practitioners.

The editors and contributors to this book are (or were) all midwives based within a higher education institution in the UK. A key focus, then, was to ensure the book meets the education requirements of student midwives for the UK regulatory body, the NMC. However, it is absolutely the case that the majority of content in this book will apply across the world, and across different health-care professions, giving the book wide-ranging appeal.

The NMC used the ground-breaking Lancet Series on Midwifery (Renfrew, 2014) to 'shape the scope and content' of the NMC Standards of Proficiency for Midwives (NMC, 2019). Set firmly within the Lancet Series, as a core characteristic of midwifery practice, is *optimising the normal biological processes of reproduction and early life.* This is reflected in the NMC Standards of Proficiency for Midwives, set firmly and centrally within the universal care which midwives provide. If midwives are to do this, having a sound underpinning knowledge of the anatomy and physiology of childbearing is crucially important. Hence, the need for this book.

Many midwifery students who come onto our programme feel incredibly nervous, though often equally excited, about learning the anatomy and physiology content.

This perhaps reflects their understanding of its importance, and also a passion to understand what can undeniably be complex content. Our hope is that through this book all readers, whether midwifery students, practicing midwives or other health-care professionals, will gain new and deeper insights into our evolving understanding of the incredible anatomy and physiological processes that enable and protect the formation and sustenance of human life.

Bearing in mind that a certain amount of terminology is unavoidable in a book such as this, we have, as far as possible, written the book in easy to understand, accessible language. In order to further help with this, we have devised an accompanying **workbook** which is packed full of activities to support learning and enable consolidation. As educators committed to inclusivity, we have chosen to make the workbook free to download. To access your workbook simply go to **www.routledge. com/9781032130842**.

As is always the case in a text such as this, we have had to make a number of key decisions as part of the writing process – and we hope you understand our reasons for doing so. Some of these key decisions are set out below.

Structure of the book – the book is structured in a similar way to how we teach the content on our midwifery programmes at Oxford Brookes. The aim is to take the reader on what we hope is a natural journey – from the foundations of life, through reproduction, maternal adaptation to pregnancy, labour, birth and the early postnatal period. It is absolutely the case that the book could have been structured in any number of ways, and that overlap is inevitable where such a wide range of content is covered. Where this occurs, we have made pragmatic decisions with where the content is included and where it is merely referred to. To help with this we refer the reader to the source chapter as appropriate within the text of the book.

Language and cultural orientation – understanding the anatomy and physiology of human childbearing relies on clear understanding of biological sex. Therefore, we made the decision to use sex-based language throughout the main text, to remove any potential for confusion. This is as recommended by the UK Network of Professors of Midwifery and Maternal and Newborn Health (2023) in their position statement, and reflects the language used in the NMC Standards of Proficiency for Midwives (NMC, 2019).

We recognise that not everyone identifies with their sex observed *in utero*/at birth. We fully respect that all those using maternal and reproductive health care and services should receive individualised, respectful care including use of the gender nouns and pronouns they prefer. In some 'Application to practice' boxes, where we are applying the anatomy and physiology content to practice-based examples, it is more appropriate to use additive language, and we have done so on occasion.

We further recognise that, to date, knowledge of anatomy and physiology has been largely based on historical work and teachings of white, male physicians who have largely viewed the world through a colonialist lens, and have, on occasion, violated women's bodies in the pursuit of knowledge. We have tried to apply

a critical, inclusive mindset to received anatomical and physiological knowledge whilst writing this book. For example, many anatomical entities were originally named after a person (often male) and may still be used despite having preferred modern terminology. We use the preferred terminology, but occasionally supply the historical term in brackets for clarity. We recognise that we will doubtless have come up short on occasion, as the science and understanding of childbearing physiology is still developing. We apologise for our shortcomings and pay tribute to all the women who have contributed to our evolving knowledge.

Application to practice boxes – throughout each section of the book we have applied the anatomy and physiology content back to practice-based examples. These aim to demonstrate how core content underpins what student and qualified midwives will observe in practice.

Interrupters – throughout each section of the book are a number of 'Interrupters'. In the most part, these refer the reader to an accompanying section of the workbook and one or more exercises to complete there to embed/consolidate learning. The idea is to encourage the reader to engage fully with this additional resource to enhance understanding of the content.

Challenge sections – in many chapters of the book we have added a 'Chapter challenge'. These sections are there to stretch students, particularly in light of the fact that many midwifery programmes in the UK teach this content to students studying at differing academic 'levels' (for example students studying at MSc level and/or on a shortened route to qualification). These sections often ask students to access research or other articles and apply their learning from the book to this reading, or vice versa.

It has been quite the journey editing this textbook with an amazing group of dedicated contributors. It has also been an absolute joy to slowly but surely see the work come together and come to life (pun intended!). We are thrilled that we have now completed this text, and very much hope that all readers will find it a useful resource whether midwifery student, educator, practitioner or from another profession entirely.

Jane Carpenter and Louise Hunter

The Foundations for Life

Giada Giusmin and Jane Carpenter

*All life begins at the cellular level. Life cannot be without cells – they are the fundamental building block of life – indeed, the foundation for life. Some organisms consist of just one cell, others of billions of cells. Most cells are tiny, requiring a microscope to view, but the largest cell is just visible to the human eye. Over two hundred different types of cells exist in the human body, all functioning in their own way to enable life to continue. Cells come together to form tissues; tissues form organs which make up the human body. Cells ensure the internal environment remains optimal at all times, working and communicating constantly to ensure this is so. We are rarely aware of our cells doing their work, and yet it is happening in every human, indeed in all life, all of the time. In order to understand anything about how the human body works, we must, then, start with the **foundations for life**.*

DOI: 10.4324/9781003227571-1

The human cell

Jane Carpenter

The cell

The cell is the most fundamental structural and functional unit of any living organism. All living organisms are made up of at least one cell, making them the essential requirement for life.

Cells that make up animals, plants and fungi are **eukaryotic**, whereas **prokaryotic** cells are found in bacteria. Eukaryotic cells contain a nucleus enclosed in a nuclear envelope, whereas prokaryotes do not. There are further differences between animal cells and the other eukaryotic cells, in particular, animal cells do not have a cell wall.

In humans, there are more than 200 different cell types, performing different functions and therefore consisting of a wide variety of shapes and sizes. The largest human cell is the oocyte, just visible to the naked eye. However, most cells are smaller and invisible to the naked eye. Indeed, in order to observe any cell in detail, an electron microscope is required.

Despite such variety in size, shape and function, there are certain features common to all or most human cells. Therefore, it is helpful to consider the generic, or **composite**, human cell first, before considering how and why our cells differ. Figure 1.1.1 shows a composite human cell.

Components of the human cell

The human cell is surrounded by a **plasma membrane**. This plasma membrane surrounds the **cytoplasm**, which is the intracellular fluid, containing a number of **organelles** – small structures carrying out various cell functions. The **nucleus** is usually found towards the centre of the cell

DOI: 10.4324/9781003227571-2

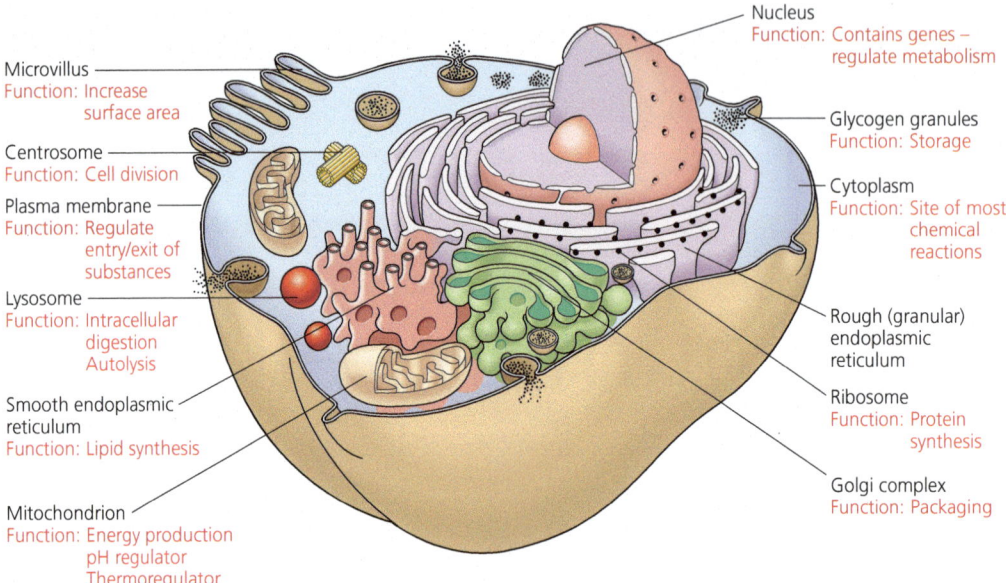

Microvillus
Function: Increase surface area

Centrosome
Function: Cell division

Plasma membrane
Function: Regulate entry/exit of substances

Lysosome
Function: Intracellular digestion Autolysis

Smooth endoplasmic reticulum
Function: Lipid synthesis

Mitochondrion
Function: Energy production pH regulator Thermoregulator

Nucleus
Function: Contains genes – regulate metabolism

Glycogen granules
Function: Storage

Cytoplasm
Function: Site of most chemical reactions

Rough (granular) endoplasmic reticulum

Ribosome
Function: Protein synthesis

Golgi complex
Function: Packaging

Figure 1.1.1 Diagram of a composite human cell
Source: Figure 2.3, p.24, Clancy and McVicar (2009)

and controls the cell's activity. Below, we consider each of these in more detail.

Plasma membrane

The human cell is enclosed in the plasma membrane (Figure 1.1.1). This separates the cytoplasm and internal cell components from the extracellular fluid.

The main component of the plasma membrane structure is the **phospholipid bilayer**. These phospholipids consist of a **hydrophilic** (water-loving) head and a **hydrophobic** (water-hating) tail. Thus, the heads naturally turn to face fluid and the tails naturally turn away from fluid. In the case of the plasma membrane, the two layers (bilayer) lie tail-to-tail, with the water-loving heads facing out towards the intra- and extracellular fluid (Figure 1.1.2).

Although the main structure of the plasma membrane is the phospholipid bilayer, up to 20% can be made up of cholesterol. Also polar, it wedges into the phospholipid

tail structure and provides strength to the membrane.

As shown in Figure 1.1.2, the membrane contains a number of additional elements – the membrane proteins. These membrane proteins are important to help the plasma membrane carry out its four key functions:

▶ **Barrier** – The phospholipid bilayer, strengthened with cholesterol, provides a physical barrier between the inside of the cell and the extracellular environment.
▶ **Regulation** – The plasma membrane is selectively permeable, determining which materials move in and out of the cell.
▶ **Communication** – Membrane proteins interact with chemical messengers to relay messages to the cell interior.
▶ **Cell recognition** – Carbohydrates on the cell surface allow cells to recognise each other.

Proteins in the cell membrane can either be **integral** or **peripheral**. Integral proteins are

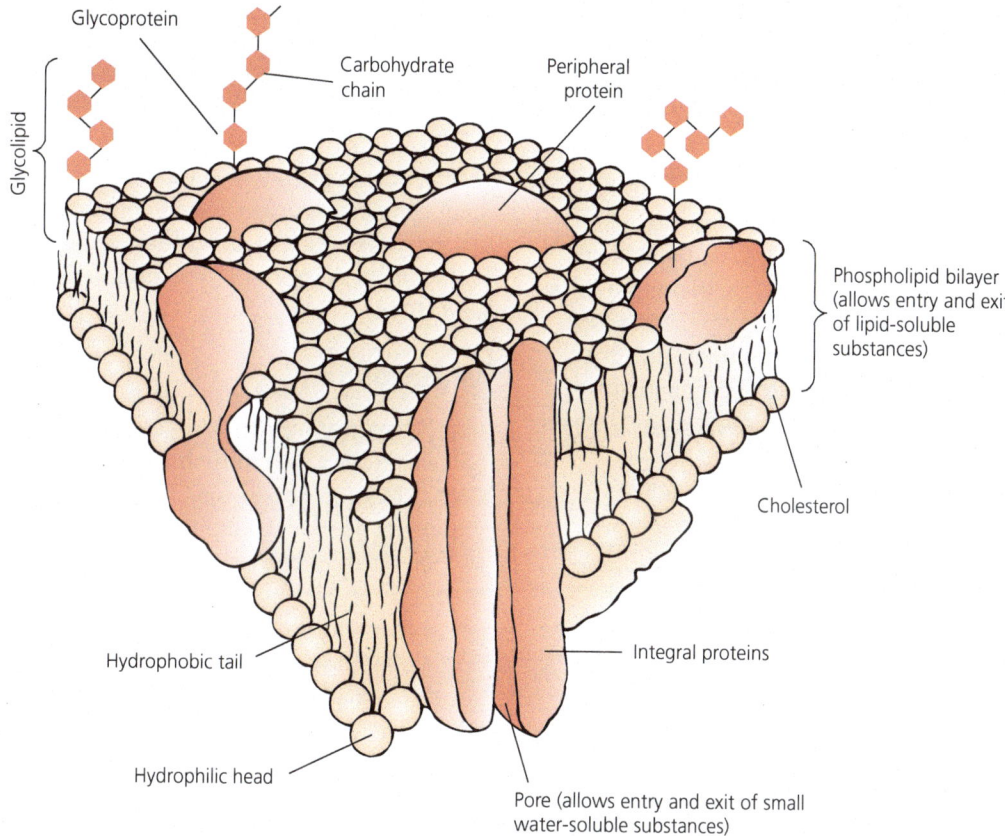

Glycoprotein

Carbohydrate chain

Peripheral protein

Glycolipid

Phospholipid bilayer (allows entry and exit of lipid-soluble substances)

Cholesterol

Hydrophobic tail

Integral proteins

Hydrophilic head

Pore (allows entry and exit of small water-soluble substances)

Figure 1.1.2 Structure of the plasma membrane
Source: Figure 2.4, p.26, Clancy and McVicar (2009)

embedded in, and often pass right through, the lipid bilayer. Peripheral proteins are not embedded in the bilayer, and instead may attach to other integral proteins, or to the bilayer itself.

Integral proteins may transport ions or small water-soluble molecules via 'channels' through their centre. Others may act as a carrier transporting substances through the bilayer, as hormone receptors enabling communication or as enzymes. Peripheral proteins are involved in maintaining cell structure and linking cells together.

Across the extracellular surface, most proteins and some of the lipids have a carbohydrate chain attached (Figure 1.1.2). If attached to a protein, this is known

as a **glycoprotein**, if attached to a lipid it is known as a **glycolipid**. These glycoproteins and glycolipids are important in creating identity markers by which cells can recognise each other – and can also recognise cells which are foreign to the body.

Cytoplasm

The cytoplasm of the human cell consists of all of the material inside the cell, but outside of the nucleus. All of the organelles of the cell are contained in the cytoplasm.

Two key components of the cytoplasm are the **cytosol** and the **cytoskeleton**. It is often assumed that the inside of the cell is something of a liquid-mush – however, this is not the case. In fact, both the cytosol and cytoskeleton give the cell structure and strength, enabling it to carry out its function.

The cytosol is the fluid component of the cytoplasm, containing the cell organelles. This usually colourless fluid can vary from a watery solution to a thick gel-like substance, pushing against the cell membrane and helping to give the cell structure. Although composed of approximately 80% water, it also contains various salts, fats, sugars and other substances to help the cell function.

The cytoskeleton is a highly organised framework of protein filaments, providing a skeletal-like structure to the cell and situating the organelles within the cell.

Cell organelles

Each cell contains a number of organelles – 'mini organs'. Many of these organelles are bound by a membrane. This is important, as by having their own membrane they can maintain an internal environment which differs from that of the cell's cytoplasm.

Nucleus

The nucleus is a membrane-bound organelle, often referred to as the 'control centre' of the cell. Most cells contain just one nucleus – although some cells, such as some muscle cells, are **multinucleate**, and red blood cells are **anucleate** (do not contain a nucleus).

The **nuclear membrane** surrounds the nucleoplasm, nucleolus and chromatin. **Nuclear pores** located at various points around the nuclear membrane allow the movement of substances into and out of the nucleus. The gelatinous **nucleoplasm** is similar to the cytosol, containing dissolved nutrients and situating the other nuclear

components. The **nucleoli** (usually one or two per nucleus) facilitate the synthesis of ribosomes. **Chromatin** is the complex of **deoxyribonucleic acid (DNA)** and histone proteins that, when condensed, form chromosomes within the nucleus. DNA contains the specific instructions for life that make each of us unique. Proteins are synthesised from DNA by **ribonucleic acid (RNA)**.

Mitochondria

Mitochondria are complex organelles containing their own **mitochondrial DNA**, **RNA** and **ribosomes**. They can be thought of as the 'powerhouse' of the cell, as their main function is the production of adenosine triphosphate (ATP) – the energy carrying molecule in cells. This is completed via aerobic respiration: the stored chemical energy in glucose reacts with oxygen and forms ATP. Therefore, the number of mitochondria in a cell will reflect its function; cells with high energy requirements, such as muscle and liver cells, are packed with mitochondria, whereas other cells may only have one or two.

Mitochondria are surrounded by an outer membrane. The inner membrane is thrown into folds known as **cristae**. These folds increase the surface area of the mitochondria increasing its ability to produce ATP.

Ribosomes

Ribosomes are the site of protein synthesis in the cell and are comprised of proteins and **ribosomal RNA**. **Free ribosomes** float freely in the cytosol, whereas **fixed** (or membrane-bound) **ribosomes** are attached to the rough endoplasmic reticulum. The ribosomes can switch between these two types, attaching and detaching from the endoplasmic reticulum as required.

Endoplasmic reticulum

This system of membranes and tubes continues out from the nuclear membrane. **Rough endoplasmic reticulum (RER)** is studded with ribosomes along its membrane surface. Proteins synthesised by these ribosomes then progress into the RER tubes, move along these and are packaged into vesicles where they are transported to the Golgi apparatus. All proteins which go on to be secreted by cells are produced by the RER. **Smooth endoplasmic reticulum (SER)** is continuous with the RER and consists of a network of tubules. Its functions include steroid and lipid synthesis, regulation of intracellular calcium levels, breakdown of stored glycogen into glucose (particularly in the liver) and drug detoxification.

Golgi apparatus/complex

The Golgi apparatus is comprised of a series of curved, flattened membranous sacs, surrounded by vesicles. The main function of the apparatus is to modify, sort and package proteins made in the RER in readiness for export from the cell.

Lysosomes

Spherical or oval in shape, and surrounded by a single membrane, lysosomes contain **hydrolytic** (digestive) enzymes. These enzymes can digest almost any molecule. Lysosomes are abundant in phagocytes – white blood cells which destroy bacteria, foreign particles and dying cells.

Perioxisomes

Perioxisomes appear like a small lysosome. They contain enzymes including **oxidases**. Oxidases use oxygen to detoxify substances, being particularly important for detoxifying **free radicals**. If allowed to accumulate in cells, free radicals can be destructive and dangerous. Perioxisomes tend to be abundant in the kidney and liver, which have important roles in detoxification.

INTERRUPTER

Using the relevant table in your workbook (or create your own), in your own words summarise the structure and function of the different cell organelles.

Extracellular substances

Extracellular substances comprise any substance outside of the cell which contributes to body mass. The **extracellular matrix (ECM)** is the non-cellular component of tissue, secreted by cells into the surrounding medium. The basic composition of the ECM is usually a gelatinous mixture of water, proteins and sugar. However, ECM composition can differ substantially within each tissue depending on its function. For example, in connective tissue such as bone, the ECM is mineralised and hardened.

Extracellular fluid (ECF) constitutes all the body *fluid* outside of the cells. It includes the blood plasma and cerebrospinal fluid, which transport substances around the body, and the **interstitial fluid**, which surrounds cells in the tissues and from which each cell draws its functional requirements. Certain cells also **secrete** extracellular substances, such as those required for digestion, or which lubricate.

Cell differentiation

There are over 200 types of cells in the human body. These **differentiated** cells perform specific functions. In order to perform this function, a particular shape and structure is required, hence the need for differentiation. For example, a nerve cell has a very different shape and structure to an epithelial cell. This is explained in more detail in Chapter 1.2.

Differentiation comes at a cost, however, as these specialised cells often cannot replenish themselves. Therefore, the body needs to maintain some undifferentiated cells so that specialised cells can be replenished. These undifferentiated cells, known as **stem cells**, can divide and/or develop into specialised cells. **Embryonic stem cells** are found only in the earliest stages of embryo development and may develop into any specialised cell. **Tissue stem cells** are found throughout life and enable replenishment of a reduced group of specialised cells. For example, blood stem cells are produced in the bone marrow, and can then develop into the various blood cell types.

Further reading

Alberts, B. *Molecular biology of the cell* (7th edition). New York: Garland Science, 2022.

Kabekkodu S.P., Chakrabarty S. et al. Mitochondrial biology: From molecules to diseases. *Mitochondrion* 2015, 24:93–8. doi:10.1016/j.mito.2015.07.008.

Picard M., Wallace D.C. et al. The rise of mitochondria in medicine. *Mitochondrion* [Internet] 2016, 30:105–16. https://pubmed.ncbi.nlm.nih.gov/27423788/.

Walters A.D., Bommakanti A. et al. Shaping the nucleus: Factors and forces. *J. Cell Biochem.* [Internet] 2012, 113(9):2813–21. https://pubmed.ncbi.nlm.nih.gov/22566057/.

CHAPTER 1.2

Tissues

Giada Giusmin

LEARNING OUTCOMES

▶ Understand the four key types of tissue found in the human body
▶ Explain the basic structure and function of these four tissue types

From cell to tissue

Even though there are around 200 types of cells differing by structure, these can be grouped into categories according to their ability to perform a common or related function. Differentiated cells together form tissues, which have a specialised function, tissues then combine with other tissues to form organs, which in turn, when grouped together, become organ systems (Figure 1.2.1).

There are four main types of tissues, and each of them includes subtypes:

▶ Epithelial tissue
▶ Muscle tissue
▶ Connective tissue
▶ Nervous tissue

Epithelial tissue

Epithelial cells cover the internal and external surfaces of organs, for example forming the lining of blood vessels and lungs, or the outer layer of the skin. Epithelial tissue cells are closely packed and the intercellular substance is minimal.

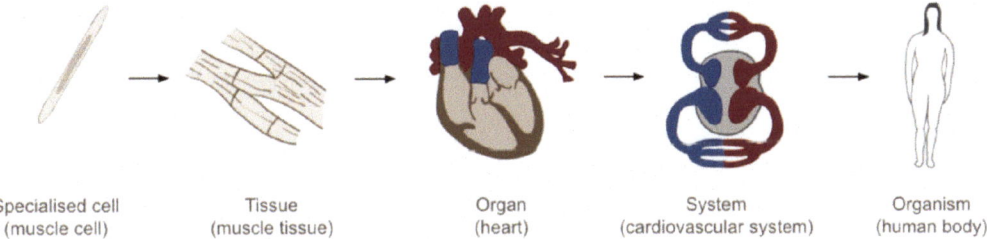

| Specialised cell (muscle cell) | Tissue (muscle tissue) | Organ (heart) | System (cardiovascular system) | Organism (human body) |

Figure 1.2.1 From cell to organism

DOI: 10.4324/9781003227571-3

The epithelium is also avascular, which means there are no blood vessels, but it is innervated. Epithelial cells are supported by nourishment coming from blood vessels present in the underlying connective tissue. The basal membrane is then responsible for the nutrients' diffusion to the layers. When there is more than one layer of epithelial cells, these are polarised, meaning they have different characteristics depending on their position. This enables the cells to take part in specialised functions such as secretion, absorption, transport, protection, filtration and sensory perception.

Epithelial cells are classified by their shape, being either **cuboidal**, **columnar** or **squamous**, and by the number of layers of cells, being either simple or stratified (Tables 1.2.1 and 1.2.2). **Simple** refers to when there is a single layer, and cells are all in contact with the basement membrane. This type is more likely to be located on absorptive or secretive surfaces. **Stratified** refers to when there are numerous layers made of cells of different shapes. This type is usually found where underlying structures need to be protected from mechanical damage.

The skin

The skin is not only a specialised epithelial layer but also the largest organ in the body. The skin can be divided into two main layers, the epidermis (superficial) and the dermis. In the **epidermis**, epithelial cells which are generated in the basal layer (where cell division occurs) are generally cuboidal. Then, as new cell layers are formed, these get pushed towards the surface, which means they are further away from the nourishment. When the cells reach the skin surface, they have become dead stratified keratinised squamous epithelium.

This means that these cells' cytoplasm has been enriched with keratin (which makes them waterproof), enabling the barrier function provided by the skin. The **dermis**, on the other hand, is made of connective tissue. The dermis contains a number of structures, such as blood and lymph vessels, nerves, hair, glands and ducts.

Muscle tissue

Myocytes (muscle cells) originate from the mesodermal layer of the embryo. These cells can generate the mechanical force necessary to move the body, or substances within the body, by contracting and relaxing.

Muscle tissue can be classified into three categories: **skeletal** muscle tissue, **cardiac** muscle tissue and **smooth** muscle tissue.

Skeletal muscle

Skeletal muscle can be attached to the bones (by tendons), for example, to control movement and posture of the skeleton, or to the skin, to control facial expressions. Skeletal muscle contractions are usually voluntary (under conscious control) as these are initiated by the central nervous system. As shown in Figure 1.2.2, skeletal muscle fibres have stripes visible using a microscope, for this reason, they are called striated.

Skeletal muscle fibres, which are organised in parallel bundles, can be divided into slow-twitch and fast-twitch fibres. Slow-twitch fibres are red in appearance because they are formed by numerous capillaries and rely upon aerobic metabolism. These can contract for a prolonged period of time. Fast-twitch fibres use anaerobic metabolism and contract much more than slow-twitch fibres, however, they tire quickly.

Table 1.2.1 Types of simple epithelium

1.2

Simple epithelium	Description	Location
Squamous	A single layer of slim cells that are very close to one another This allows diffusion to occur smoothly	• Alveoli of the lungs • Blood and lymph vessels (endothelium) • Glomeruli of the kidney • Endocardium in the heart
Cuboidal	A single layer of cube-shaped cells tightly adjacent to one another Usually involved in absorption and secretion	• Kidney tubules • Thyroid
Columnar	A single layer of tall cells which, as the cuboidal epithelium, is involved in secretive and absorptive functions Can also have microvilli or cilia on its top surface	• Small intestine (with microvilli to enhance the absorption of nutrients) • Trachea (with cilia to move mucus upward)
Pseudostratified columnar	As the name suggests, this epithelium appears to be stratified but, in fact, is made of a single layer of irregularly shaped columnar cells These are all in contact with the basement membrane	Upper respiratory tract where it might have cilia on the top surface

(*Continued*)

Table 1.2.2 Types of stratified epithelium

Stratified epithelium	Description	Location
Cuboidal	Cuboidal cells arranged in multiple layers The main function is protection	Ducts of: • Sweat glands • Mammary glands • Salivary glands
Columnar	Columnar cells arranged in multiple layers The main function is to protect	• Ducts of some glands • Male urethra
Squamous	Made of multiple layers of cells, which are usually columnar, close to the basement membrane The closer these get to the top surface, the thinner they become, until they shed Their main function is to protect from mechanical damage	• Mouth • Oesophagus • Vagina
Transitional	A type of epithelium that allows the organs to stretch It appears cuboidal when relaxed and squamous when stretched	Bladder and other organs of the urinary system

1.2

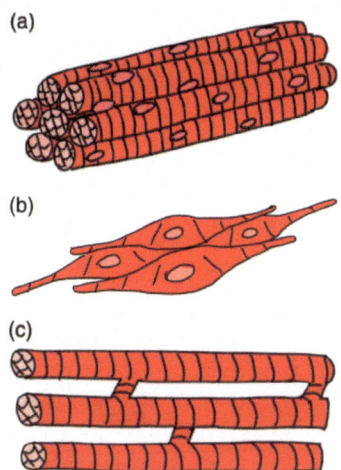

(a)

(b)

(c)

Figure 1.2.2 Three types of muscle cells. a) Skeletal, b) Smooth, and c) Cardiac

Smooth muscle

Smooth muscle is called smooth because there are no visible striations. It is under involuntary control, as it is innervated by the autonomic nervous system (see Chapter 3.3). However, smooth muscle is not just controlled by the autonomic nervous system, but also hormones and metabolites that affect its contractility.

It is usually found in the vascular, digestive, respiratory and urinary systems, as well as the uterus, i.e. mostly hollow organs. Cell junctions are responsible for linking the smooth muscle cells and allowing them to contract slowly for a long period of time.

Smooth muscle is important for maintaining the function of some essential body systems. For example, in order to maintain stable blood pressure, the smooth muscle layer of the blood vessels contracts and relaxes when required. When the smooth muscle contracts, the internal diameter of the blood vessels is reduced (vasoconstriction) and the blood pressure increases. On the other hand, when the smooth muscle relaxes, the internal diameter of the blood vessels is increased and the blood pressure is reduced (vasodilation).

As the smooth muscle contracts and relaxes, creating synchronised waves, this generates peristaltic movement, which allows unidirectional flow of the contents within the lumen (hollow centre) of the organ. For example, this occurs after eating a meal, when peristaltic contractions allow the ingested food to move through the bowel to be digested.

Cardiac muscle

Cardiac muscle (made of myocytes, heart muscle cells) is only found in the walls of the heart and is under involuntary control and therefore, cannot be consciously controlled by an individual. Cardiac muscle is structurally similar to skeletal muscle, with striations visible under a microscope. However, rather than being in parallel bundles, cardiac muscle fibres branch. As shown in Figure 1.2.2, these are microscopic joints, called intercalated discs, which join adjacent cardiac muscle cells. These junctions are important as they enable coordinated contractions of the heart so that myocytes do not need to be stimulated individually.

Connective tissue

The main functions of connective tissue are to connect and provide support to body structures, as well as facilitate the diffusion of nutrients and oxygen from the vascular system and return waste products back to it. It also works as a fuel reserve and as insulation to the body – body organs are insulated and protected by fat, which also provides a fuel reserve. It is not surprising that connective tissue is the most abundant

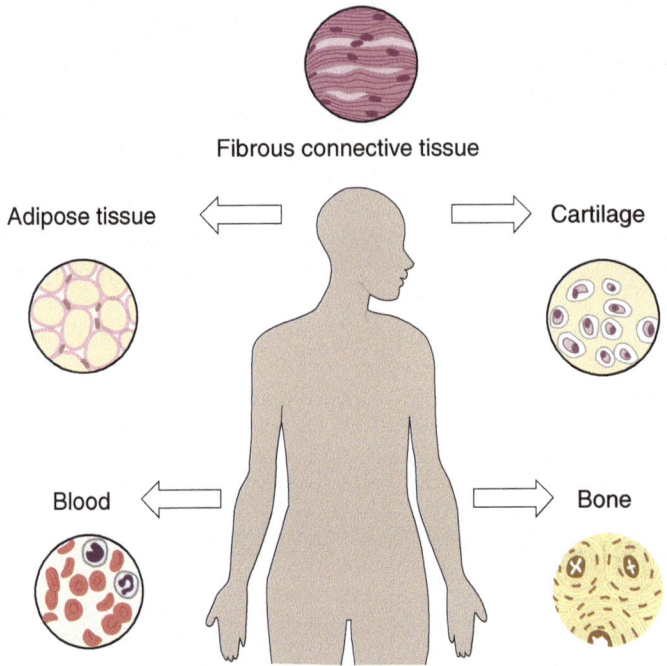

Figure 1.2.3 Different types of connective tissue

tissue in the body, and apart from the blood, it is found in all organs.

The cells of connective tissue include:

▶ Fibroblasts, large cells which produce collagen and elastin fibres
▶ Adipocytes, also known as fat cells
▶ Macrophages, mast cells and leukocytes, which will be discussed in the immune system chapter (see Chapter 3.8)

Connective tissue can generally be classified into **connective tissue proper**, further divided into loose and dense (or fibrous) connective tissue, and **special connective tissue**. Loose connective tissue is the most abundant and its function is to link and support other tissues, such as blood vessels under the skin. Dense connective tissue is made by tightly packed collagen fibres giving strength and structure. Dense connective tissue is generally found as a protective covering of some organs such as the brain; or when

forming ligaments which connect bone to bone. Special connective tissue includes blood and lymphatic fluid (further described in Chapters 3.1 and 3.8, respectively), bone and cartilage (further described in Chapter 3.5), reticular connective tissue, usually found in the lymphatic system and adipose tissue. Figure 1.2.3 shows some of the different types of connective tissue.

Nervous tissue

Nervous tissue is comprised of nerve cells, called neurons, cells of the neuroglia (Figure 1.2.4). The neurons' main function is to initiate and conduct electrical signals to control and regulate all body functions. In order to do this, neurons are formed by:

▶ Dendrites (which receive and respond to electrochemical signals)
▶ A cell body
▶ Axons (which transmit the signal to the

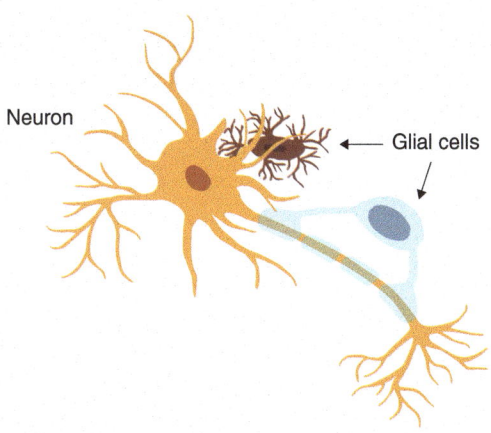

Neuron

Glial cells

1.2

Figure 1.2.4 Nervous tissue

next neuron, often covering considerable distances)

As neurons are so specialised once developed, they rarely undergo further mitotic division. For this reason, during fetal and childhood development, there is an

additional number of neurons compared to the actual number required. Throughout life, neurons then become dysfunctional and die, leading to a marked neurological decline later on in life.

To maintain neuron function, glial cells are necessary for providing support and nourishment. These also help with the propagation of the electrical impulses in the neurons; however, these are non-conducting.

Glial cells, unlike neurons, will carry on replicating throughout life.

INTERRUPTER

Use the boxes in the tissue section of your workbook, or draw your own, to summarise the structure and function of each of the different types of tissue.

Homeostasis

Giada Giusmin

Homeostasis

Homeostasis is the state in which all the organs and physiological systems work together to maintain a constant internal environment. Even when conditions in the external environment change, the internal constancy, despite some minor variations, is kept within narrow limits. This is regulated by the endocrine system, the nervous system and behavioural factors.

Examples of homeostasis in the human species include maintaining stable electrolyte concentrations to regulate pH and water balance as well as blood pressure, and also thermoregulation.

In order to maintain the homeostasis of a specific variable, three main components are necessary (Figure 1.3.1):

▶ The receptor, which detects the change in the variable and sends the input to the next component.
▶ The control centre, which is responsible for setting the range in which the variable needs to be maintained. This component is also necessary for analysing the stimuli against the set range and regulating the response.
▶ The effector system, which is in charge of reinstating the stability by acting on the control centre's signals to correct the deviation from the range.

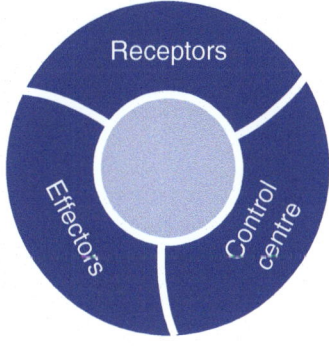

Figure 1.3.1 The three components for homeostatic control

DOI: 10.4324/9781003227571-4

Negative feedback loop and thermoregulation

In order to maintain homeostasis, the main mechanisms used are **negative feedback loops**. In this case, once a variable is lower or higher than the set range, negative feedback ensures that this variable is raised or lowered to return to homeostasis. Once constancy has been achieved thanks to the effector system, this feeds back to the regulator and the stimulus ceases to exist. A perfect representation of this is thermoregulation.

In the human body, a relatively constant internal temperature is required. A key reason for this is to protect the enzymes responsible for biochemical and metabolic functions. These enzymes are vulnerable to varying internal temperatures, as this can denature their protein structure. Homeostatic processes prevent this from happening, by maintaining the internal temperature within a tight range.

As shown in Figure 1.3.2, a rise or a drop in temperature will be detected by specialised nerve endings on the skin. This information will then be communicated to the hypothalamus, the temperature control centre, located in the brain. Following the receipt of this information, the hypothalamus will then stimulate the effector system to set in motion mechanisms that can lower or raise the body temperature. For example, if our body temperature is low, our muscles will involuntarily contract to cause shivering which will cause the production of heat (and we will be likely to add an extra layer of clothing!). In addition to this, our blood vessels will become narrower (vasoconstrict) to prevent heat loss by reducing the blood flow to the skin.

Once the body temperature has returned to normal, specialised nerve endings will cease sending signals to the hypothalamus, and the effector system will then stop activating mechanisms to raise or drop

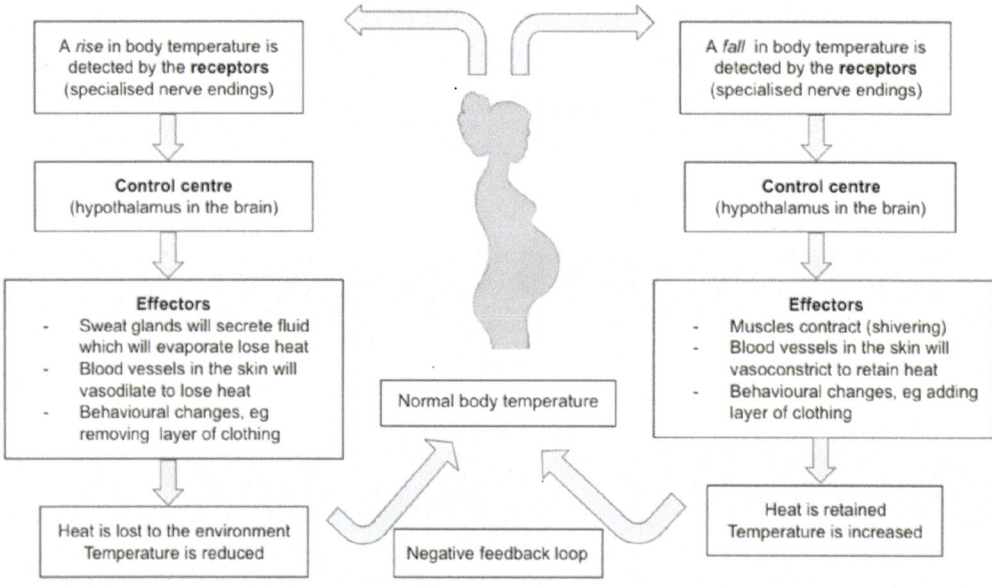

Figure 1.3.2 Thermoregulation

the temperature. This will lead the skeletal muscles to stop shivering, in case of an initially low temperature, or if the initial temperature is high, this will put a stop to the production of sweat.

Acid-base homeostasis

Understanding the acid-base balance is important for midwives as an imbalance in this homeostatic process can severely affect an individual's well-being.

The pH scale was designed at the beginning of the twentieth century to determine the acidity of a solution in order to detect any changes that could cause imbalances, and possibly ruin the properties of this solution.

The pH scale goes from 0 to 14 (Figure 1.3.3), and solutions with a pH of less than 7 are considered acidic (left of the scale), whereas if the pH is above 7 (right of the scale) they are considered basic (alkaline). At a pH of 7, the solution is described as neutral, an example of this is pure water.

In order to determine if a solution is acidic or alkaline, the pH scale is based on the relative concentration of hydrogen (H^+) and hydroxide (OH^-) ions in various fluids. It is important to note that the pH scale is logarithmic, which means there is a tenfold change at every pH point. Therefore, a solution with a pH of 4 contains ten times the hydrogen ions contained in a solution with a pH of 5. At a pH of 7, the number of hydrogen ions is equal to the hydroxide ions.

The pH level of body fluids is generally tightly controlled (homeostatic) and is carefully regulated by some buffering chemicals found in the body fluids. Their function is to take up hydrogen and hydroxide ions in order to maintain the pH within a very narrow range. However, this can only happen if the respiratory and renal systems are working properly to excrete the excess acids and bases.

A critical example of homeostasis is the blood pH level, which must be between

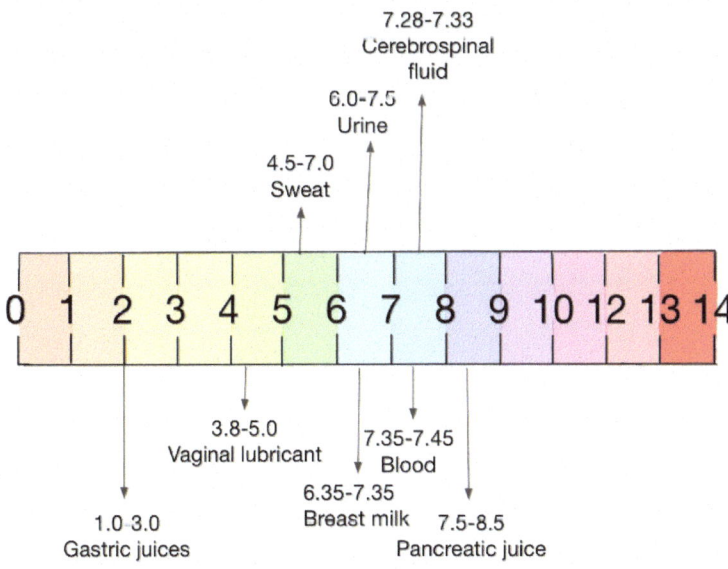

Figure 1.3.3 Examples of body fluids and their pH
Source: Image modified from Clancy and McVicar (2009)

7.35 and 7.45 in order to prevent cell death. As CO_2 increases, hydrogen ions (H^+) make the pH more acidic, lungs help the excretion of CO_2 during respiration. The brain will detect the rising level of H^+ in the blood and then stimulate the lungs to breathe out CO_2, which in turn will reduce the H^+ level. On the opposite side, if the blood pH is too basic, the brain will slow down the breathing process to retain CO_2 and increase H^+ levels. The renal system is also involved in blood pH homeostasis by having the kidneys regulate the excretion of H^+ and bicarbonate when needed.

In conclusion, there are many ways in which the body maintains homeostasis, mostly by using negative feedback loops. However, when maintaining homeostasis is not the primary goal, our body can also use positive feedback loops to ensure other vital functions.

Positive feedback loop and haemostasis

A **positive feedback loop** describes the mechanism by which the stimulus amplifies the response by the control centre, rather than trying to maintain homeostasis. Therefore, as long as the initial stimulus continues, the response will increase. This can be observed during labour when the production of oxytocin keeps increasing as long as the fetal head stretches the cervix and then the pelvic floor (see Chapters 4.2 and 4.3). The production of oxytocin stops shortly after the baby is born, and there is no further pressure on the soft tissues of the pelvis.

Blood clotting also follows a positive feedback loop. Once a blood vessel has been injured, chemical signals are emitted to attract platelets. The more platelets arrive, the greater the signal to attract more platelets to the injured area. This continues until the clot is sufficiently large to stop the bleeding and hence, obtain haemostasis.

Reproduction and Fetal Development

Ginny Mounce

Reproduction is essential for life itself; all life on earth, and therefore our very existence depends on the processes by which new organisms are formed. In the human body the systems of reproduction fulfil this function with astounding complexity, ensuring survival of our species across generations. For individuals, reproduction itself is not necessary for a successful or complete life course, although physiological health is impacted by reproductive system functioning.

This section describes the processes of human reproduction, from a cellular through to system level, by which reproductive cells are formed and then brought together to form a new individual.

DOI: 10.4324/9781003227571-5

Mitosis and meiosis

Ginny Mounce

LEARNING OUTCOMES

▶ Understand the key elements of the cell cycle

▶ Define mitosis, and detail the different stages of the mitotic process

▶ Define meiosis, and detail the different stages of the meiotic process

The cell cycle

Cellular activities (see Section 1) maintain the life of cells on a daily basis. However, as cells age, are damaged or become exhausted, they are replaced by a process of cell division where cells reproduce themselves. The cell cycle is the name of the orderly sequence of events which occur when cells replicate and make new cells.

There are two types of cell division; somatic (body) cell division called **mitosis**, and reproductive cell division called **meiosis**. In mitosis, the nuclear and cytoplasmic division results in two identical daughter cells. Each daughter cell has duplicate **chromosomes** of the original cell.

In humans, body cells have 23 pairs (sets) of chromosomes (46 in total). In cell biology, since **n** is the number of sets of chromosomes in a cell, human somatic cells are described as **diploid** (2n), with *dipl* meaning 'double'. **Meiosis** (described below) is reproductive cell division that creates sex cells, or **gametes**, which are **haploid** (n) and have 23 chromosomes, with *hapl* meaning 'single'.

Somatic cell division occurs continuously as the cells and tissues of the body grow or are replaced. However, the cell cycle, although continuous, is usually described as a series of events to aid understanding. There are two main phases: **interphase**, when the cell is not dividing, and the **mitotic (M) phase**, when the cell is dividing. A cell spends the majority of its lifetime in interphase; growing, replicating its chromosomes and manufacturing other components in preparation for cell division. Unsurprisingly, interphase is a period of high metabolic activity. Interphase has three named stages: G_1, **S** and G_2.

The overall sequence of events in the cell cycle is: G_1 phase, S phase, G_2 phase, mitosis and cytokinesis (Figure 2.1.1).

DOI: 10.4324/9781003227571-6

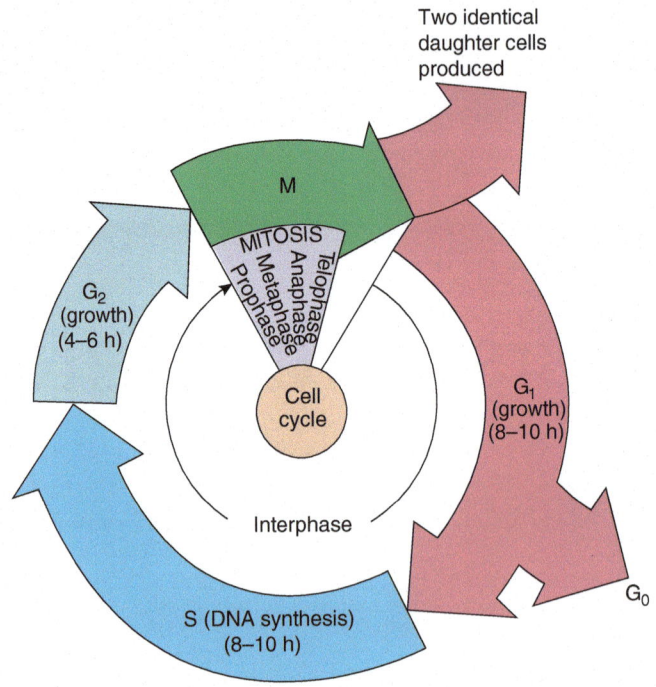

Figure 2.1.1 The cell cycle
Source: Figure 2.15b, p.43, Clancy and McVicar (2009)

Interphase

The interval called **G₁ phase** (named as this is the **G**ap between chromosome duplication) is when the cell components and organelles *other* than chromosomes are duplicated. Most normal cellular activities occur during G₁. A typical somatic cell cycle might be 24 hours, and G₁ could last 8–10 hours (although this varies from minutes to many hours depending on cell type). The **S** (named for **S**ynthesis) **phase** is where the cell's DNA, which makes up its chromosomes, is replicated. This ensures the daughter cells have an identical genetic make-up as the original cell. In our typical example, the S phase might last 8–10 hours. At this point, the cell contains an extra copy of genetic material. Note that some cells, for example many nerve cells, stay in the G₁ state for a very long time, perhaps never entering the S phase. These cells are said to be in the G₀ state. All cells that enter the S phase will continue to cell division.

The **G₂ phase** is the shortest; in our example around 4–6 hours. Here, replication is completed, and cell growth and synthesis of enzymes and other molecules continues as preparation for mitotic cell division. A characteristic of interphase is that individual chromosomes appear as a granular mass, called **chromatin**. This is just the way that the chromosome molecules are packed; as large, fairly diffuse loops of DNA and protein molecules. During interphase, the chromatin and nucleolus are visible inside a defined nuclear envelope (see Table 2.1.1).

Later, at the end of the G₂ stage, the chromatin filaments condense into rod-shaped structures called **chromatids**. Because of the chromosomal replication during the S phase, each chromatid has an identical sister chromatid, and these are held together by a **centromere**. This gives the chromosomes at this stage their characteristic x shape. The mitotic phase follows interphase.

Mitotic phase

The events of the mitotic (M) phase of the cell cycle can be easily seen under a light microscope because the chromatin has condensed into visible x-shaped chromosomes. Mitotic events are nuclear division (mitosis) and cytoplasmic division or **cytokinesis**. When the process is complete, two identical daughter cells are formed.

Mitosis

In mitosis, the replicated DNA (remember that during interphase the chromosomes were duplicated) is partitioned exactly into two separate nuclei. Like the rest of the cell cycle the mitotic process is continuous, but for clarity it is understood as having phases: **early prophase**, **late prophase**, **metaphase**, **anaphase** and **telophase**. Cytokinesis, which is the equal division of the cell's contents after two new nuclei are formed, occurs during late anaphase or early telophase stages.

Table 2.1.1 shows the sequence of events in the mitotic phase of the cell cycle, showing how a somatic cell divides to produce two daughter cells, each having 46 identical chromosomes (23 pairs).

2.1

Table 2.1.1 Events of the mitotic phase of the somatic cell cycle

Stage	Diagram	Activity
Early prophase	Mitotic spindle starts to form; Chromosomes start to condense; Nucleolus is gone!; Centrosome	Chromatin fibres condense and shorten into visible filaments called chromatids Each replicated identical chromatid pair is joined at a constricted region called the centromere This forms 46 x-shaped pairs (of chromosomes) Outside each centromere is a protein complex called the **kinetochore** Centrosomes (structure containing the centriole) have divided and start to be pushed apart
Late prophase (Prometaphase)	Nuclear envelope breaks down; Chromosomes fully condensed	Nuclear envelope disintegrates and nucleolus disappears All 46 chromosomes (with sister chromatids) move to the centre The lengthening microtubules push the centrosomes to opposite poles (ends) of the cells The **mitotic spindle** starts to form as: 1. Non-kinetochore microtubules extend inwards towards chromosomes 2. Kinetochore microtubules extend inward and attach to kinetochores 3. Star-shaped microtubules, called **asters** radiate outwards from the spindle The spindle's role is to separate the sister chromatids to opposite poles of the cell

(Continued)

Table 2.1.1 (Continued)

Stage	Diagram	Activity
Metaphase	Chromosomes line up at metaphase plate	The centrosomes of chromosomes are aligned at the exact centre of the mitotic spindle, by the kinetochore microtubules That is, all 46 chromatid pairs are aligned on this mid-point region, known as the **metaphase plate**
Anaphase	Kinetochore microtubules pull chromosomes towards poles Microtubles push poles apart	Centromeres split, allowing one chromatid of each pair to move to opposite sides of the cell Kinetochore microtubules pull each chromatid away from the metaphase plate by the centromere, giving a 'V' shape to each chromatid The separated chromatids are each now called **daughter chromosomes** Midway between the centromere an indentation of the plasma membrane begins to develop; the **cleavage furrow** (see cytokinesis below)
Telophase	Spindle disappears Nuclear membrane re-forms Chromosomes start to decondense Nucleolus reappears	Chromosomal movement stops Identical chromosomes (at opposite poles of the cell) uncoil, becoming threadlike chromatin filaments again Nucleoli and nuclear envelope reappear Mitotic spindle disintegrates The cleavage furrow develops, pulling the plasma membrane further inwards

Cytoplasmic division/ cytokinesis

The final stage of mitotic division is the division of the cytoplasm and organelles into the two daughter cells. This phase begins during anaphase (see Table 2.1.1). Actin microfilaments, found just near the cell's plasma membrane, form a contractile ring that pulls the plasma membrane inward. This constricts the cell at the middle (this is the cleavage furrow) like a belt, and eventually splits into two separate cells. Each cell has an equal share of cytoplasm.

Note that the plane of cleavage is at right angles to the mitotic spindle; ensuring that the two daughter cells are segregated correctly. Newly formed daughter cells then enter the interphase of their own cell cycle.

Meiosis

As introduced above, **meiosis** is a special type of cell division, with the purpose of producing sex cells, or **gametes**. In sexual reproduction the union of these gametes – one from each parent – produces a new organism. Human meiosis occurs in the gonads, and the gametes produced are sperm and ova (see Chapter 2.4).

It is vital to note here that if each gamete was diploid (2n with 23 *pairs* of chromosomes), as all somatic cells are, then the union occurring in sexual reproduction would double the number of chromosomes produced. This does *not* happen because each meiotic cell cycle in the gonads produces gametes which are haploid (n) containing a single set of 23 chromosomes.

As in somatic cell division, cells first undergo interphase, during which DNA replication occurs. Meiosis has two distinct and successive phases; **meiosis I** and **meiosis II** and can be thought of as two separate cell divisions.

Meiosis I begins once the replication of chromosomes is complete. It has four phases: prophase I, metaphase I, anaphase I and telophase I. Meiosis I is the first round of cell division, in which the goal is to **separate homologous pairs**. Homologous pairs are chromosomes (one from each parent, giving 23 pairs) that are very similar to one another and have a similar size and shape. Therefore, at the end of cell division of meiosis I there are two haploid daughter cells.

During **meiosis II**, the goal is to **separate sister chromatids**. The two haploid cells divide in sequences similar to that of mitosis. The sister chromatids line on the equatorial plane and split at their centromeres, moving to opposite poles of the cell. The overall result is four haploid cells which are genetically different, i.e. not identical daughter cells (as in mitosis). The four phases of meiosis II are prophase II, metaphase II, anaphase II and telophase II.

In Table 2.1.2, we outline the sequence of events in meiosis, showing how a single diploid (2n) parent cell produces four haploid daughter cells (n), all genetically different.

Table 2.1.2 Events of meiosis

Stage	Diagram	Activity
Meiosis I = Separating homologous pairs		
Prophase I	Starting cell is diploid (2n = 4) Homologous chromosomes pair up and exchange fragments (crossing over)	The chromosomes (with sister chromatids) start to become arranged in **homologous pairs** at the cell's centre (see Chapter 2.2 for further explanation of homologous pairs) The pairing up of the chromatids like this is called **synapsis** In these pairs, there are now four chromatids which together are termed a **tetrad** 'Crossing over' of tetrads during synapsis allows portions of genetic material to be exchanged between the homologous chromosomes This exchange is the mechanism by which genes are **recombined**, and the resulting daughter cells (gametes) are genetically different This stage is important in the genetic variation of humans

(Continued)

Table 2.1.2 (Continued)

Stage	Diagram	Activity
Metaphase I	Homologue pairs line up at the metaphase plate	The homologous chromosome pairs are lined up side by side on the metaphase plate The kinetochore microtubules at each pole extend inward and attach to kinetochores of the chromosome pair opposite
Anaphase I	Homologues separate to opposite ends of the cell Sister chromatids stay together	The centromeres <u>do not</u> split, instead, the homologous pairs separate Each one of the pair (sister chromatids still held by their centromere) moves to the opposite pole of the cell to the other The action of kinetochore microtubules draw the chromosomes to each pole The cleavage furrow begins to develop
Telophase I	Newly forming cells are haploid ($n = 2$) Each chromosome has two (non-identical) sister chromatids	Telophase I, which includes cytokinesis, is similar to the same stages in mitosis – the chromosomes have moved to opposite poles Nucleoli and nuclear envelope reforms Spindle fibres disintegrate The cleavage furrow develops, pulling the plasma membrane further inwards and dividing the cytoplasm The two cells are **haploid** (they have single chromosomes, but two sister chromatids each) – they are non-identical

(Continued)

Table 2.1.2 (Continued)

Stage	Diagram	Activity
Meiosis II = separate sister chromatids		
Prophase II	Starting cells are the haploid cells made in meiosis I Chromosomes condense	These phases are similar to those of mitosis; but the difference is that the starting point is two **haploid non-identical cells**: Chromatin fibres condense to sister chromatids and the nuclear envelope disappears Centrosomes move to opposite poles
Metaphase II	Chromosomes line up at metaphase plate	Centromeres of each chromatid pair line up on metaphase plate Spindle microtubules reform – see the kinetochore microtubules attach to the kinetochore of each centromere

(Continued)

2.1

Table 2.1.2 (Continued)

Stage	Diagram	Activity
Anaphase II	Sister chromatids separate to opposite ends of the cell	Centromeres divide, drawing chromatids to opposite poles of the cells Cleavage furrow develops
Telophase II	Newly forming gametes are haploid Each chromosome has just one chromatid	The chromosomes have moved to opposite poles Nucleoli and nuclear envelope reforms Spindle fibres disintegrate The cleavage furrow develops, pulling the plasma membrane further inwards and dividing the cytoplasm equally The net result is **four non-identical haploid daughter cells** (23 chromosomes each)

Table 2.1.3 Key definitions used in mitosis and/or meiosis

2.1

Term	Definition
Centromere	A constricted region of a chromosome, holds sister chromatids together
Chromatin	The material of which the chromosomes of eukaryotes are composed
Crossing over	Exchange of DNA between paired homologous chromosomes
Diploid (2n)	'n' is the number of chromosome sets of a cell Diploid (2n), means 'double' or two sets of chromosomes in a cell 2n Human somatic cells have 23 pairs of chromosomes (one of each chromosome from each parent)
Gamete	Reproductive cell Female gametes are eggs (ova) Male gametes are sperm
Haploid (n)	'n' is the number of chromosome sets of a cell Haploid (n) means a single set of chromosomes in a cell Human gametes have 23 single chromosomes
Homologous chromosomes	Homologous pairs are chromosomes (one from each parent, giving 23 pairs) that are very similar to one another and have a similar size and shape
Nucleolus	Spherical structure in the nucleus
Sister chromatids	Before cell division, each chromosome is replicated, giving rise to two sister chromatids – a sister chromatid is one of the identical halves of the replicated chromosome

Overall, meiosis starts with one diploid parent cell and ends with four haploid daughter cells; these sex cells are genetically unlike the parent cell and genetically unlike each other. The mechanism responsible for this genetic diversity is the **crossing over** of the tetrads, which occurs during prophase I of meiosis.

Some of the main key terms used in descriptions of mitosis and meiosis throughout this chapter are defined in Table 2.1.3.

These sections have described how genetic information is distributed in diploid body cells, and how genetic material is replicated from cell to cell through the mitotic cycle. We have also explained that reproductive cell division, called meiosis, produces haploid gametes, necessary for maintaining the correct number of chromosomes in each generation. We have also seen how meiosis creates genetic diversity because the gamete cells are genetically dissimilar to each other.

The next section looks at how genetic traits are inherited, i.e. passed from one generation to the next.

INTERRUPTER

Mitosis and meiosis are fundamental concepts in anatomy and physiology. Spend time annotating the equivalent mitosis and meiosis tables in your workbook. Use your own words to describe what is happening, including identifying the key differences between mitosis and meiosis.

Genetics, genetic disorders and epigenetics

Ginny Mounce

Basic genetic concepts

Earlier in this section we described the production of new cells by mitosis and meiosis. Both involve replication of the structures called **chromosomes**. These contain functional units called **genes**, which carry specific instructions for **protein synthesis** in order for the body to function. **Genetics** is the name given to the study of individual genes and their **heredity** – meaning understanding the significance of their passing from one generation to the next. This is clearly relevant for midwives, as some genetic changes or disorders are associated with birth defects, developmental disorders or diseases. Understanding how such conditions occur,

DOI: 10.4324/9781003227571-7

how they can be identified, prevented or treated, increasingly includes knowledge of genetics.

Below we introduce the main concepts of genetics including **genomics**, which is the study of *all* of a person's genetic components (not just their genes). A person's total set of cellular genetic instructions is called their **genome**.

Introduction to chromosomes and DNA

The nucleus of human cells contains chromosomes. These are long, coiled molecules of deoxyribonucleic acid (DNA) plus proteins that carry genomic information. One chromosome contains hundreds or thousands of genes; with each gene being a tiny segment of DNA arranged in a linear order. It is the chemical structure of the DNA in each gene that provides the information, or '**genetic code**', used by cells to specify biological traits, generally by synthesising proteins for cell functions.

Because of the coding function of genes, chromosomes are said to contain an individual's **genetic blueprint** – the instructions for life. Humans are known to have around 20,000 different protein-coding genes. However, the vast majority of DNA (possibly as much as 99%) is non-coding. This was historically known as 'junk DNA' but it is becoming established that much DNA has other, some as yet to be determined, functions.

Deoxyribonucleic acid (DNA)

DNA is one type of nucleic acid, the other being **ribonucleic acid (RNA)**. Both share structural similarities although RNA, unlike DNA, is mainly single-stranded. The individual unit or building block of these nucleic acids are monomers, called **nucleotides**. Each nucleotide consists of a **base**, a **pentose sugar** and a **phosphate group**.

DNA molecule

The DNA molecule is a polymer made up of two intertwined strands, arranged as the famous '**double helix**' (twisted ladder) shape. Each strand of DNA is a chain of repeated nucleotides. In DNA, the nucleotide bases project from the sugar-phosphate backbone towards the other strand. Each nucleotide pairs with a corresponding base projecting inwards from the opposite strand, creating a shape reminiscent of the rungs of a ladder. Hydrogen bonds keep the pairs together (Figure 2.2.1). There are four types of nucleotide bases which pair in specific ways: **adenine** (A) pairs with **thymine** (T), and **cytosine** (C) pairs with **guanine** (G). It is the sequence of these bases along the backbone which encodes the information for making amino acids and building proteins.

The pentose sugar in DNA is **deoxyribose** while in RNA it is **ribose**. Additionally, in RNA, the base **uracil** (U) takes the place of thymine (T). RNA has an important function in protein synthesis (described later).

DNA structure

We have stated that chromosomes are long structures made up of single DNA molecules surrounded by proteins. As previously described, most of the time when a cell is not dividing (i.e. during interphase) the 46 chromosomes appear as a granular mass called chromatin. Seen under great magnification, this has an appearance like 'beads-on-a-string', where the 'beads' are strands of DNA wrapped around protein molecules called **histones**. Each repeated unit of DNA and histone is called a **nucleosome**. The histones' function is to fold nucleosomes into more compact

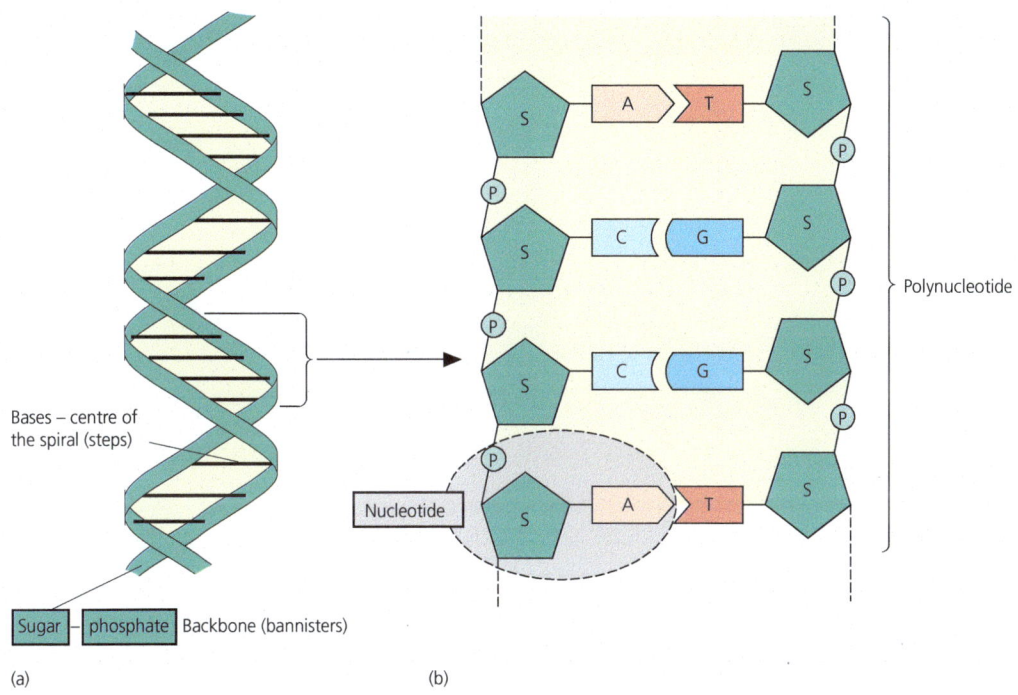

Bases – centre of
the spiral (steps)

Polynucleotide

Nucleotide

Sugar – phosphate Backbone (bannisters)

(a) (b)

Figure 2.2.1 a) The double-helical structure of DNA. b) Magnified view of DNA components:
S, sugar (deoxyribose); P, phosphate; T, thymine; A, adenine; C, cytosine; G, guanine
Source: Figure 2.13, p.40, Clancy and McVicar (2009)

structures called chromatin fibres, and en
masse these make up the larger threadlike
loops of chromatin (Figure 2.2.2). This is
how the lengthy chromosome molecules,
said to be around three feet in length if fully
'unravelled', are able to be packed into a
single nucleus.

As described in Chapter 2.1, in a cell
cycle, just before cell division, the DNA
and histones replicate and become more
condensed. The duplicated chromatin fibres
form a pair of identical rod-shaped **sister
chromatids**. A constricted area, named the
centromere, joins the chromatid sisters.
It is only after replication and condensing
during cell division that chromosomes
take on this appearance, which is their
characteristic X-structure.

DNA and protein synthesis

Protein synthesis is a highly complex
process, and full exploration is outside the
scope of this book. However, a summarised
description is given below, and shown
diagrammatically in Figure 2.2.3.

Protein synthesis occurs via the processes
of **transcription** and **translation**. Three
successive pairs of bases in nucleic acids
(DNA or RNA) are called base triplets or
trinucleotides. A **codon** is the name given
to a unit of triplets that encode for one
of 20 amino acids, which build proteins,
or code to stop protein synthesis (called
stop signals). A sequence of codons in a
segment of DNA (a gene) therefore governs
which protein is synthesised by that gene.

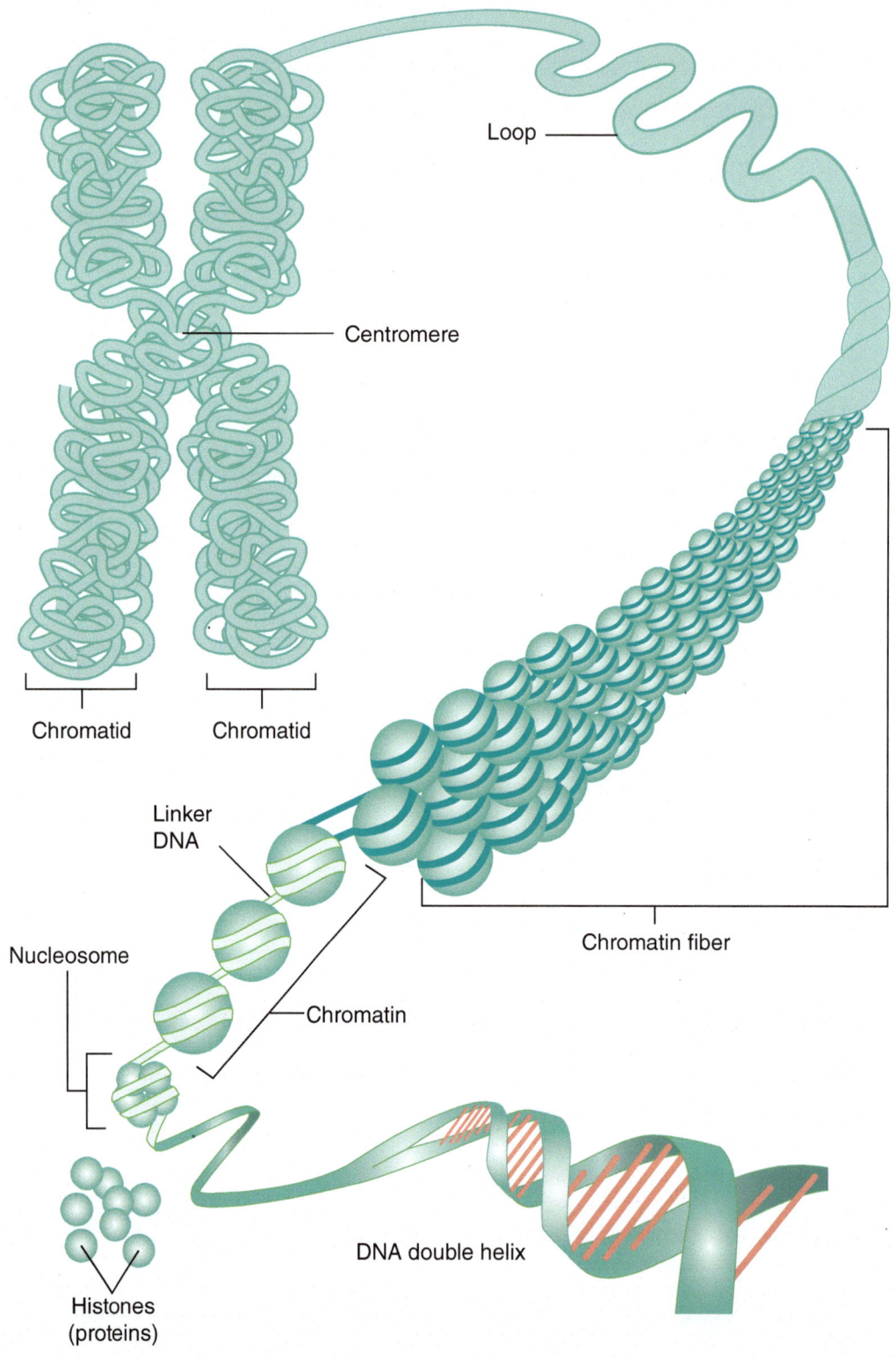

Loop

Centromere

Chromatid   Chromatid

Linker
DNA

Nucleosome

Chromatin

Chromatin fiber

DNA double helix

Histones
(proteins)

Figure 2.2.2 Structure of a chromosome in a dividing cell

(a)

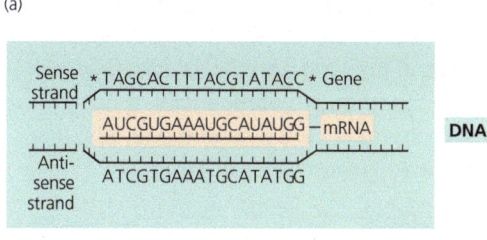

(b)

(c)

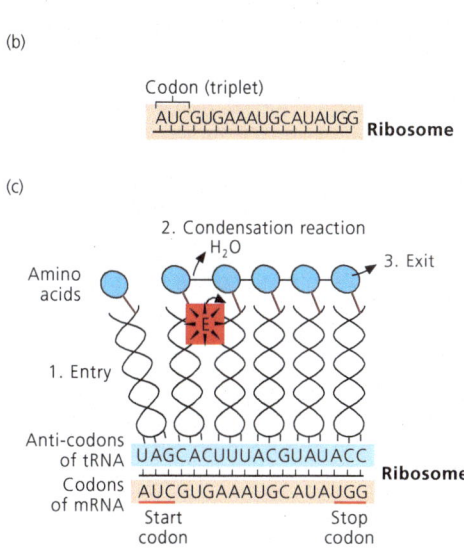

Figure 2.2.3 Protein synthesis. (a) Transcription: messenger RMA (mRNA) synthesis alongside the DNA strand in the nucleus. Note the gene is composed of the triplets from *to* on the sense strand. (b) mRNA passes out of the nucleus to become attached to ribosomes. (c) Translation: transfer RNA (tRNA) brings the amino acids to the ribosome. E, energy from the breakdown of ATP into ADP + Pi + energy. Note that tRNA anticodons are the original triplets on the sense strand of DNA, which code for the specific amino acids. Pi inorganic phosphate
Source: Figure 2.14, p.41, Clancy and McVicar (2009)

For protein synthesis to occur, in the nucleus, DNA strands temporarily separate. The 'unzipped' DNA codons are a template for the formation of a complementary strand of **messenger RNA (mRNA)**. The strands of DNA then reunite. The mRNA leaves the nucleus and attaches to ribosomes where its genetic message is **translated**. Ribosomes move along the mRNA and produce amino acids according to the sequence of codons, i.e. the codons serve as a pattern for making a specific protein. There are 61 codons that specify amino acids and three are used as stop signals to end translation.

Chromosomes

Each of the 46 chromosomes (23 pairs) contain similar genes, arranged in similar order, to the other in the pair. They are all known as **homologues** or **homologous chromosomes**. The chromosome pairs 1–22 are also alike in terms of appearance and size and are known as **autosomes**. The twenty-third pair is known as the **sex chromosomes**. The sex chromosomes are designated **X** and **Y**; females have a pair of X chromosomes (which look the same) and males have a single X and a single Y chromosome (which look different). Additionally, the X chromosome is approximately three times larger than the Y chromosome and includes many more genes.

The genes for traits, such as eye colour, are located at the same position, or **locus**, in homologous chromosome pairs. However, there may be some differences in the DNA sequence for particular genes in these chromosome pairs (since they come from two parents). The name for versions of the genetic sequence at a given locus is an **allele.** An example might be one allele of the gene that codes for lip shape being broad lips, while another allele is for thin lips. A person who has two identical alleles for the broad lip gene is said to be **homozygous** for that gene and will have 'broad lips'. But if they have different alleles (broad lip and thin lip) they are **heterozygous** for that gene. The relationship between the two alleles determines how the lip trait is **expressed** (observed) and passed on to the next generation. How these relationships affect gene expression are the principles of **inheritance**, which is explained later.

Karyotype

An individuals' chromosomes viewed under a microscope from a somatic cell can be sorted into the 23 homologous pairs based on their size and morphology. The autosomes (chromosomes 1–22) are numbered in approximately descending size order, with chromosome 1 being the largest (although chromosome 21 is actually the shortest). The sex chromosomes are pair 23. A **karyotype** is an individual's whole chromosome sequence and is often viewed as a chart with the chromosome pairs ordered from 1 to 23 (see Figure 2.2.4). Staining further identifies chromosome pairs, as every chromosome has distinct, characteristic **banding** patterns, where there are areas of tightly coiled DNA and proteins. Some sources liken this to a 'barcode'.

The position of centromeres is also used to tell chromosomes apart. The largest, chromosome 1, is **metacentric**, meaning the centromere is at the middle. Most human chromosomes such as chromosome 5 (pictured) are **submetacentric**, which means the centromere is not quite at the middle and the chromosome arms are

clearly of unequal length. In all cases, the short or 'petite' arm is called the 'p' arm and the long arm the 'q' arm. Five chromosomes are **acrocentric**, meaning the centromere is very near one end, resulting in one very much shorter arm.

A further recognisable region of chromosomes is called the telomere. This is a protective 'cap' at the end which becomes progressively shorter with cell division. Eventually, when telomeres become too short, the cell dies.

The naming of chromosome arms into 'p' and 'q', and further subdivision into regions and within this into bands, is the classification system used to identify or analyse parts of a chromosome during genetic testing. As shown in Figure 2.2.4 the combination of sex chromosomes (pair 23) identifies if this is a male or female human (if XY then male, and if XX female).

Genotype to phenotype

As introduced earlier, every nucleated somatic (body) cell contains the same 46 chromosomes, arranged as 23 pairs (2n).

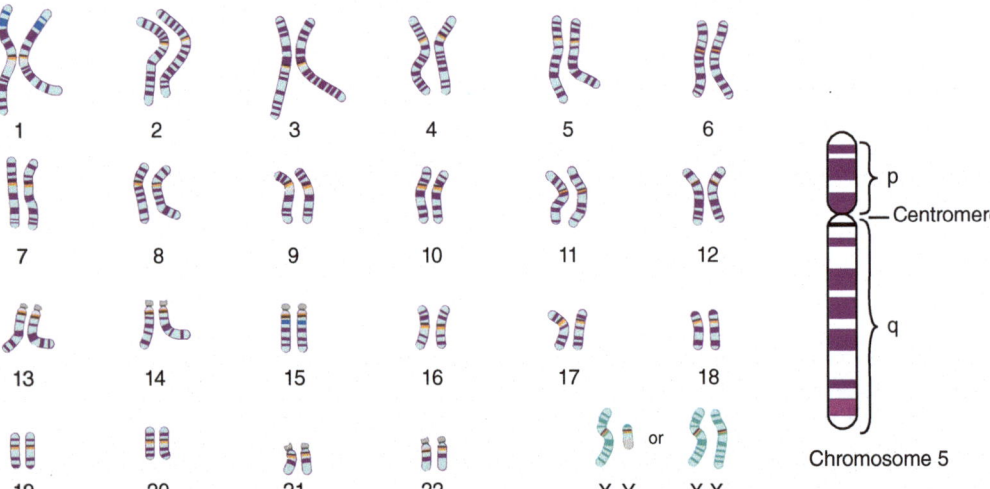

Figure 2.2.4 A human karyotype

Earlier, we showed that gametes, or sex cells (eggs and sperm), contain a single set (n) of chromosomes. During reproduction, the sperm and egg cells fuse and the genetic material is combined, resulting in a new organism with a diploid set of chromosomes (2n). Therefore, one member of each chromosome pair is acquired from the biological mother and the other from the biological father. This means that individuals will resemble both of their parents because they inherit traits from each.

However, every individual is unique. They have their own genetic makeup of alleles on their chromosomes, called their **genotype**. In fact, most of the genes belonging to an individual will have codons that differ from another individual by 1–3 letters. In large part, this is due to the genetic recombination which occurs during crossing-over in meiosis I, and also because the fertilisation of a single egg by a single sperm leads to multiple genetic variations.

The outward expression of an individual's genotype, observed as physical traits such as eye colour or other characteristics such as risk of disease, is known as the **phenotype**. Most traits are not usually the result of the expression of a single allele as phenotype is influenced not only by which alleles are present, but in interactions between multiple alleles, other genes and with the environment. In other words, a person's destiny is not entirely determined by the genes they have inherited. This emphasises the importance of lifestyle choices and environmental factors in maintaining good health. Nevertheless, there are general principles of **heredity** which govern how genes are inherited and traits expressed, explained in *Modes of inheritance* below.

Occasionally, changes or mutations in genetic sequences, which may arise spontaneously or be inherited, result in illness or variations in heritable characteristics that have adverse effects. These are genetic disorders, which are described next.

Genetic disorders

Generally, changes in a persons' genetic code will have no adverse consequences, but sometimes the effect is harmful. **Genetic disorders** are abnormal changes or mutations of a persons' genome that cause disease. Mutations may be inherited from parents and are present at birth, an example being cystic fibrosis, while others are caused by acquired mutations in a gene or group of genes that occur during a person's life, such as some cancers.

Because of genetic inheritance, many diseases or susceptibility to disease, run in families. This is why knowledge of family history is important for identifying potential conditions arising from inherited disorders. Individuals, most often those with potential or already known serious genetic mutations, can use genetic testing to identify their likelihood of acquiring disease or, if they are planning parenthood, of passing disease to children. The health professionals who offer advice on these possible problems are called **genetic counsellors**. Screening programmes to identify possible genetic disorders of a fetus during pregnancy are routinely part of antenatal services, and prenatal testing is also available to diagnose major conditions. Pre-implantation screening of gametes before implantation is also possible during assisted reproductive treatments, meaning some screening is carried out before pregnancy.

There are three main types of genetic disorder: **chromosomal**, **single gene** (or **monogenic**) and **multifactorial**.

Chromosomal disorders

Chromosomal disorders are due to abnormal changes in chromosome number (either too many or too few), or to alterations in the structure. The majority of all chromosomal abnormalities occur during meiosis, when errors in cell division or duplication result in sperm or egg cells with incorrect numbers or arrangements of chromosomes. **Non-disjunction** is when a chromosome pair fails to separate during meiosis and gives rise to an imbalanced number of chromosomes in gametes. A resulting fertilised cell will therefore contain any such abnormalities which, because they are happening for the first time, are called '*de novo*' errors. Less frequently, structural chromosomal abnormalities can be inherited from parents, or arise after conception.

The majority of miscarriages which happen in the first trimester of pregnancy are due to chromosomal abnormalities.

Numerical chromosome disorders

Cells with the normal number of 46 chromosomes are called **euploid**, while cells with missing or extra chromosomes are called **aneuploid**. Abnormal chromosome numbers can relate to single chromosomes or whole sets.

Polyploidy is the term for cells with an extra set of chromosomes. This occurs either when an abnormal diploid gamete is fertilised or by polyspermy when more than one sperm fertilises an egg. Any resulting polyploid embryo is generally not viable, although rarely infants have survived for a few days after birth. Disorders where cells have a missing chromosome are called a **monosomy** and those with an extra chromosome are called a **trisomy**. Historically, chromosomal disorders were named for the person who first identified them, but now are labelled according to the main chromosome affected.

The vast majority of conceptions with incorrect numbers of autosomal chromosomes will not survive to birth, although some do. In living infants, the disorders can have severe and life limiting consequences, often affecting brain function, although severity varies. If the aneuploidy is not present in all cells but found in only a proportion, then it is called a **mosaicism,** and the effects may not be as severe. For example, the most commonly occurring human aneuploidy is believed to be trisomy 16, which is always lethal unless mosaic.

Fully aneuploid autosomal disorders that may be non-fatal are, in order of frequency at birth, **trisomy 21** (formerly Down syndrome), **trisomy 18** (Edwards syndrome) and **trisomy 13** (Patau syndrome). Aneuploid disorders of the sex chromosomes are usually less severe. In fact, the only survivable monosomy is **XO syndrome** (formerly Turner syndrome) in females where there is a missing X chromosome, rather than the usual two. However, only about 1% of pregnancies with this monosomy lead to a live birth, and only half of these are a 'true' monosomy. More relatively common are the male sex chromosome aneuploidies **trisomy XXY** (Klinefelter syndrome), where there is an extra copy of chromosome X, and **trisomy XYY** (Jacobs syndrome), where the extra chromosome is Y.

The presence of aneuploidy can be identified by chromosomal analysis by a karyotype obtained from a cell sample. See Table 2.2.1 for the incidence and features of the major numerical chromosome disorders.

Structural chromosomal abnormalities

These are changes to chromosomes which make them structurally incomplete, differently shaped or when segments are

Table 2.2.1 Major human numerical chromosome disorders

Type of aneuploidy	Example (former named disorder)	Incidence	Possible symptoms in affected individuals
Polyploidy	Triploidy All cells have an entire extra set of chromosomes	1–3% of all conceptions	Fatal unless mosaic Multiple physical effects, molar pregnancy
Trisomy	Trisomy 21 (Down syndrome)	1/700 births	Distinctive facial features (protruding tongue, slanting eyes, round head), single palmar crease, short stature, developmental delays, intellectual disability, malformations of heart, ears, hands and feet
	Trisomy 18 (Edwards syndrome)	1/3000 births	As trisomy 13, plus small head and jaw, clenched fists and overlapping fingers, abdominal skin flaps
	Trisomy 13 (Patau syndrome)	1/5000 births	Intellectual disability, heart defects, underdeveloped face and adrenal glands, fused finger/toes, cleft lip and palate
	47, XXY (Klinefelter syndrome)	1/1000 male births	Hypogonadism (gonadal defects appearing at puberty), infertility, long legs, breast growth, intellectual disability
	47, XYY (Jacobs syndrome)	1/1000 male births	Few symptoms, above average height, risk of learning disability
Monosomy	45, X0 (Turner syndrome)	1/2500 female births (1/5000 mosaicism)	Short stature, heart defects, webbed neck, ovarian failure, genital hypoplasia, underdeveloped sex characteristics

moved to another location or chromosome. Again, most arise during meiosis and early cell development when DNA segments are broken and reattached. This results in chromosomes with extra parts or some missing parts, segments duplicated, inverted, inserted or formed in a ring.

As with numerical chromosomal disorders, the effects of these rearrangements may be significant when expressed phenotypically. However, if the overall chromosome set (like the ingredients in a recipe) remains as intended, i.e. if there is no net loss or gain of genetic material, then the disorder is called a **balanced rearrangement** and rarely causes a problem for an individual. This also means it may not be known

to them, but during meiosis to create gametes the rearrangement may become **unbalanced** and so passed onto the next generation in pregnancy. Rearrangements that are unbalanced will have extra or missing genetic material and are associated with various consequences including miscarriage, stillbirth or birth defects.

Structural changes that are unbalanced will include deletions, duplications, insertions and ring chromosomes. Other rearrangements may be balanced, such as **inversions** and **translocations**, although both can also be unbalanced. Inversion is often of a single chromosome; a chromosome breaks in two places, either including the centromere or not, rotates 180 degrees and is reinserted. Translocations are when locations of segments of chromosomes are moved. There are two main types: **reciprocal** and **Robertsonian** translocations. During reciprocal translocation, parts of non-homologous chromosomes are exchanged; generally these rearrangements are balanced. In Robertsonian translocations, the whole long arms of acrocentric chromosomes are fused together. See Table 2.2.2 for the main forms and features of structural chromosome disorders.

Table 2.2.2 Forms of human structural chromosome disorders

Change	Description			Examples
Deletion	Portion of single chromosome deleted (loss of genetic material)			**Cri du chat syndrome (5p-):** Missing terminal piece on p arm of chromosome 5
				Distinctive high-pitched cry (like a cat), intellectual disability, delayed development, microcephaly, hypotonia
				Incidence 1/50,000 births
				Williams/Williams-Beuren syndrome: Deletions from q arm of chromosome 7
				Distinctive facial changes (broad forehead, underdeveloped chin), intellectual disability, outgoing personality
				Incidence 1/7,500 births
Duplication	Portion of single chromosome duplicated (gain of genetic material)			**Charcot–Marie–Tooth disease type 1A:** Duplications of genes on chromosome 17
				Causes severe muscle wasting
				A rarer sub-type is **Roussy–Lévy** with essential tremor and ataxia

(Continued)

Table 2.2.2 (Continued)

Change	Description			Examples
Inversion	Portion of single chromosome broken off, turned upside down and reattached (no overall loss/gain)			Usually does not cause problems Often chromosome 2
Translocation	Portion of chromosome broken off and reattached to another chromosome (possible overall gain if unbalanced)	Reciprocal Robertsonian		**Reciprocal:** portions from two chromosomes are exchanged Usually balanced and does not cause problems **Robertsonian:** acrocentric chromosomes break at the centromere and long arms attach to each other If unbalanced, possibilities are trisomies, e.g. trisomy 21 (translocation causes 3% Down syndrome)
Rings	Chromosome breaks and end join together as rings (possible overall loss)			Very rare, syndromes cause marked growth delay
Insertion	Portion of chromosome deleted from original location and inserted into another chromosome			Very rare, overall gain/loss of genetic material

2.2

APPLICATION TO PRACTICE

Robertsonian translocations

These are the most common translocation in humans, occurring in around 1 in 1000 live births. They only involve the five **acrocentric** chromosomes which are 13, 14, 15, 21 and 22. Usually, the translocations are of non-homologous chromosomes, including for example 13 and 14, 14 and 21, or 14 and 15. Chromosomes break at the centromere and the two long arms then fuse, making one chromosome. The short (p) arms also fuse together, but after several cycles of cell division are soon lost (Figure 2.2.5).

This may have little obvious consequence because typically genes in the p arms of acrocentric chromosomes are not unique, i.e. while the total number of chromosomes in a cell is now only 45, all the significant genetic material is still present. This individual (who has the balanced form of the translocation and is a carrier) will show few symptoms, but if they become a parent their child may receive an unbalanced copy of the Robertsonian translocation. If so, the consequences are likely to be fatal or severe.

An inherited form of trisomy 21 (which we discussed earlier in numerical chromosomal disorders) can arise when chromosome 21 is involved in a Robertsonian translocation since it is possible that any children will inherit three copies of chromosome 21. Parents who have a baby with Down syndrome can use a karyotype to identify if they are a Robertsonian translocation carrier; if so, the chances of them having other affected children are much higher than with *de novo* forms.

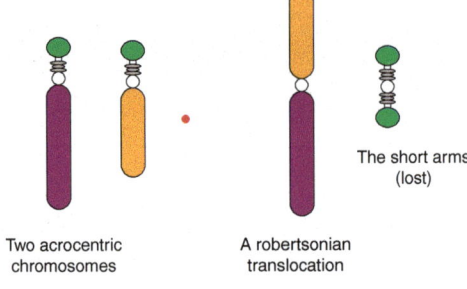

Two acrocentric chromosomes

A robertsonian translocation

The short arms (lost)

Figure 2.2.5 Example of Robertsonian translocation

Single-gene disorders

These are also known as **monogenetic** disorders as they relate to health problems caused by problems or mutations of one single gene.

From understanding DNA and protein synthesis, you know that the codon sequences are the instructions of the gene. Therefore, alterations to the structure or order of the DNA code will affect these instructions. This may lead to a loss or change in the production of proteins, including enzymes, and in their function. Loss of specific cell function can lead to disease. In Figure 2.2.6 you can see an illustration of how altering the genetic code might lead to disease.

A real example of this is found in the sickle-cell haemoglobin gene. In this gene defect, just one nucleotide is altered compared to the standard, but this changes one of the 147 amino acids in the beta haemoglobin protein chain (the sixth amino acid becomes valine compared to glutamate) of red blood cells. The consequences of this single nucleotide mutation are significant; molecules of sickle-cell haemoglobin are misshaped and function poorly, leading to lower blood oxygen levels and causing sickle-cell disease.

2.2

(a) Consider this sentence:

THE OLD CAT WAS TOO FAT

This is an understandable sentence. By analogy, if this was genetic code, its translation would be acceptable to a cell.

Rearranging the words:

THE FAT CAT WAS TOO OLD

In this genetic code, the translation would still be acceptable, but the meaning of the original sentence (by analogy a protein synthesized by the cell) has been lost. The function associated with that sentence is no longer available, but has been replaced with the new one, which may or may not be to a cell's advantage, or may even be a disadvantage.

Alternatively:

THE OLD CAT WAS TOO FTA

The original meaning has been lost, and been replaced with a nonsensical sentence. By analogy, this new code (i.e. protein) will not have any action in the cell.

(b) Using this principle to illustrate gene mutation, the following is a piece of genetic code:

GCA ACC CAG CUU CAC UCA UCC GGC ACG

In the next sequence, a gene mutation called a substitution has occurred, in which a base at one point in the original has been changed into another:

GCA A*A*C CAG CUU CAC UCA UCC GGC ACG

In the next sequence, a gene mutation called an insertion has occurred in the original, in which an extra base has been inserted into the sequence:

GCA ACC *G*CA GCU UCA CUC AUC CGG CAC G..

Compare these to the original above.

Figure 2.2.6 Alterations of genetic code may lead to disease
Source: Figure 19.11, p.536, Clancy and McVicar (2009)

Single-gene disorders are fairly common, believed to occur in approximately 1 in 50 people. The severity and features of the diseases they cause depends on the gene affected and other factors. Mutations of individual genes are not always the same either, meaning that the same disorder can have somewhat different phenotypes. Examples of other well-known monogenetic disorders are cystic fibrosis, Tay-Sachs disease, myotonic dystrophy, phenylketonuria and Duchenne muscular dystrophy.

Because they involve alterations to a single gene, monogenetic disorders are relatively well understood. Many gene mutations that cause disease can be identified by a genetic test. Mutations may arise spontaneously in gametes, so the offspring will have the disorder but not the parents, or they can be passed on (inherited) to children. Patterns of inherited traits and characteristics are observed in families. This can often be predicted as the way single-gene disorders are inherited are usually determined by the main modes of inheritance: **dominant**, **recessive** and **sex-linked** (which we first mentioned when discussing alleles above). These were first established by the scientist Gregor Mendel in the nineteenth century, so you may hear them described as Mendelian genetics. The knowledge of these hereditary principles is very relevant to the work of midwives, particularly in the antenatal period. Pregnancy screening and medical history taking is pivotal for understanding genetic disorders and in anticipating likely traits for the offspring of two parents.

Modes of inheritance

Before considering the different modes of inheritance, it is helpful to remember that individuals have two copies of most genes, one copy inherited from each parent, with alleles which are homozygous or heterozygous. Charts such as **genetic diagrams** and **Punnett squares** are used to illustrate these various modes of inheritance.

The genes of autosomal chromosomes (numbers 1–22) have two main patterns of inheritance: **autosomal recessive** and **autosomal dominant**.

Autosomal recessive inheritance

In this pattern, two copies of a gene (an allele) are required to be present in an individual if the trait or disorder is expressed. That means that the allele must be homozygous for it to be seen. Common autosomal recessive conditions include cystic fibrosis, haemochromatosis, thalassaemia, albinism and sickle-cell disease.

Figure 2.2.7 is a genetic diagram of how an autosomal recessive monogenetic disorder could be inherited from parents who are **carriers** for the condition. In this example, the parents are each heterozygous for the **recessive** disorder, and so carry the condition but it is not expressed. However, when these parents reproduce, a number of outcomes are possible. The disorder being recessive means that if the offspring alleles are heterozygous, the allele carrying

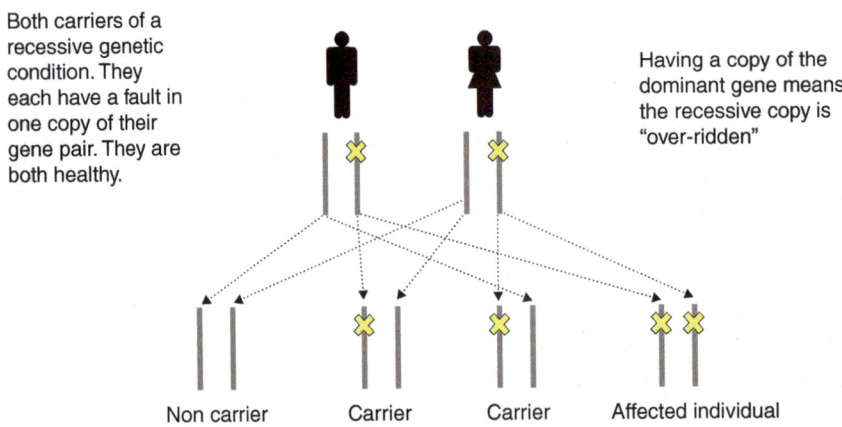

Both carriers of a recessive genetic condition. They each have a fault in one copy of their gene pair. They are both healthy.

Having a copy of the dominant gene means the recessive copy is "over-ridden"

Non carrier   Carrier   Carrier   Affected individual

Figure 2.2.7 A genetic diagram for autosomal recessive inheritance such as cystic fibrosis

the recessive disorder is 'over-ridden' by the normal allele, and the disease is masked. If the offspring alleles are homozygous for the affected gene, this will produce the disease. If the offspring alleles are homozygous for the normal gene, they will be unaffected by the condition.

We can also use a Punnett square chart to predict the possible combinations of inheritance of genetic disorders. In Figure 2.2.8, the autosomal recessive disorder is cystic fibrosis and possible offspring combinations from alleles of male gametes (written on the left) and alleles of female gametes (written at the top) are shown. The allele that codes for cystic fibrosis is symbolised as **c**, while the allele that codes normally is symbolised as **C**. In this case, there is a one in four chance (25% chance) that offspring from these parents will result in expression of the condition cystic fibrosis. It is important to note that this chance is the same each and every time offspring are produced. Regardless of whether the first offspring is a carrier, or has the condition, the chances of being a carrier, or having the condition,

are exactly the same for each and every subsequent offspring.

INTERRUPTER

Your workbook has plenty of versions of Punnett squares to fill in for different modes of inheritance depending on dominance. Work through these to understand possible patterns of inheritance for difference conditions.

Autosomal dominant inheritance

In this pattern, only one single copy of a gene (an allele) is required to be present for the trait or disorder to be expressed – as it is **dominant** and so will override the other allele. A well-known and devastating neurodegenerative disease which is autosomal dominant is Huntington's disease. Children who have one parent with a heterozygous Huntington gene (Hh) will have a 50% chance of inheriting the disease. Predictive testing is particularly significant for this disease, as symptoms do not usually appear until mid-reproductive age, when parents may have already started families. A Punnett square for Huntington's disease is shown in Figure 2.2.9 where the father of the offspring has the heterozygous Huntington gene (Hh).

You can see that offspring who are heterozygous for the Huntington gene will be affected by the condition. It is not possible for a person to simply be a carrier of the disorder; a person can pass it on but will also be affected. The risk of inheriting the disorder is 50%.

We mentioned earlier that every individual genotype is unique, and this means that people do not have the exact same symptoms of diseases, even from inherited single-gene disorders (including

Father		Mother	
		C	c
	C	CC (1:4 normal)	Cc (1:4, carrier)
	c	Cc (1:4, carrier)	cc (1:4, cystic fibrosis)

Figure 2.2.8 A Punnett square for autosomal recessive inheritance such as cystic fibrosis, where both parents are carriers for the condition

Father	Mother	
	h	h
H	**Hh** (1:4 affected)	**Hh** (1:4, affected)
h	hh (1:4, normal)	hh (1:4, normal)

Figure 2.2.9 A Punnett square for autosomal dominant inheritance such as Huntington's disease where one parent has the condition

monozygotic twins). One genetic concept called **penetrance** is important to introduce here. This relates to the 'all or nothing' expression of genotype, which means that not all people who inherit a particular combination of alleles for a gene will show the symptoms. Penetrance is described numerically, e.g. as 80% if 80 people out of 100 with the mutation develop the disease. If all individuals who inherit the variant for a gene develop the disease it is said to have complete (100%) penetrance. Autosomal dominant disorder neurofibromatosis type 1 is an example of this, while another, autosomal dominant mutations of the BRCA1 breast cancer gene has incomplete penetrance (80%). Another term, **expressivity**, is used to describe the variation in intensity of symptoms displayed by a phenotype; most are **variably expressive**.

A single-gene disorder may also give rise to different symptoms, which can be observed as different diseases amongst families. This is called **pleiotropy**, and is seen in, for example, autosomal dominant Marfan syndrome.

Sex-linked inheritance

The sex chromosomes (the 23rd pair) determine the biological sex of an individual. Females have two X chromosomes while males have one X and one Y chromosome.

We can use a Punnett square again to illustrate how sex of offspring is determined at fertilisation (Figure 2.2.10). Haploid male gametes will contain either a X or a Y chromosome, while haploid female gametes can only contain a X chromosome. The chance of producing either a male or female offspring, therefore, is 50%.

Father	Mother	
	X	X
X	XX (female)	XX (female)
Y	XY (male)	XY (male)

Figure 2.2.10 A Punnett square to illustrate how offspring sex is determined at fertilisation

The X chromosome is much larger than the Y chromosome and contains genes that are absent from the Y chromosome that code for several non-sexual traits or disorders. This creates a pattern of inheritance which is due to the genes found only on the X chromosome, so are known as X-linked genes. The **X-linked inheritance** pattern differs in how males and females are affected. Although there are a few rare Y-linked disorders these can only be passed from men to sons; they usually cause male infertility and so will only ever be inherited via assisted reproduction, we will not consider these further.

As males have only one X chromosome, any X-linked gene that carries a disorder will result in disease; it does not matter if it is inherited in a dominant or recessive manner. This is because there is no ability of genes in a second X chromosome to compensate for the faulty ones. On the other hand, females will only be affected if they inherit two copies of a recessive mutated X-linked gene. X-linked dominant conditions such as Rett syndrome will affect females even if only one copy is present, although these are very rare. All this means that daughters do not usually show symptoms of X-linked disorders but may be carriers. Males cannot pass X-linked disorders onto their sons (because a male gamete has only a Y chromosome).

Haemophilia is an example of a X-linked recessive disorder. This disease causes low or absent blood clotting functions and prolonged bleeding. Figure 2.2.11 uses a Punnett square to illustrate the inheritance of such a X-linked recessive condition if the male parent (father) has the condition. Figure 2.2.12 uses a Punnett square to illustrate the inheritance of a X-linked recessive condition if the female (mother) is a carrier.

For a male parent affected with the condition, daughters will become carriers of haemophilia, while sons will be unaffected.

	Mother	
Father	X	X
X°	X°X (female carrier)	X°X (female carrier)
Y	XY (male unaffected)	XY (male unaffected)

Figure 2.2.11 A Punnett square to illustrate inheritance of an X-linked recessive condition, if the male parent (father) has the condition. X° denotes carrier for the recessive gene

2.2

	Mother	
Father	X	X°
X	XX (female unaffected)	XX° (female carrier)
Y	XY (male unaffected)	X°Y (male affected)

Figure 2.2.12 A Punnett square to illustrate the inheritance of an X-linked recessive condition if the female (mother) is a carrier. X° denotes carrier for the recessive gene

A female parent who is a carrier of the haemophilia disorder will have a 25% chance of producing an affected male child and 25% chance of producing a carrier female.

Contrary to what has previously been explained, in some recessive X-linked conditions, female carriers may exhibit mild symptoms of the disease. This is due to alterations in the physiological mechanism called **X-chromosome inactivation**.

Normally, one of the two X chromosomes in female cells are silenced to prevent their over-expression. This occurs randomly, but if the normal genes are suppressed more than they should then features of the genetic disorder may be observed in the female carriers. This is seen with Duchenne muscular dystrophy, which is a severe and progressive muscular weakness that usually affects boys.

Multifactorial genetic disorders

Sometimes genetic disorders are more complex and multifactorial, caused by changes to multiple genes and influenced by the environment. They do not necessarily follow Mendelian patterns of inheritance, although often clustering of disease is observed in families. The lack of definite inheritance patterns means that it is harder to predict the risk of a disease being passed on.

Disorders which are controlled by a combination of genes are called polygenic and they are passed on through polygenic inheritance. Predicting their observed characteristics is difficult because there are so many variations of characteristics between extremes amongst individuals. An example of a normal polygenic trait is skin colour (which has many observed variations).

Often all the specific genes that are involved in polygenic disorders are unknown, but it is becoming apparent that environmental factors often affect them. More and more genes are being identified as candidates for these disorders. Examples of multifactorial genetic disorders are neural tube defects, cleft lip and palate, most congenital heart diseases, schizophrenia, and type 1 and 2 diabetes.

APPLICATION TO PRACTICE

Genetic testing

There are various tests and screening tools available to diagnose genetic disorders by the analysis of DNA from cell samples. A **karyotype** (Figure 2.2.4) is one method of analysis, others include **DNA sequencing**, **microarray analysis** and **karyomapping**. The purpose of genetic testing is mainly to provide information about the possible development or treatment of disease. In maternity, genetic tests usually take the form of newborn/pregnancy screening, prenatal or pre-implantation diagnosis and pre-pregnancy screening for parents with a family history or predisposition to a disorder.

Newborn/pregnancy screening

Pregnancy screening programmes use blood tests and ultrasound scanning to predict the risk of the carried fetus having a genetic condition. Screening tests are not fully diagnostic and are usually confirmed with one or more other tests. Routine newborn screening for several inherited conditions is undertaken by analysis of blood cells collected via a heel prick test before a baby is ten days old.

Prenatal diagnosis

This tests the genes or chromosomes of a baby before birth. It is offered when there is an increased risk the baby has a genetic or chromosomal disorder, such as when antenatal screening shows the likelihood is higher. Not all possible inherited disorders can be diagnosed, but the main chromosomal disorders such as trisomy 21 and 18 are. Methods include testing cells from the amniotic fluid (amniocentesis) or chorionic villus sampling (CVS).

Pre-implantation genetic diagnosis

These tests are carried out on human embryos created via assisted reproduction, usually *in vitro* fertilisation before they are transferred into a woman's uterus (i.e. before pregnancy). Specific single-gene disorders and major chromosomal disorders can be diagnosed by analysing cells from the early embryo, meaning couples can decide to avoid transferring an embryo with a disorder. There are strict criteria for single genes that can be tested for, and embryos cannot be rejected based only on sex.

Pre-pregnancy screening

Screening tests may be offered to people who have a family history or other increased risk of passing on a genetic condition and therefore, such tests are completed during the preconceptual period. Examples include testing prospective parents for the cystic fibrosis gene. The results, possibly including production of a Punnett chart or similar, can give couples an idea of the likelihood of their offspring inheriting a condition.

Epigenetics

The 'epi' in **epigenetics** relates to the Greek meaning 'on' or 'above'. The term epigenetics is used to describe changes to the ways genes work that goes beyond (or sits above – 'epi') the genetic code.

Epigenetic changes affect how cells read genes but does not involve alterations to the underlying DNA sequence. This is termed '**gene expression**' and is commonly understood as the turning of genes 'on' or 'off'. So, while there is no change in the genotype, there is a change in phenotype. Some epigenetic changes happen naturally during a lifespan, influencing how cells differentiate, but they can be damaging. They are of particular interest in health care because they are influenced by factors such as age, behaviour and environment. Epigenetic effects can be minor, but they can also be severe, for example leading to expression of cancer. They may also be reversible, which means that positive lifestyle choices made by individuals can improve their health prospects by altering gene expression. The changes are also heritable, so effects can have consequences for future generations, such as children and grandchildren. In pregnancy, environmental factors such as a woman's diet can affect epigenetic changes in the baby which can last into adulthood.

Conditions such as cancers, neurological and metabolic disorders have been linked to epigenetics. Another epigenetic phenomenon is **genomic imprinting**. Here, genes are expressed differently if inherited from the mother or father, but the genetic code is unaltered. Mutations of imprinted genes cause both Angelman syndrome (a disorder inherited from the mother) and Prader-Willi syndrome (a disorder inherited from the father), but these have the same genetic cause.

There are at least three types of epigenetic changes:

1. **DNA methylation** in which attachment of methyl groups to DNA turns genes 'off' (and demethylation turns them 'on').

2. **Histone modification** where tightly wrapped histones mask reading of the gene, so it is turned 'off' (more loosely wrapped histones turn them 'on').

3. Gene **silencing** by actions of non-coding RNA in preventing the formation of proteins.

APPLICATION TO PRACTICE

Epigenetics: DNA methylation and smoking

Epigenetic effects can be reversible, as shown by DNA methylation of the 'AHRR gene' in smokers. AHRR methylation tends to be lower in smokers (meaning the gene can be 'turned on') than in non-smokers. Lung-cancer mortality rates are far higher in those with low AHRR methylation and differences are greater in those who smoke more or for a longer time. However, importantly, when individuals stop smoking, AHRR methylation increases again and may return to similar levels to those of non-smokers.

Male and female reproductive systems

Ginny Mounce

LEARNING OUTCOMES

▶ Describe the male reproductive organs and spermatogenesis
▶ Describe the female reproductive organs and their functions
▶ Understand the female reproductive cycle, from oogenesis and follicle development to ovulation
▶ Understand the hormonal control of the female reproductive cycle

Introduction

Female and male sex cells, called gametes, each contain an individual's genetic information. Female gametes are egg cells, or **ova**, and male gametes are **sperm**. The structures that produce gametes are called the **gonads**. In females, these are the **ovaries**, and in males they are the **testes**. For successful human reproduction, gametes must be produced, stored, nourished, developed and brought together. The reproductive system includes all the organs, glands and passageways involved in these actions. The functions of the reproductive system in both sexes are regulated by hormones, mainly released from the gonads. This chapter introduces the male reproductive system first, before turning to the more complex female physiology.

Male reproductive system

The purpose of this reproductive system is to manufacture male gametes (sperm) and hormones, mainly testosterone, and to nourish and deliver sperm to the reproductive tract of a female.

DOI: 10.4324/9781003227571-8

Male reproductive organs

The primary organs are the testes (male gonads), plus the system of ducts which transport sperm from the testes via the penis to the exterior (Figure 2.3.1).

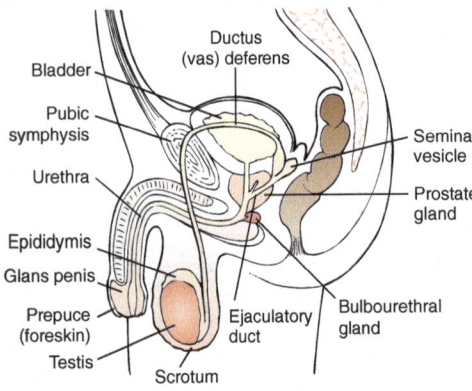

Figure 2.3.1 Main structures of the male reproductive system
Source: Figure 18.2(a), p.486, Clancy and McVicar (2009)

Testes

A pair of oval shaped organs, 4 cm by 2.5 cm, lie outside the pelvic cavity, suspended in a pouch of skin called the **scrotum**. The external location of the testes is important for maintaining the temperature (3°C lower than body temperature) necessary for optimal sperm production. In extreme cold conditions, the testes are pulled closer to the body for warmth by contractions of the scrotum's muscle fibres.

Each individual testis has a fibrous, white connective tissue outer called the **tunica albuginea** (literally a 'white coat'). Inward extensions of the tunica albuginea form large numbers of divisions called lobules. Inside each of these lobules are between one and four highly coiled tubules, named **seminiferous tubules** (Figure 2.3.2). These are the location of **spermatogenesis**, the creation of sperm. During spermatogenesis

(see below), sperm cells – **spermatocytes** – develop from germ cells in the seminiferous tubules.

Sertoli cells, embedded in the seminiferous tubules, are large specialist cells which nourish and protect the developing spermatocytes. Clusters of Sertoli cells at the basement membrane form dense junctions that are a blood-testis barrier, separating spermatogenic cells from the whole-body circulation. The barrier also separates the fluid in the lumen of the tubule from general interstitial fluid, maintaining the unique composition (high levels of amino acids, androgens and potassium ions) needed for sperm development.

Clusters of interstitial **(Leydig)** cells of the surrounding testicular tissue produce male hormone androgens, particularly testosterone. The seminiferous tubules in each lobule then open into the rete testis network area, which connects to the reproductive duct system.

The duct system

Sperm are transported to the exterior via a system of ducts: the epididymis, ductus deferens, ejaculatory ducts and urethra (Figure 2.3.1).

The first part of the duct system after the rete testis is the curved **epididymis**, which first hugs the superior part of each testis and then runs posterolaterally to it (Figure 2.3.2). This duct is highly coiled and if straightened would be around 6 metres in length. Immature sperm develop **motility** as they pass through the epididymis, a process that can take around 20 days. Sperm may then remain stored in this region for a month or more. During male sexual arousal and ejaculation, peristaltic contraction of the walls of the epididymis expel the sperm into the ductus deferens.

The wider and less convoluted **ductus deferens** runs upwards along the posterior

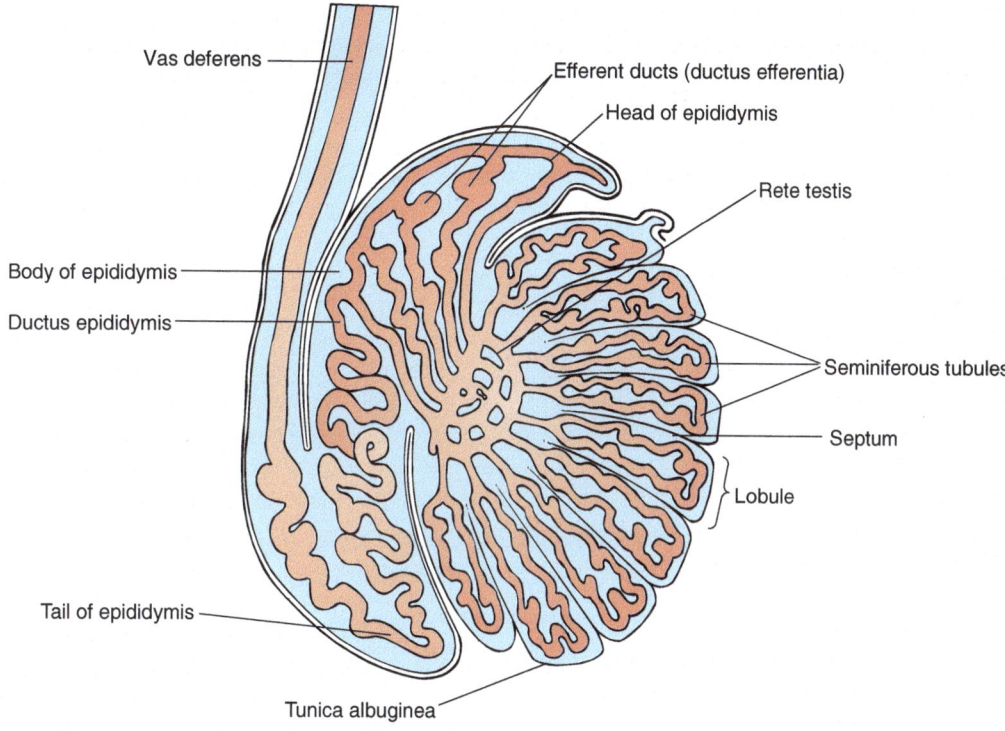

Vas deferens

Efferent ducts (ductus efferentia)

Head of epididymis

Rete testis

Body of epididymis

Ductus epididymis

Seminiferous tubules

Septum

Lobule

Tail of epididymis

Tunica albuginea

Figure 2.3.2 Sagittal section of a testis
Source: Figure 18.5(a), p.489, Clancy and McVicar (2009)

border of each epididymis, through the inguinal canal where it enters the pelvic cavity. This section of duct is enclosed by a connective sheath, called the spermatic cord, which also encloses blood vessels and nerves supplying the testes. In the pelvic cavity, the duct passes over the upper part of the bladder, loops around the ureter and descends behind the posterior bladder wall. Just in front of the prostate and seminal glands it widens to an ampulla region. The smooth muscle layers of the duct transport sperm by peristalsis, and like the epididymis, sperm can remain stored here for months. Sperm which are not ejaculated are eventually reabsorbed.

Next, the sperm enter the **ejaculatory duct**, which passes through the prostate gland where it merges with the urethra, still surrounded by prostate tissue. Just before ejaculation, sperm and seminal vesicle

secretions are moved into this prostatic urethra region by peristaltic contractions of smooth muscle. At ejaculation, sperm and seminal fluid are pushed powerfully and rapidly forward to the external urethral opening, aided by smooth muscle contractions of the ducts, seminal glands and walls of the prostate. Peristaltic contractions act on the bladder and internal urethral sphincter, causing them to contract at the same time, preventing semen from passing into the bladder. The contraction of the prostate acts as a clamp, preventing urine passing through.

The **urethra** is the final passageway of the male duct system, leading to the exterior, and is shared between the reproductive and urinary systems. The **penis** is the tubular male external genitalia which contains the urethra. The urethra transports both sperm and urine but, as described above, never at the same time. It is around 20 cm in length from the base of the urinary bladder to the tip of the penis, where the external urethral orifice is found.

Accessory glands and semen

The main accessory glands in males are the paired **seminal vesicles** and **bulbourethral glands**, and single **prostate gland** (Figure 2.3.1). These glands secrete fluid into the ejaculatory ducts and urethra which, combined with sperm, form the liquid called **semen**. The seminal vesicles empty thick, yellowish secretions into the ejaculatory ducts, making up around 60% of the seminal fluid volume. At ejaculation, small ducts from the prostate release a milky coloured and slightly acidic secretion which accounts for about a quarter of the seminal fluid. The bulbourethral glands open into the spongy urethra region and produce thick, clear alkaline mucus which helps to lubricate the penis tip and neutralise any urinary acids left in the urethra. This contributes about 5% of the seminal fluid.

Semen, then, is a milky-white mixture of 2–5 ml seminal fluid (including various secretions from the epididymis as well as accessory glands) and sperm (at a concentration of 50–150 million sperm per millilitre). Each ejaculate contains:

- Fructose, providing sperm with easily metabolised energy, needed for motility.
- Prostaglandins, which can stimulate muscle contractions in both the male and female tract.
- Fibrinogen, which temporarily clots semen in the vagina (thought to help maintain its position there).
- Alkaline secretions from seminal vesicles, which help to make semen slightly alkaline (pH 7.2–7.6) overall (despite the acidic contribution from prostate glands). This combats the more acidic conditions of the urethra and

vagina, which is hostile to the rather delicate sperm.

- Several enzymes, including a protease which helps to break down mucus in the female tract.
- A protein, seminal plasmin, which has antibacterial properties.

Spermatogenesis

While in females the mitotic division of germ cells to produce gametes (oogenesis – see below) begins in embryonic development, the equivalent process in males – **spermatogenesis**, the creation of sperm – begins during puberty (the time, generally between ages 10 and 15 years, when the reproductive organs in both sexes develop and become functional), and continues throughout a males' lifetime. Each day millions of sperm are produced.

Spermatogenesis starts with germ cells called **spermatogonia**, found in the basement membrane of the seminiferous tubules in the testes (Figure 2.3.2). From birth until puberty spermatogonia proliferate by mitotic cell division (see Chapter 2.1). At puberty, **follicle stimulating hormone** (FSH) is secreted from the anterior pituitary gland (found at the base of the brain), triggering subsequent mitotic divisions of the germ cell to produce two functionally different but chromosomally identical daughter cells:

- **Type A daughter cells**, which remain at the basement membrane, continuing mitotic division to maintain the germ cell population.
- **Type B daughter cells**, which are pushed away from the basement membrane towards the lumen of the seminiferous tubule. These cells are destined to become sperm. At this point they are called **primary spermatocytes**.

As the primary spermatocytes advance towards the middle of the tubule, they undergo **meiosis**, producing four haploid daughter cells (see Chapter 2.1). **Meiosis I** of the primary spermatocyte produces two haploid **secondary spermatocytes**. Meiosis II leads to the production of **spermatids** (Figure 2.3.3).

There are now four early spermatids, each with half the genetic material, as the germ cells. At this stage spermatids are not functional gametes. They are immature, small and non-motile. Their excess cytoplasm, which gives them a rounded shape, is phagocytised by the Sertoli cells (see above) aiding their transformation. A tail is formed, and the resulting spermatozoa are compacted and streamlined. The maturing spermatozoa, detached from the supporting cells and released into the lumen of seminiferous tubules, are still not fully motile.

The final stage of spermatogenesis, called **spermiogenesis**, is the gradual physical maturation to adult sperm. As sperm exit the seminiferous tubules and are directed along the various ducts of the male reproductive system, they develop into adult sperm with increased motility and ability to fertilise. Approximately three million spermatozoa are matured each day, and their complete development takes around 70 days.

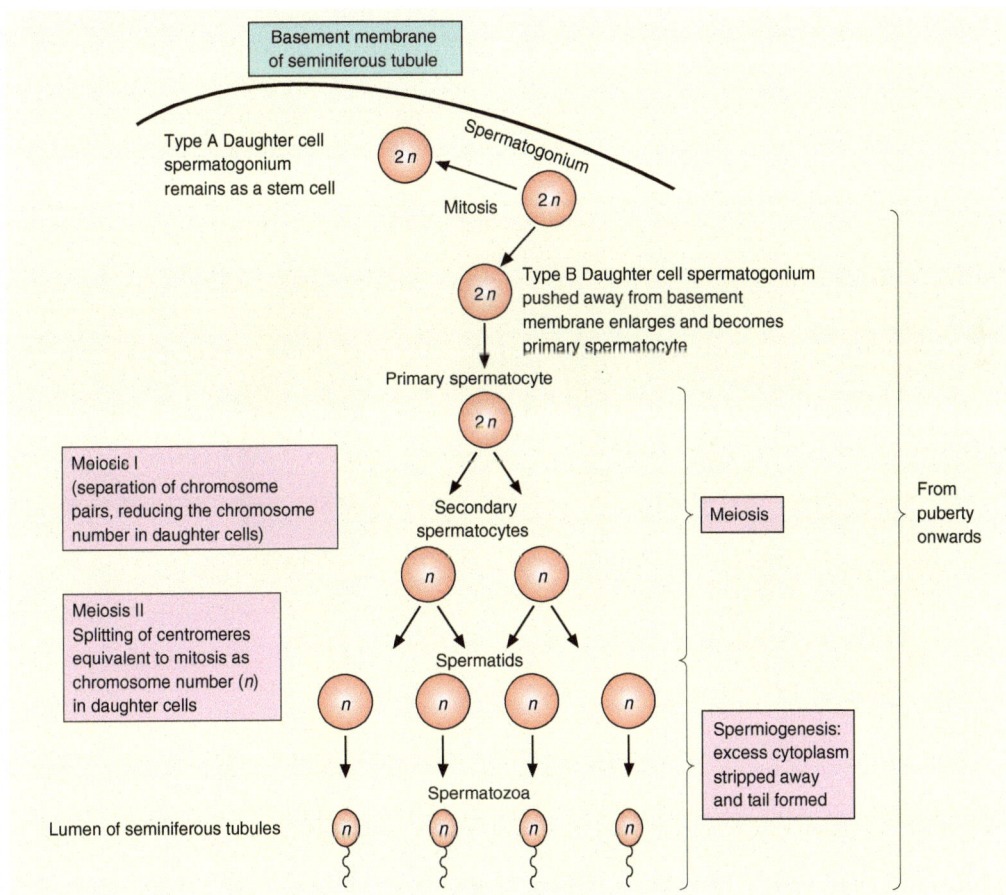

Figure 2.3.3 Spermatogenesis: Events in the seminiferous tubules; 2n = diploid; n = haploid
Source: Figure 18.11, p.501, Clancy and McVicar (2009)

Sperm

Spermatozoa (singular form is **spermatozoon**) or sperm (Figure 2.3.4), the male gamete, contains the genetic information necessary for reproduction. A mature sperm cell is microscopic, being around 65 μm in length, and 20 times smaller than an oocyte. It has a distinct streamlined shape, consisting of three sections: a head, mid-piece and tail. Its structure is highly adapted to its purpose: to reach and fertilise a female gamete.

Mature sperm can propel themselves quickly, by means of their tail. This is a flagellum, a cellular organelle which causes movement by its whip-like motion – sperm are the only human body cells with this feature. Their movement requires metabolic energy in the form of adenosine triphosphate (ATP), generated at a high rate by specialised 'spiral mitochondria' in the mid-piece of the sperm. As sperm do not store the energy needed for this purpose, or have many other cell organelles, they do not survive for long outside the male reproductive tract – about 48 hours. Nutrients and sugar, mainly fructose, are absorbed by sperm from the surrounding seminal fluid. The headpiece of sperm contains the nucleus, compacted genetic material (DNA), capped by an area called the acrosome. This is a vesicle similar to a lysosome, containing enzymes and other proteases that will help the sperm penetrate and fertilise an oocyte (see Chapter 2.4).

Unsurprisingly, perhaps, many of the several million sperm formed each day in adult males will be morphologically or physiologically abnormal, for example having giant heads or low motility. Examples of common sperm abnormalities found in a sample of semen and their possible causes are shown in Table 2.3.1.

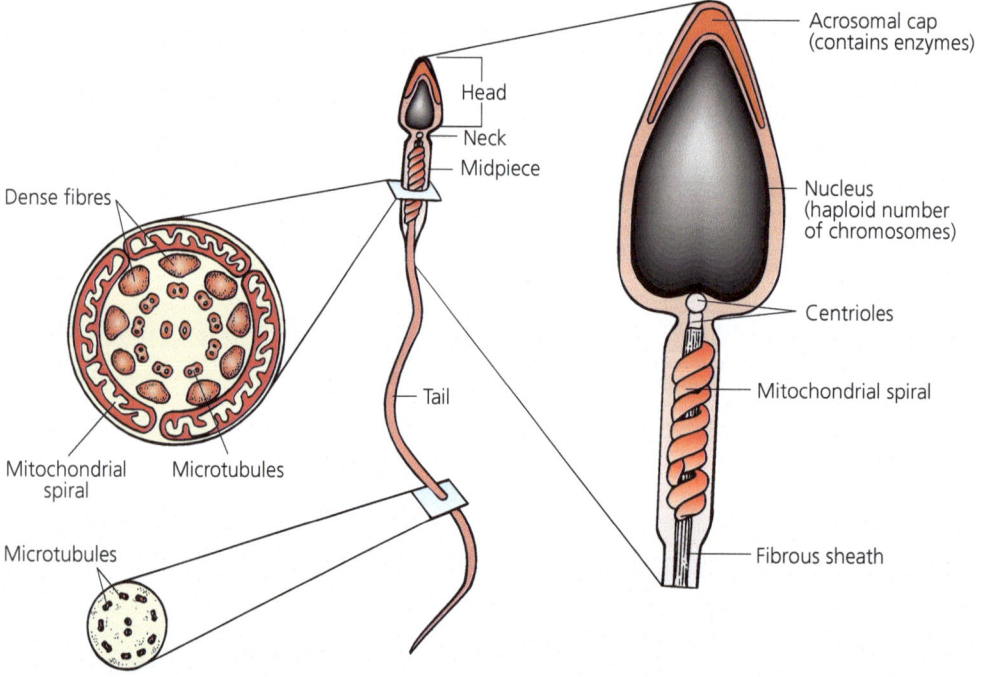

Figure 2.3.4 Structure of sperm
Source: Figure 18.12, p.502, Clancy and McVicar (2009)

Table 2.3.1 Sperm abnormalities

Sperm abnormality	Description	Possible cause
Azoospermia	No measurable sperm in ejaculate	Testicular failure (Klinefelter syndrome, orchitis, chemotherapy, hypogonadism), duct obstruction (congenital, orchitis, trauma), successful vasectomy, genetic, unknown
Oligozoospermia	Low sperm count	As above, plus varicocele, hydrocele, toxins, drugs, obesity
Idiopathic oligospermia	Low sperm count with no identified underlying cause	Unexplained
Teratozoospermia	Abnormal shaped sperm, e.g. round headed, no tails, two heads	Unexplained, associated with genetic conditions, toxins
Asthenospermia	Reduced sperm motility	Inherited metabolic diseases, toxins
Agglutination	Sperm adhered to each other	Presence of anti-sperm antibodies, infection

Sexual intercourse – male physiology

Semen is generally introduced into the female reproductive tract during sexual intercourse, or coitus. This is a complex event of physiological and psychological responses for both partners. The female physiology is described below. From the male perspective:

▶ Sexual arousal with visual or tactile stimulation leads to erection of the penis.
▶ Arteries dilate, rapidly fill with blood and enter the spongy tissue.
▶ The resulting expansion of vascular channels compresses the veins which prevents venous return and maintains the erection.
▶ After entry into the vagina, rhythmic stimulation of the penis causes peristaltic contractions of the duct systems, moving sperm forward along the urethra.
▶ Secretions from the accessory glands add seminal fluid to the sperm.
▶ Eventually, the skeletal muscles eject the semen from the urethra (into the vagina) during ejaculation.

▶ Sperm ascend the reproductive tract and may reach and fertilise a secondary oocyte (see Chapter 2.4).

The body wide release of tension is the pleasurable sensation of the male (and female) **orgasm**. Post orgasm, blood drains from the penis which becomes flaccid and leaves the vagina.

Female reproductive system

The female external genitalia and internal female reproductive organs, consisting of the ovaries, uterine tubes, uterus and vagina, are described below.

External female genitalia

The female reproductive tract is exposed at the external opening of the vagina into a space called the **vestibule**. This space also contains the **external urethral orifice**, where urine is excreted. The vestibule is bordered by structures collectively known as the **vulva**. The vulva functions as sensory tissue during sexual arousal and intercourse, in directing the passing of urine and in protecting the internal reproductive tract from infection.

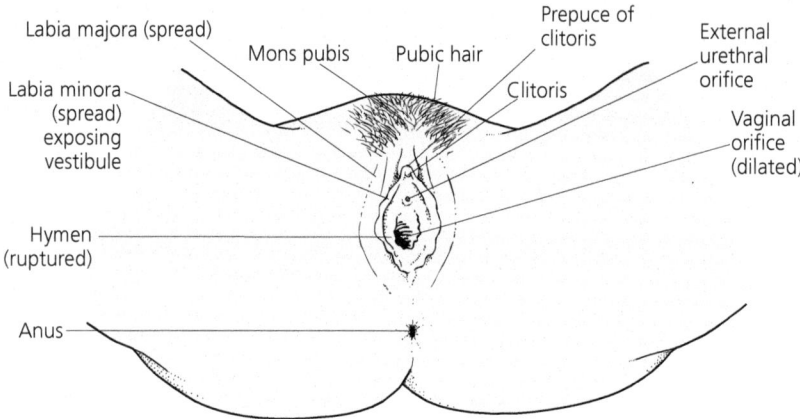

Figure 2.3.5 External female genitalia
Source: Figure 14.6, p.258, David Sturgeon (2018)

Figure 2.3.5 shows the main anatomical structures of the vulva, with the woman positioned lying on her back with her legs raised and apart. The vestibule is usually enclosed by two folds of hairless skin, the **labia minora**, themselves lying within two hair-bearing external skin folds, the **labia majora**. The urethral opening and vaginal entrance may only be visible when the folds of the labia minora are gently parted.

The **clitoris**, formed of erectile tissue and nerve endings, is located under a hood of tissue formed by anterior fusion of the labia minora. The merging of the labia minora posterior to the vaginal opening forms a fold of tissue, the **fourchette**. The vestibule area is kept moist by secretions from the **greater and lesser vestibular glands**, and secretions from sebaceous glands lubricate the inner surface of the labia majora.

The labia majora are bounded by the **mons pubis** (a pad of subcutaneous fat covering the symphysis pubis) anteriorly and **perineal body** (see Chapter 4.6) posteriorly.

Blood supply to the external genitalia is via pudendal arteries and veins. Motor and sensory nerve supply is via branches of the pudendal nerve which innervate the external genitalia, skin and anus (as well as the perineum and pelvic floor muscles).

Internal female reproductive organs

The main internal structures of the female reproductive tract are contained within the pelvic cavity, where they are protected from external elements. These are the **ovaries** (gonads), **uterus**, **cervix**, **vagina** and **uterine tubes**. Figure 2.3.6 indicates their positions relative to each other in a classic cross-sectional view. The vagina lies behind (posterior to) the bladder and urethra. The uterus, uterine tubes and ovaries are all above (superior to) the bladder and vagina. Additionally, they are all in front of (anterior to) the rectum and colon, the final passageways of the digestive tract and the most posterior structures in the pelvic cavity.

APPLICATION TO PRACTICE

As shown in Figure 2.3.6, the passages of the urethra, vagina and rectum are all very closely situated. A sound understanding of the location and function of each of these can help to

(a)

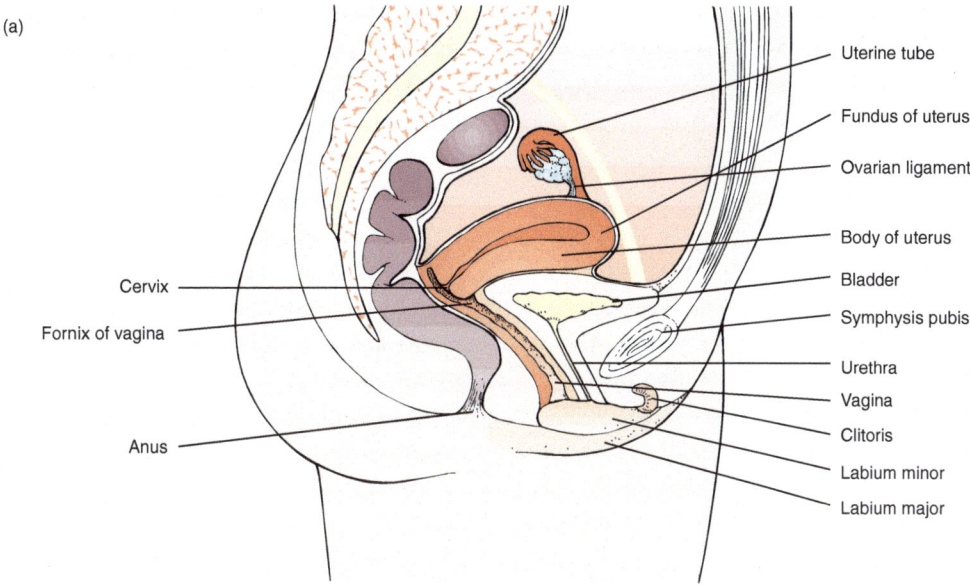

Uterine tube
Fundus of uterus
Ovarian ligament
Body of uterus
Bladder
Symphysis pubis
Urethra
Vagina
Clitoris
Labium minor
Labium major

Cervix
Fornix of vagina
Anus

(b)

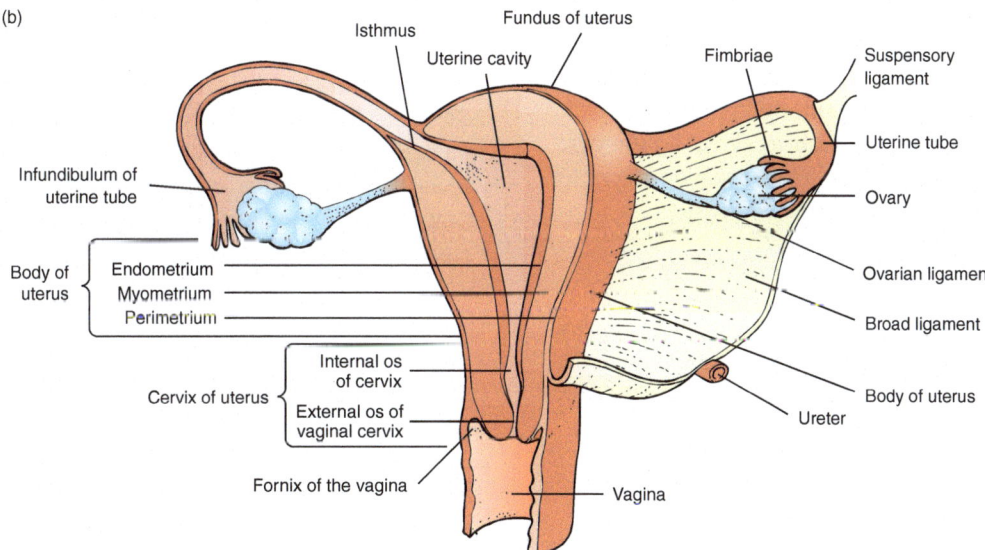

Isthmus
Fundus of uterus
Uterine cavity
Fimbriae
Suspensory ligament
Uterine tube
Ovary
Infundibulum of uterine tube
Body of uterus
Endometrium
Myometrium
Perimetrium
Ovarian ligament
Broad ligament
Cervix of uterus
Internal os of cervix
External os of vaginal cervix
Body of uterus
Ureter
Fornix of the vagina
Vagina

Figure 2.3.6 The female reproductive organs: a) sagittal section; b) frontal section
Source: Figure 18.7, p.494, Clancy and McVicar (2009)

inform understanding of the physiological processes of pregnancy, childbirth and recovery. For example, note how the bladder sits inferior to the uterus, and anterior to the vagina. In pregnancy, the uterus enlarges and so compresses the bladder, resulting in increased frequency of urination. Conversely, a bladder full of urine pushes the uterus upwards, and can impede the advancing fetus during labour. This is one reason why careful monitoring of urine output is important.

All of these main structures are held in place in the pelvic cavity by various abdominal ligaments. The most significant is the **broad ligament** (shown in Figure 2.3.6b), a flat sheet of ligament which encloses the surfaces of the uterus, uterine tubes and ovaries anteriorly and posteriorly, extending laterally to the pelvic walls. It can be helpful to think of the broad ligament as being rather like a sheet thrown, or draped, over their surface. The broad ligament also encloses the uterine blood vessels, nerves and lymph vessels, and controls side-to-side movement and rotation of organs. Other supportive uterine and ovarian ligaments are themselves located within the broad ligament. The **round ligament** arises from the uterine horns and passes via the inguinal canal to tissues of the external genitalia. This maintains the posterior position of the uterus. Stretching of this ligament during pregnancy can cause discomfort. **Uterosacral ligaments**, **cardinal ligaments** and **pubocervical ligaments** also play an important role in situating the uterus within the pelvic cavity.

The uterus

A pear-shaped, hollow, muscular organ, the uterus receives, protects and nourishes the fertilised egg (ovum) as it develops through the embryonic stage into the fully formed fetus. In labour, its muscular structure produces contractions to aid birth. Pre-pregnancy, the uterus is around 7–8 cm in length, 4–5 cm at its widest and 4 cm thick. A pregnant or gravid uterus gradually increases in size to be around five times larger. The uterus projects onto and joins the vagina and connects laterally to the uterine tubes. It has a good blood supply from interconnected branches of the uterine artery; this supports its ability to provide and renew a suitable environment for ovum implantation and possible development of a placenta.

It is usual to think of the uterus as having three distinct anatomical regions: **fundus**, **body** and **cervix** (Figure 2.3.6b). The fundus is the rounded top portion, just above the entry of the uterine tubes at the uterine horns. The main part of the uterus is the body, the lower aspect of which narrows to a region known as the isthmus. A structurally distinct lower 3 cm part extends downwards from the isthmus; this is the cervix. It projects about 1.25 cm into the vagina.

The uterus is made up of three main layers. The **perimetrium** is the outer, serous layer covering the fundus and, posteriorly, the uterine body and isthmus. The **myometrium** is the middle layer of thick, smooth muscle, making up 90% of the uterine mass. Muscle fibres are positioned longitudinally, obliquely and circularly within the myometrium and coordinated contractions of these in labour facilitate childbirth (see Chapter 4.2). The **endometrium** is the collective name for cells lining the uterine cavity. The innermost functional endometrial layer undergoes regular proliferation and morphological changes during the menstrual cycle in response to hormonal changes. If there is no pregnancy, this layer is shed during menstruation.

The normal position of the uterus outside of pregnancy can be described as **anteverted** (rotated forward, towards the anterior surface of the body) with respect to the vagina, and **anteflexed** (flexed (or bent) towards the anterior surface of the body) with respect to the cervix (Figure 2.3.6a). Less often, the uterus is tilted backwards at the cervix (**retroflexed**) toward the sacrum. This has no clinical significance, and in late pregnancy most become anteflexed. Usually, the anterior and posterior walls of the uterus are described as being in apposition, meaning very close together, so little space is actually present (not as it may appear in many diagrams).

2.3

The **cervix** connects the uterus and vagina via a restrictive passageway, the cervical (endocervical) canal. The lower portion of the cervix, which projects into the vagina, is known as **ectocervix** (Figure 2.3.7). The spaces surrounding the cervix in the vagina are called the fornix, with the portions between the anterior and posterior vaginal walls called, respectively, the anterior and posterior fornix. The ectocervix has a rounded end, which curves inwards to the **external os** (opening) of the cervical canal. The **internal os** is where the narrow cervical canal opens into the cavity of the uterine body.

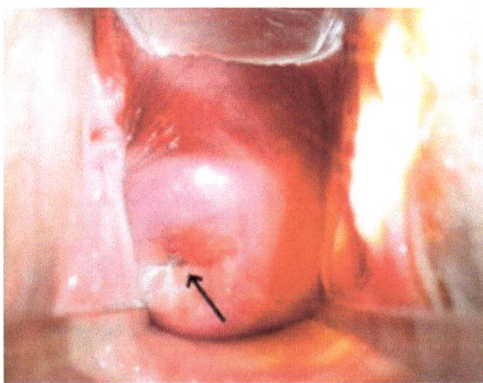

Figure 2.3.7 The ectocervix and external os (identified with an arrow)

The cervix acts as both a passageway and a barrier. Access through the endocervical canal is restricted by the narrow external os and by thick mucus secretions from columnar epithelial cells. The uterus above the cervix is thus protected from ascending infection. Around the time of ovulation, under the influence of oestrogen, cervical mucus becomes thinner and more alkaline (hospitable to sperm). This allows passage through the external os which, also due to the effects of oestrogen, opens slightly. At other times in a menstrual cycle and in pregnancy the thicker and more acidic mucus prevents sperm entering the uterus. In childbirth, the cervix softens, shortens and dilates in order to allow descent of the baby through the birth canal.

The vagina

The vagina is the short passageway connecting the cervix to the exterior. It is a thin walled, distensible fibromuscular organ of 7–10 cm in length. The vagina projects upwards and backwards, at an approximately 45° angle from the vestibule. Its muscular walls and many transverse folds of vaginal epithelium (called **rugae**) allow for expansion, so that during childbirth the vagina can expand to accommodate the descending fetus. Outside of pregnancy, it functions as a passageway for the monthly flow of menstrual blood. During sexual intercourse, the vagina receives the erect penis. Ejaculated sperm pass from the vagina, through the cervix into the uterus, where they may later meet and fertilise an oocyte (see below).

The stratified squamous epithelium lining the vagina is a defensive layer, lubricated by cervical mucus. The vagina itself does not contain any glands. It does contain antigen-presenting dendritic cells which process foreign antigens, such as viruses. The bacteria that naturally colonise the vagina (the vaginal flora) metabolise the nutrients from the cervical mucus, producing lactic acid. Consequently, these colonies, usually dominated by lactobacillus, contribute to maintaining the acidic environment of the vagina. The low pH (<4.5) is protective against infection by common pathogens. While an acid pH is also harmful to sperm, the composition of semen neutralises this effect. Disruptions to the environmental composition of the vagina, by other bacteria or changes in pH, can give rise to problems such as candida yeast infection.

Uterine tubes

The two uterine tubes extend c.10 cm from either side of the uterus, each towards an ovary (Figure 2.3.6). The slightly wider portion where each joins the uterus is a thick-walled isthmus. Two thirds of each uterine tube is the ampulla portion. The distal end is funnel-shaped, called the **infundibulum**, which ends in 'finger like' projections called **fimbriae**. Although the infundibulum of both tubes is open to the pelvic cavity, the fimbriae surround and drape over the ovary, aiding in the collection of any oocytes the ovary releases. The uterine tubes therefore function as a channel to transport oocytes from the ovaries to the uterus, as well as being the site of fertilisation.

The uterine tubes consist of three layers. The internal surface contains columnar epithelial cells, either secretory or with cilia (hairlike projections). The middle part is smooth muscle arranged in thick rings covered by longitudinal sections. The outer layer is a serous membrane. The epithelial secretions of lipids and glycogen provide both ovum and sperm with nutrients. An oocyte is transported towards the uterus by the twin effects of peristaltic contractions of the smooth muscle layer, and the rhythmic movement caused by beating of epithelial cilia. Events of fertilisation are described further in Chapter 2.4.

Ovaries

Ovaries are the primary female reproductive organs; they are the gonads where gametes (egg cells) are produced. They also produce the hormones progesterone, oestrogens, inhibin and relaxin (see below).

Ovaries are paired organs, roughly almond shaped, found at the lateral walls of the pelvic cavity on each side of the uterus just below the level of the uterine tubes. They have a grey or whitish nodular appearance. Although well supported in their location by ligaments, the ovaries are fairly mobile, particularly in women who have had children.

Sexual intercourse – female physiology

Sexual stimulation of the female causes the clitoris to swell with blood and become highly sensitive. The vestibular bulbs (tissue masses deep into the labia, either side of the opening) also become erect, narrowing the orifice. The labia become engorged, enhancing pleasurable sensations. Mucus release from the cervix and greater vestibular glands moistens the vaginal area, reducing friction and easing the entrance of the erect male penis. Female orgasm causes muscle spasms that move the cervix towards the vagina, aiding passage of sperm into the cervical canal.

The female reproductive cycle

In reproductive age females, the development and release of oocytes involves an approximately monthly series of changes that coincide with adjustments in the uterus in preparation to receive a fertilised oocyte. If this does not happen and if pregnancy does not occur, then the changes are reset, and the cycles start again. The overall term for these events is the **female reproductive cycle**. Within this cycle are two cycles at play – the **ovarian cycle** and **uterine cycle** – both of which are controlled by hormones.

Before covering the ovarian and uterine cycles, we will introduce **oogenesis**, the development of mature female gametes from germ cells in the ovaries.

Oogenesis

Oogenesis, like spermatogenesis, involves meiotic division of germ cells to create gametes – in this case egg cells (**oocytes** or **ova**).

In females, all the mitotic division of germ cells (**oogonia**) to **primary oocytes** (daughter cells) is completed during embryonic development. By five months gestation a female fetus may have around seven million primary oocytes. This number falls to approximately two million at birth due to degeneration, in a process called **atresia**. By puberty, the number of primary oocytes has fallen further to around 400,000. Before birth, all remaining primary oocytes in an ovary have begun cell division by meiosis, but they only reach the prophase stage of meiosis I (see Chapter 2.1). At this point they are said to be in a state of **suspended development**.

From puberty onwards, each month several primary oocytes are stimulated by the action of FSH to continue their meiotic development. However, generally only one primary oocyte each month completes meiosis stage I; resulting in a single **secondary oocyte** (paused at the metaphase stage of meiosis II). Instead of a second secondary oocyte forming, a tiny **polar body** is formed which is discarded DNA (Figure 2.3.8). The functional secondary oocyte is expelled from the ovary at **ovulation**, passing into the uterine tube. If penetrated by a sperm, then meiosis II of the oocyte is completed and it is renamed an **ovum**, a mature female gamete (with half the number of chromosomes). With the completion of meiosis II comes creation of a second polar body. Both of the meiotic divisions result in unequal distribution of cytoplasm; the secondary oocyte is very much larger than the three tiny polar bodies. All the polar bodies degenerate. This process overall means that for females, each meiotic division leads to creation of just one, much larger ovum, and two polar bodies.

Follicle development and ovulation

In the ovary, the primary oocytes are enclosed by a layer of follicular cells; together the structure is called an **ovarian follicle**. The most immature, found at the outer cortex region, are called **primordial ovarian follicles**. These are continuously being activated (by mechanisms not fully understood), meaning that in ovaries there is a pool of follicles at various stages of development.

Primary ovarian follicles develop as the oocyte inside enlarges, with follicular cells proliferating to produce several new layers, known as **granulosa cells**. A clear glycoprotein layer called the **zona pellucida** develops in between the primary oocyte and granulosa cells.

The outside layer of granulosa cells continues to grow and thicken, and the follicle is now a **secondary follicle** (or antral follicle). This process occurs over many months, controlled by an ovarian growth factor. Further growth continues until the deepest granulosa cells start to secrete follicular fluid. This accumulates between the inner and outer layers, forming a distinct fluid filled central region, the **antrum**. This doubles the size of the follicle, which is now known as a **tertiary follicle** (Figure 2.3.9). Tertiary follicles are now ready to be acted upon by the hormones of the ovarian cycle, as described in the following sections.

Only a few tertiary follicles are present at the start of an ovarian cycle. By day 5 usually just one, stimulated by FSH, becomes the largest. This is known as the **dominant** (or Graafian) **follicle**. Rapid growth continues for around 10–14 days until it measures 15–20 mm in diameter.

2.3

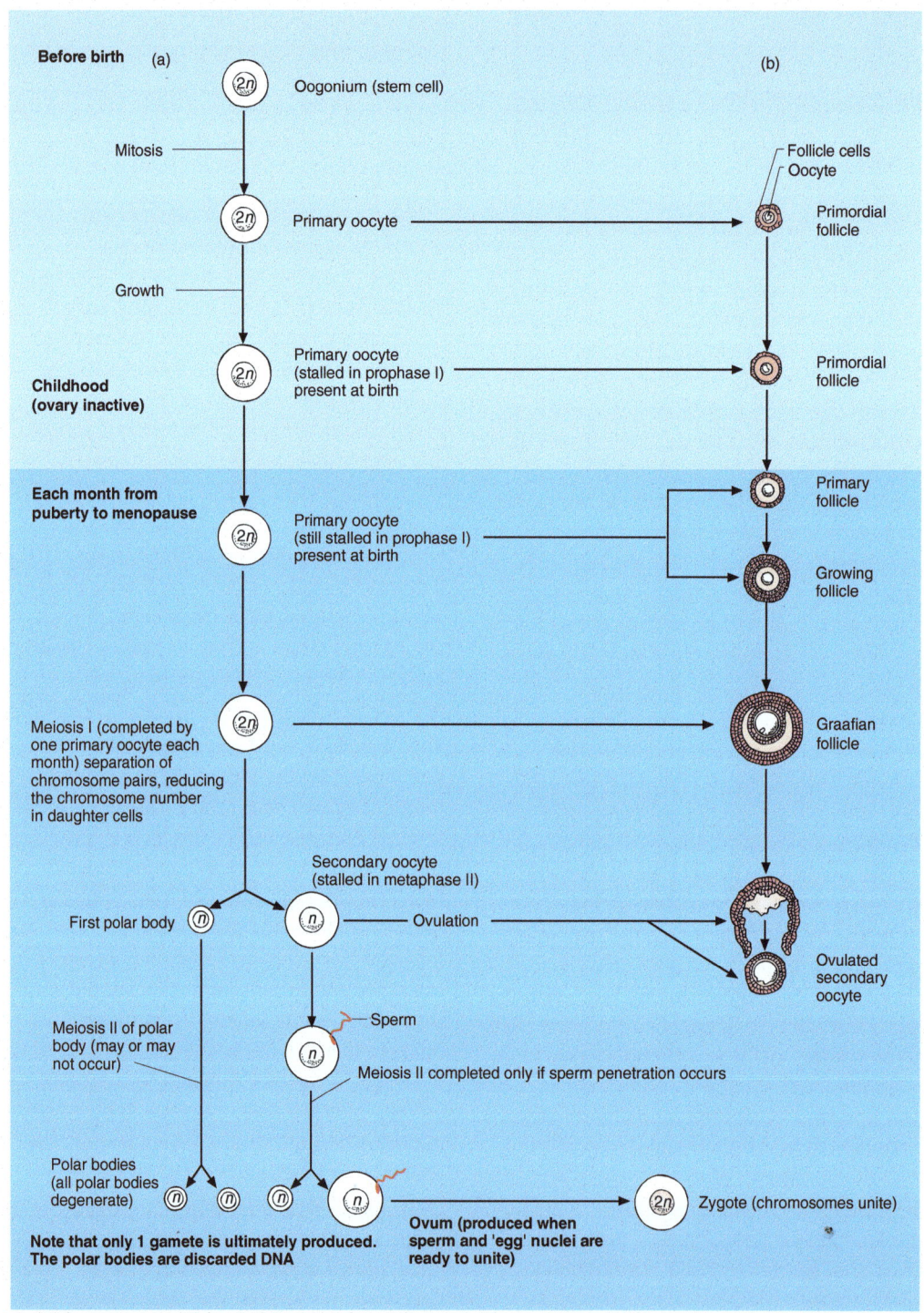

Figure 2.3.8 a) Process of oogenesis (2n = diploid, n = haploid); b) Follicle development in the ovary

Source: Figure 18.13(a), (b), p.504, Clancy and McVicar (2009)

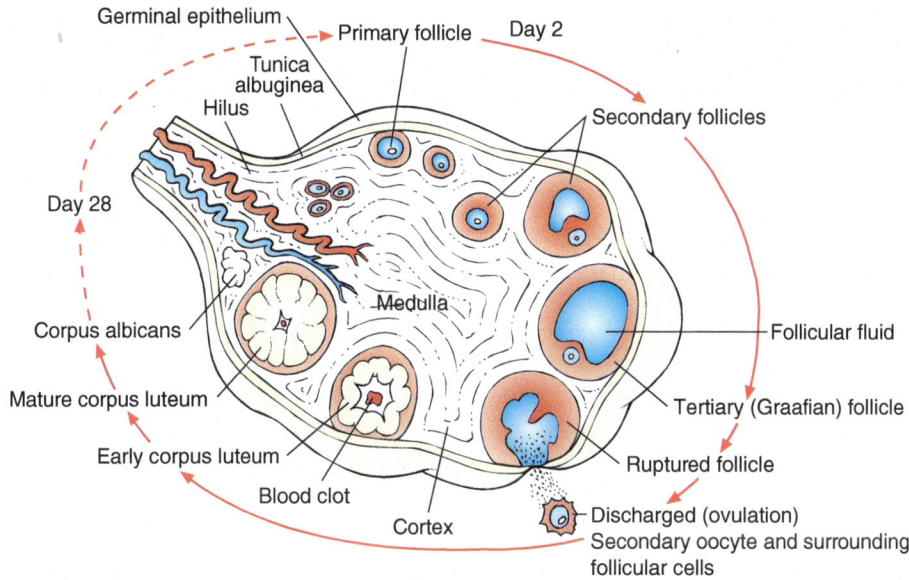

Germinal epithelium
Tunica albuginea
Hilus
Primary follicle
Day 2
Secondary follicles
Day 28
Medulla
Follicular fluid
Corpus albicans
Mature corpus luteum
Early corpus luteum
Blood clot
Cortex
Tertiary (Graafian) follicle
Ruptured follicle
Discharged (ovulation)
Secondary oocyte and surrounding follicular cells

Figure 2.3.9 Development of an ovarian follicle
Source: Figure 18.8 (a), p.495, Clancy and McVicar (2009)

The primary oocyte within this follicle, surrounded by a ring of granulosa cells called the **corona radiata**, projects into the antrum. The dominant follicle moves towards the edge of the ovary, and with a surge of luteinising hormone (LH), the tertiary follicle releases the secondary oocyte into the pelvic cavity.

The now empty ruptured **dominant follicle** initially collapses, but the remaining granulosa cells, still influenced by LH, proliferate to form the **corpus luteum** (yellow body). Its yellow colour is from the cholesterol used to make the hormone **progesterone**. If fertilisation occurs, the corpus luteum will remain and produce progesterone and other hormones until the placenta takes over. If fertilisation does not occur then the corpus luteum will degenerate after around 12 days, forming an area of white fibrous tissue called the **corpus albicans** (white body).

Although many primary follicles are developed, only a few tertiary follicles are activated each month, so a woman is likely to release only 500 or so secondary oocytes in a lifetime. Over time, and increasingly as she approaches 40 years of age, the pool of available primordial ovarian follicles decreases, and her ovaries become less responsive to hormones, which in turn means fewer eggs are released. As her ovarian cycles become less regular and decline further, and generally before she reaches 50, her reproductive capacity is limited. **Menopause** is the term for the complete cessation of the monthly cycles.

The female reproductive cycle in depth

The ovarian and uterine cycles of the female reproductive cycle operate synchronously; if they do not, then successful ovulation and implantation cannot occur. A cycle is typically of 25–35 days duration, but for the purposes of clarity here we assume a cycle to be 28 days. Both cycles are maintained due to the action of hormones, described in Table 2.3.2. A summary diagram of the two cycles, and how they work in synchrony,

Table 2.3.2 Hormones of the female reproductive cycle

Hormone	Source	Initiation	Main effects
Gonadotrophin releasing hormone (GnRH)	Hypothalamus, continuous pulses	Increased by oestrogens, decreased by progesterone	Stimulates FSH synthesis and secretion, stimulates LH synthesis
Follicle stimulating hormone (FSH)	Anterior pituitary gland	Stimulated by GnRH, inhibited by inhibin	Stimulates follicle development, oestrogen production, oocyte maturation
Luteinising hormone (LH)	Anterior pituitary gland	Stimulated by GnRH, and surge initiated by high GnRH and oestrogen	Stimulates ovulation, creation of corpus luteum, progesterone production
Oestrogens	Ovarian follicles (granulosa and theca cells), corpus luteum	Stimulated by FSH	Stimulates LH secretion and increases GnRH pulses (at high levels), maintains secondary sex characteristics and behaviour, stimulates endometrial growth
Progesterone	Ovarian follicle (granulosa cells), corpus luteum	Stimulated by LH	Maintains endometrial growth and secretion, reduces GnRH pulses
Inhibin	Ovarian follicles (granulosa cells)	Developing follicles	Inhibits FSH secretion
Relaxin	Corpus luteum	Stimulated by LH	Inhibits uterine contractions

is shown in Figure 2.3.10. An in-depth description of both cycles follows.

INTERRUPTER

Fill in the gaps in the hormones of the female reproductive cycle table in your workbook (or make your own) to help embed this knowledge.

Ovarian cycle

The three phases of the ovarian cycle support the growth and maturation of a secondary oocyte in preparation for fertilisation and reproduction under hormonal control.

Follicular phase

In the **follicular phase** there are low levels of circulating oestrogens and progesterone because there is no pregnancy. This promotes the frequency of pulses of **gonadotropin releasing hormone** (GnRH) from the hypothalamus, which in turn stimulates FSH and LH production from the anterior pituitary gland. Secretion of FSH causes several tertiary follicles in the ovaries to grow. These begin to secrete **oestrogens** (**oestradiol**, oestrone and oestriol). Rising levels of oestradiol cause a surge in LH. When oestradiol reaches a certain peak, FSH secretion is inhibited. This causes a slowing in growth of the tertiary follicles, except the dominant follicle. The dominant follicle secretes **inhibin** which further suppresses FSH. The dominant follicle prevails and forms a bulge near the surface of the ovary and soon becomes competent to ovulate.

The follicular phase of the ovarian cycle overlaps with the **menstrual** and **proliferative phases** of the uterine cycle (see below).

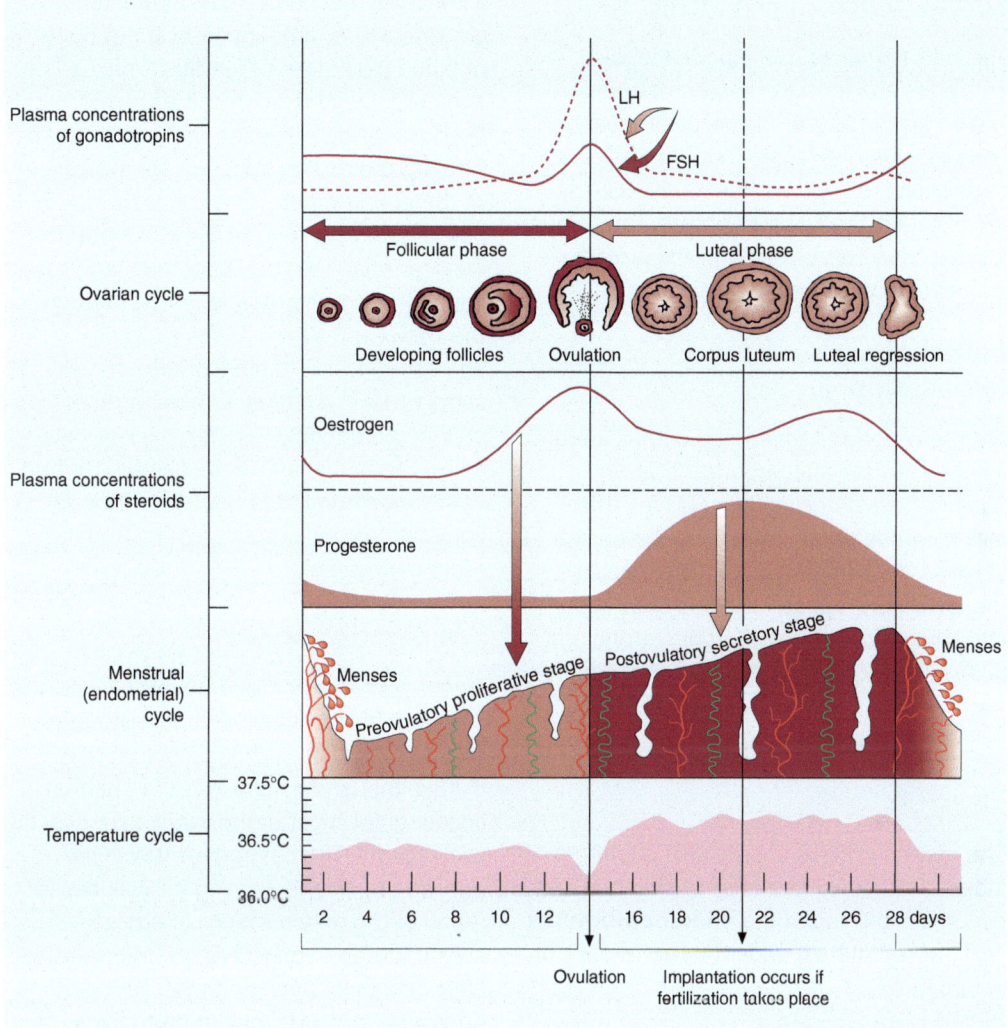

Figure 2.3.10 Summary diagram of the female reproductive cycle
Source: Figure 18.15, p.507, Clancy and McVicar (2009)

Ovulation

By around day 14, levels of oestrogens have peaked, as have the frequency of GnRH pulses, giving rise to a massive surge in LH from the anterior pituitary gland. This LH surge occurs around day 12–13, and triggers three main events:

▶ Completion of meiosis I by the dominant follicle. Meiosis II begins.
▶ A rupture of the dominant follicular wall.

▶ Ovulation, at around day 14. This is the expulsion (release) of the secondary oocyte along with its corona radiata cells from the ovary.

The LH surge starts around 36 hours before ovulation. This rise may be detected by urine tests and used to predict ovulation for those seeking pregnancy. The oocyte will be carried towards and into the uterine tube, and may then meet a sperm and be fertilised (see Chapter 2.4).

Luteal phase – with fertilisation

The cells of the residual ruptured follicle proliferate and form the corpus luteum. The corpus luteum produces oestrogen and progesterone for around two weeks to develop the endometrium of the uterus, which awaits the fertilised oocyte. The corpus luteum continues its role until the placenta is adequately developed to take over.

Luteal phase – without fertilisation

If there is no fertilisation, the corpus luteum will degenerate after around 12 days, because levels of circulating LH fall. The failing corpus luteum becomes the corpus albicans. As its secretory activity declines, the levels of progesterone and oestrogen fall rapidly. Low levels of progesterone and oestrogen allow release of GnRH again, which in turn causes release of FSH. The ovarian cycle starts again.

Uterine cycle

The uterine cycle is usually split into three stages to explain the series of changes that occur to the lining of the **endometrium** (the lining of the uterus) under hormonal control.

Menstrual phase

This marks the start of a reproductive cycle. **Menstruation** or **menses** (or colloquially a 'period') is the vaginal discharge of blood and secretions which lasts around five days. The first day of menstruation is traditionally counted as day 1 of a woman's menstrual cycle. A female's first menses tends to be around two years after the start of puberty and is called the **menarche**, although ovulation is not usually dependable for a further year or more.

Menses occurs because of the degeneration and shedding of the functional layer of the endometrium. Over a period of around five days, the entire layer detaches, amounting to about 50 ml of blood plus other tissue fluid, mucus and cells. Degeneration comes about because falling progesterone levels release prostaglandins that constrict spiral arteries of the endometrium. This causes a lack of oxygen, and the tissues die. The blood from weak arterial walls and degenerating tissues are shed from the uterine cavity, through the cervix and vagina to the exterior. The basal layer of the endometrium, supplied by the deeper straight arteries, is unaffected but only 2–5 mm thick at this point. Menstruation can be painful, termed **dysmenorrhoea**, due to uterine muscle contractions, inflammation or related to other conditions.

Proliferative phase

This is sometimes called the preovulatory phase as it occurs between menstruation and ovulation. As such it occurs on days 6–13, although this phase is the one that accounts for most of the variation in overall cycle length. The oestrogens which are released by the developing follicles cause repair of the endometrium. The basal cells undergo mitotic division to form a new functional layer. Epithelial cells and endometrial glands multiply, arterioles lengthen and further growth restores the endometrium. It doubles in thickness to 4–10 mm. The 'proliferative' label refers to this endometrial proliferation.

The action of oestrogens means the endometrium at this stage has grown thick. It is vascular, containing small spiral arteries arising from the muscle layer of the uterus, and contains many glands that produce a mucus rich in glycogen.

Secretory phase

This postovulatory phase until the next menses is the least variable in length, lasting 14 days. In a 28-day cycle, this involves days 15–28.

For as long as the corpus luteum is present, secreting hormones, the growth and development of the endometrium continues. Progesterone is the dominant hormone in this respect; it promotes the maturation of the uterine lining in preparation for the possible implantation of an embryo. The blood supply is enhanced, with further lengthening and spiralling of arteries into the functional layer. Uterine glands become secretory, with their peak activity around 12 days post ovulation. The endometrium reaches its maximum thickness of around 12–18 mm. However, this functional lining will then begin to break down, unless there is implantation of an embryo and pregnancy.

APPLICATION TO PRACTICE

Physiological birth control

The purpose of all methods of birth control, or contraception, is to prevent pregnancy. Different forms of contraception are described in Chapter 5.1.

Physiological birth control, also called natural planning or rhythm or fertility awareness methods are based on knowledge of the cyclical changes that we have described in this section, to avoid intercourse during times of peak fertility (when fertilisation is most likely). In general, this is the time around ovulation since fertilisation typically occurs within a day or so of ovulation. As sperm may survive for two days in the vagina and a secondary oocyte is viable for around 24 hours, this means that avoidance should be a 3–4-day window around predicted ovulation.

Some detection of ovulation is required for this to be reliable, since many women do not have a textbook 28-day cycle. Indicators of ovulation are therefore used to predict 'safe' times. This can be done by:

▶ Commercially available ovulation detection kit (tests urine)
▶ Monitoring basal body temperature (dips around the time of ovulation)
▶ Identifying changes in cervical mucus (thinner and less stretchy during ovulation)

Unsurprisingly, using a combination of these predictive methods is far more effective than one alone. It has been shown as being over 99% effective with perfect use of temperature monitoring, cervical secretions and calendar calculations.

One absolutely key point for midwives is to recognise that ovulation occurs before the first menstruation following pregnancy. At any time, it is unreliable to rely on the absence of menstruation alone as a method of birth control.

Further reading about all forms of contraception, including options following pregnancy, is available from the Faculty of Sexual and Reproductive Healthcare:
www.fsrh.org/standards-and-guidance/fsrh-guidelines-and-statements/

CHAPTER CHALLENGE

Nearly all female gynaecological disorders are in some way caused or affected by imbalances in the reproductive hormones described in this section. Knowledge of the menstrual cycle can be very useful for understanding possible treatments or lifestyle changes which may be offered to those suffering.

One common and chronic endocrine condition in women of reproductive age is polycystic ovarian syndrome (PCOS), thought to affect 6–10% globally (Bozdag et al., 2016). The features of PCOS vary but may include absent or irregular menstrual cycles, infertility, hirsutism, acne and obesity. A number of criteria have been developed to identify PCOS, but in general a diagnosis is offered if two out of three of the following are present:

▶ Clinical and/or biochemical signs of hyperandrogenism
▶ Oligo-anovulation or anovulation
▶ Polycystic ovaries

PCOS is still not completely understood and its exact cause is unknown. However, some of its features are explained by its associated hormonal imbalances.

For this challenge:

▶ Find out more about hyperandrogenism and what it means. Identify both biochemical and clinical features of hyperandrogenism.

▶ Apply this knowledge to the reproductive cycle to explain some of the other features of PCOS.
▶ Suggested treatments for PCOS can include weight loss, sometimes in combination with the drug metformin. Explain why this is a suggested treatment, and what effect weight loss may have on PCOS.
▶ Finally, explain why infertility is a common symptom of PCOS. What treatment options are available for women suffering PCOS who are trying for pregnancy?

Reference

Bozdag G., Mumusoglu S. et al. The prevalence and phenotypic features of polycystic ovary syndrome: A systematic review and meta-analysis. *Hum. Reprod.* [Internet] 2016, 31(12):2841–55. https://pubmed.ncbi.nlm.nih.gov/27664216/.

Reproduction and embryology

Ginny Mounce

LEARNING OUTCOMES

▶ Explain the stages of fertilisation
▶ Understand the basic development of an embryo from unfertilised egg to week 8

Every individual human develops from just a single cell, which is a fertilised egg (the fusion of a male and female gamete). Here, we describe the events of fertilisation, or conception, which bring this about; followed by the early stages of human development before birth.

Fertilisation

For successful fertilisation, a sperm must reach a secondary oocyte within 12–24 hours of ovulation as the oocyte will not be viable for longer.

Although released into the pelvic cavity, the secondary oocyte is surrounded by sticky follicular fluid and remains near to the ovary, where it is captured by the fimbriae of the uterine tube. Here, it is carried further along the tube itself by fluid currents that are created through the movements of cilia lining endothelial cells. Further actions of peristalsis cause the oocyte to travel towards the fundus of the uterus.

Sperm introduced into the vagina around this time, possibly attracted to chemicals emanating from the oocyte, ascend the uterus, propelled by motion of their tails. Prostaglandins released by sperm cause uterine contractions that also aid their movement. Ejaculate contains millions of sperms but less than 1%, only a few hundred or so, reach the uterine tube and the oocyte. The distance the sperm must

DOI: 10.4324/9781003227571-9

travel is relatively far (around 12 cm), many are destroyed by the acidic environment of the vagina and others cannot pass through the cervical mucus (although, under the influence of oestrogens this becomes thinner and less acidic around the time of ovulation and more of a barrier at other times). Sperm may reach the oocyte within minutes, but they are incapable of fertilising it before undergoing a final series of changes called **capacitation**. This only occurs after a few hours' exposure to the environment of the female reproductive tract.

Capacitation

The exact mechanisms of capacitation are unknown but are thought to involve substances released from the **peg cells** of the uterine tube and cervical mucus. Adult sperm are already motile but following capacitation their flagella beat more vigorously and their plasma membrane becomes capable of fusing with the plasma membrane of a secondary oocyte. Generally, only one sperm will fertilise the oocyte, but many become able and many are involved in the events of fertilisation.

At this point it is useful to remember, from Chapter 2.3, that the secondary oocyte is surrounded by the protective cloud of **corona radiata** cells. Below these cells is the thick glycoprotein **zona pellucida** layer covering the oocyte's plasma membrane. You will also recall that the secondary oocyte is arrested at the metaphase stage of meiosis II, and that the first polar body, created at meiosis I, is present. The relatively large oocyte contains all the organelles and other apparatus needed for nourishment and development of the post-fertilised ovum (see Figure 2.4.1).

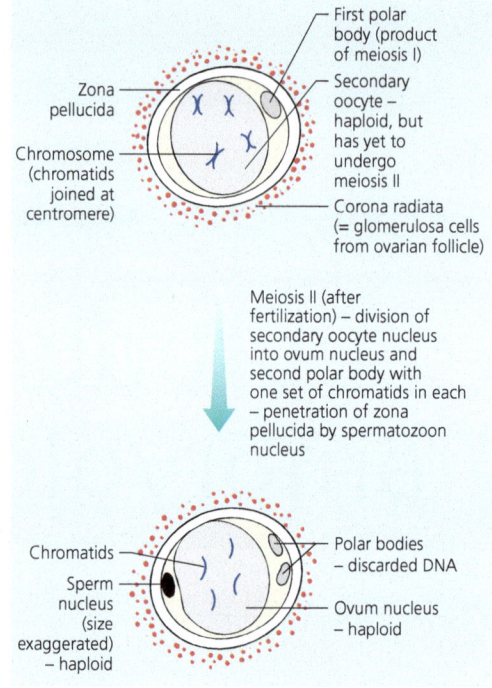

Figure 2.4.1 Overall structure of oocyte at ovulation
Source: Figure 19.2, p.523, Clancy and McVicar (2009)

Penetration and fusion

When a sperm cell makes contact with the oocyte a glycoprotein sperm receptor in the zona pellucida, called ZP3, binds to specific proteins on the sperm head. This triggers the important **acrosomal reaction**, which is the release of acrosome contents (recall Chapter 2.3), which are proteolytic enzymes, including hyaluronidase and acrosin. These break apart the bonds between the follicle cells and enable many sperm to digest a path through the zona pellucida as they are pushed forward by their beating tails. Only the first sperm cell that reaches and makes contact with the plasma membrane of the oocyte fuses with it. This fusion, termed syngamy, triggers the metabolic events of oocyte activation (which completes fertilisation, Figure 2.4.2).

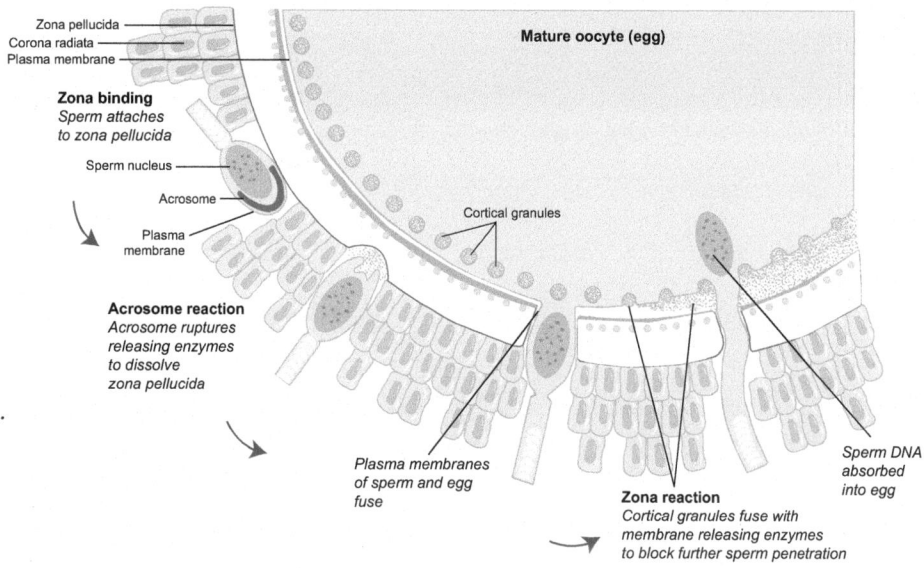

Figure 2.4.2 Stages of fertilisation
Source: Figure 2.4, p.40, Knight (2016)

Fertilisation and oocyte activation

At fusion, and almost immediately (within 1–3 seconds), depolarisation of the oocyte cell membrane stops **polyspermy** (fusion by more than one sperm). This is known as the fast block to polyspermy. Depolarisation also triggers a huge intracellular release of calcium, and this has several effects:

▶ Promotes the **cortical reaction**, which is when vesicles near the cell membrane release their contents (exocytosis) of zonal inhibiting proteins (ZIPs). These inactivate the ZP3 proteins and harden the zona pellucida. This combination prevents any further fertilisation and is known as the slow block to polyspermy.

▶ Completion of meiosis II. This forms a large *fertilised* secondary oocyte, now called an **ovum**, and a much smaller second polar body. Polar bodies later degenerate.

▶ Activation of protein synthesis and growth of the ovum.

The nuclear material of the ovum reorganises into a female **pronucleus**. The nucleus of the sperm cell swells and forms a male pronucleus, while the rest of the sperm degenerates (Figure 2.4.3). The male and female pronuclei of the ovum come together and fuse, forming a **diploid nucleus** with chromosomes mixed together. The resulting cell, now called a **zygote**, therefore has the full complement of 46 (23 pairs) chromosomes; this means both the maternal and paternal characteristics are present. Fertilisation is complete.

APPLICATION TO PRACTICE

Twins

Usually, one secondary oocyte is released from an ovary at ovulation. If two oocytes are released (possibly one from each ovary) and fertilised by two different sperm, then there will be two zygotes (Figure 2.4.4).

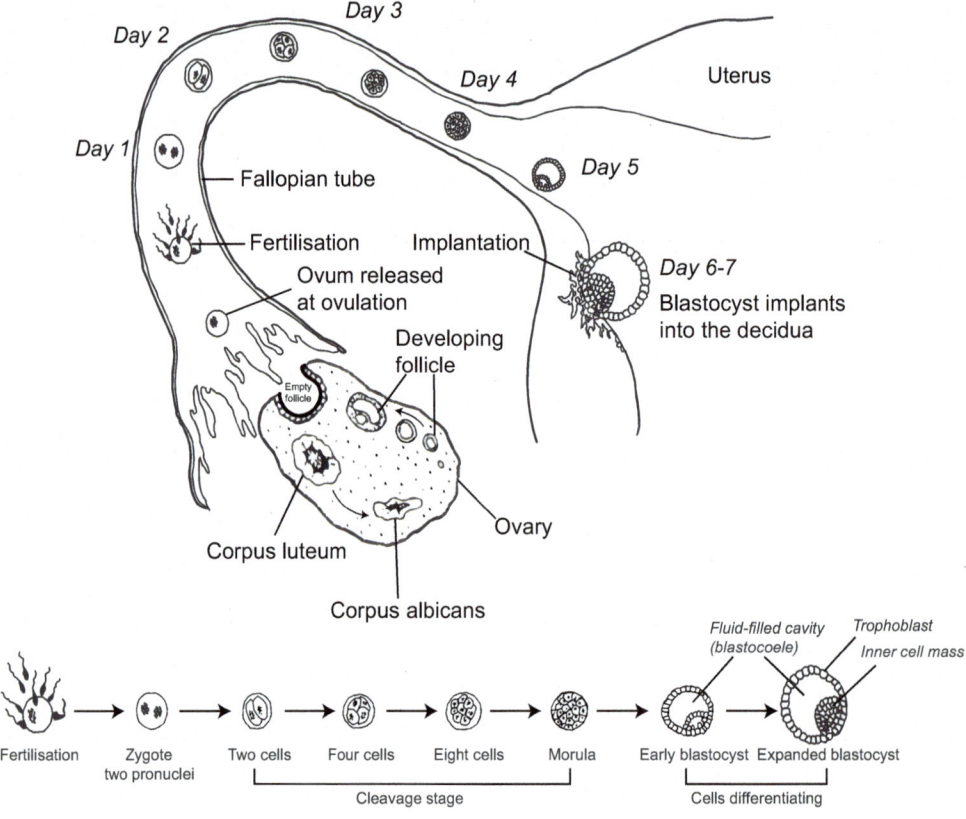

Figure 2.4.3 From fertilisation to implantation showing stages of embryo development
Source: Figure 3.5, p.57, Knight (2016)

These will develop into dizygotic (fraternal) twins. They are genetically dissimilar, because of the mixing of chromosomes during meiosis, and may not be the same biological sex. In the UK, approximately 15 births per 1000 are of twins.

More uncommonly, twins may develop from one zygote, and are called monozygotic or 'identical' twins. Here, the developing zygote separates, forming two different embryos. Because they arise from the same ovum and sperm, they have the same genetic material as each other, and will of course be the same biological sex. The zygote separation usually occurs within the first eight days after fertilisation, at the cleavage stage or pre-gastrulation (see Chapter 2.4). If it occurs later on, or is not fully completed, then this may lead to conjoined twins.

Embryology: Implantation and embryo development

The process of fertilisation, as we described in the previous section, is complete with the formation of a zygote. We now present the development of the **embryo** from this zygote, its implantation and the subsequent stages of growth in early pregnancy.

Embryology is the study of the developing embryo and covers the time span of 0–8 weeks after fertilisation. At nine weeks, the embryo has formed all the main

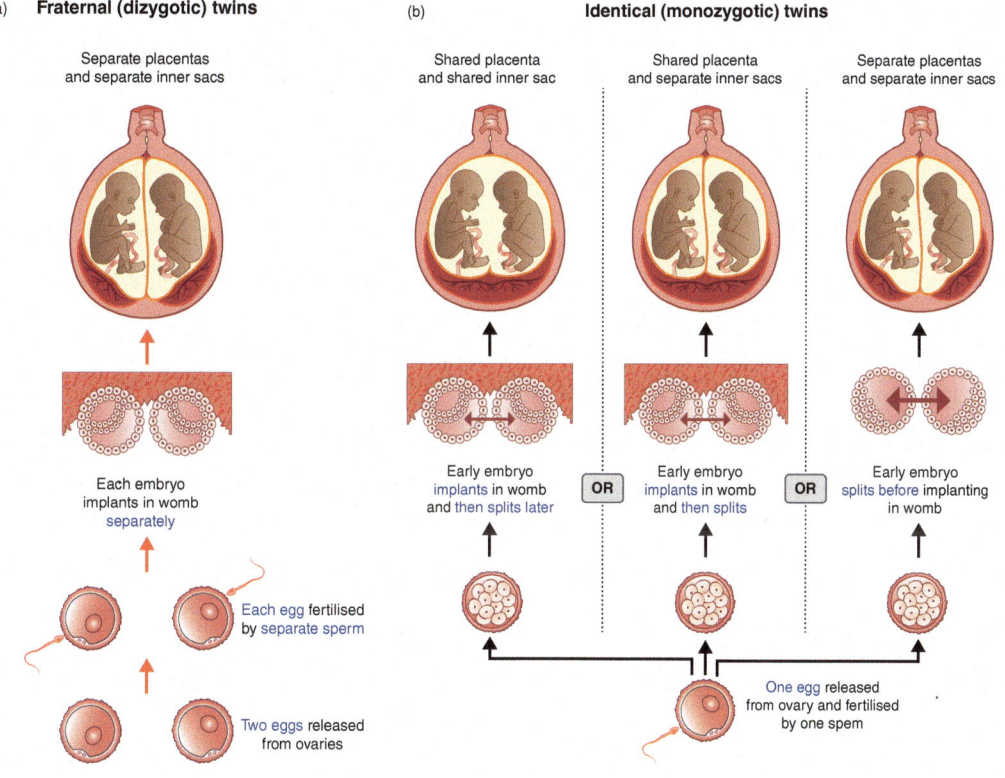

Figure 2.4.4 Development of twins: a) dizygotic twins; b) monozygotic twins

systems and organs; it is officially known as a **fetus**. Chapter 2.5 describes further development and early fetal life after nine weeks.

All this development is remarkable, and it is worth noting the complexities at each stage. An estimated 40–60% of human embryos do not survive, often failing before the first biochemical signs of pregnancy.

Immediate post fertilisation: Cleavage to blastocyst

Usually an egg and sperm will fertilise in the **ampulla** region of a uterine tube, although it can occur nearer or even in the uterine cavity. Over the first two days, as the zygote moves along the tube, mitotic cell division occurs, producing first two

cells and then four cells and so on. The first division is completed around 30 hours post fertilisation. Each cleavage division produces identical, undifferentiated cells, known as **blastomeres**. The number of blastomeres double every 12–15 hours but the zygote does not change in overall size. These early cell divisions without growth are termed **cleavage**. The outside layer is still the zona pellucida (the thick glycoprotein coat surrounding the ovum) and this helps the zygote to pass smoothly along the uterine tube without being recognised as an invader by the immune system. By around the third day, a number of cleavage divisions have occurred and the zygote now appears as a solid ball or cluster of cells with a recognisable berry-like appearance, called a **morula** ('a mulberry'). Typically, on the fourth day, the morula reaches the uterine cavity.

The blastomeres continue to divide, and by around day 5–6 they become variable in size and shape as they form into a **blastocyst**. This is a hollow ball with a fluid-filled cavity called a **blastocoel**. There are two distinct cellular regions surrounding the blastocoel, which are:

▶ An **inner cell mass** – these cells cluster at one end of the blastocyst and form into the developing embryo (eventually the fetus).

▶ The outer layer called the **trophoblast** – these cells contact the uterine endometrium (lining of the uterine cavity) and provide the embryo with nutrients. These cells will eventually go on to form the placenta and chorion.

Implantation

At around day 6–7, the blastocyst has reached the uterine cavity, and remains near but not attached to the endometrium for a day or so. The trophoblastic cells release enzymes to form a hole in the zona pellucida, allowing the blastocyst to hatch from, or shed, this layer. Now, the blastocyst cells are exposed to the glycogen and nutrient-rich uterine fluid secreted from the endometrial glands. Absorption of these nutrients accelerates blastocyst growth. When fully grown, the blastocyst makes contact with the endometrium, initiating implantation.

Almost all embryos implant near the fundus or upper body of the uterus. If implantation occurs outside the main uterine cavity, such as in the uterine tubes or cervix, then this is an **ectopic** pregnancy. Over 95% of ectopic pregnancies are tubal. Ectopic pregnancies are unviable and may be life threatening if left untreated. Around 16000 UK ectopic pregnancies are diagnosed each year, which is approximately 1–2% of the total.

It is the trophoblast cells of the blastocyst that make contact with the uterine lining, and more specifically those cells surrounding the inner cell mass are the ones that touch and adhere to the endometrium. In other words, the blastocyst rotates so that the inner cell mass is furthest away from the uterine cavity. Cell division is rapid, and the trophoblast layer now attached at the endometrium becomes many layers thick and changes:

▶ The trophoblast layer nearest the inner cell mass remains intact, forming another layer called the **cytotrophoblast** (*cyto = cellular*).

▶ The outer trophoblast layer nearest the endometrium undergoes other changes. It loses the cell membranes between individual cells, and in doing so forms a new layer of cytoplasm containing many nuclei. This is called the **syncytiotrophoblast** (see the area of syncytiotrophoblast cells day 7 and 8 in Figure 2.4.5, note no cell walls).

2.4

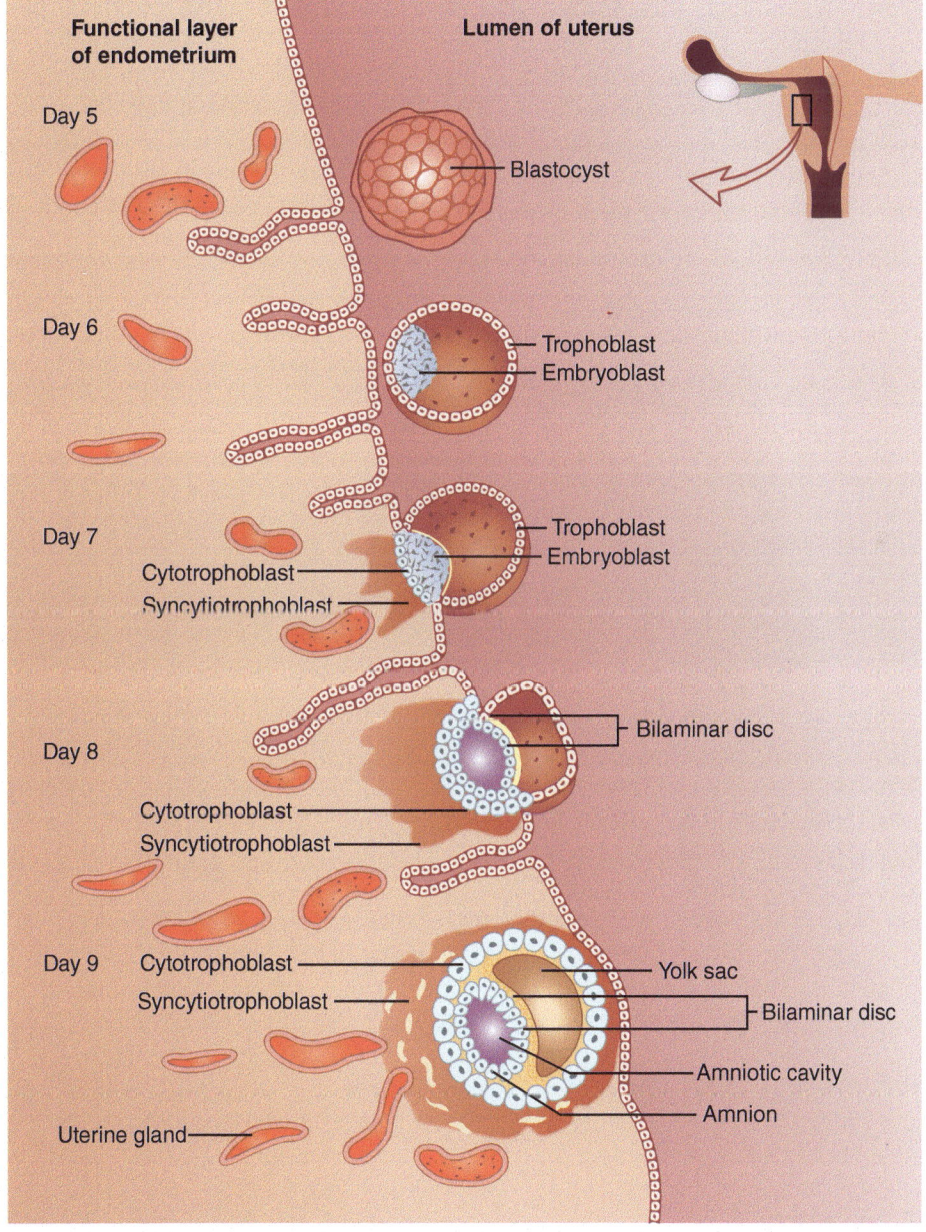

Functional layer of endometrium

Lumen of uterus

Day 5 — Blastocyst

Day 6 — Trophoblast / Embryoblast

Day 7 — Trophoblast / Embryoblast
Cytotrophoblast
Syncytiotrophoblast

Day 8 — Bilaminar disc
Cytotrophoblast
Syncytiotrophoblast

Day 9
Cytotrophoblast — Yolk sac
Syncytiotrophoblast — Bilaminar disc
— Amniotic cavity
— Amnion
Uterine gland

Figure 2.4.5 Stages of embryo implantation (days 5–10)

Together, the cytotrophoblastic and syncitiotrophoplastic layers become the **chorion**, the fetal portion of the placenta (see Chapter 2.5).

By secreting the enzyme **hyaluronidase**, the syncytial trophoblastic cells dissolve the connections between the epithelial cells, eroding a path further into the endometrium and releasing nutrients that are absorbed by growing cells. This is the same enzyme used by spermatozoa to break down bonds between follicular cells of the ovum to allow fertilisation. Some sources may describe this as the embryo 'burrowing' into the endometrium as at first, these actions cause breakdown of the endometrial surface, but this is soon repaired by rapid endometrial migration and division. Once the lining is reformed, the blastocyst is no longer in contact with the uterine cavity (Figure 2.4.5, day 9). The cellular damage as the blastocyst embeds can lead to a small blood loss which is sometimes noticed by women, sometimes called an **implantation bleed**, particularly those anticipating pregnancy.

From day 8–9, the trophoblastic cells start to extend around the capillaries in the endometrium. As the vessel walls break down, uterine blood pools in channels called **lacunae**. The extensions of the trophoblast extend further away from the main blastocyst in 'finger like' projections known as **villi**. These are of increasing complexity and size, and further erosion of larger vessels causes greater flow of blood through the lacunae. While this is happening, the inner cell mass separates from the trophoblast, forming a fluid-filled **amniotic cavity**. At day 9, the two cellular layers of the inner cell mass now start to be organised as a superficial layer facing the amniotic cavity, and a deeper inner layer is exposed to the blastocoel. As the inner layer of cells migrate around the blastocoel, this forms the yolk sac.

It is now that the syncytiotrophoblast cells begin to synthesise and secrete hormones, notably **human chorionic gonadotrophin** (hCG). This has actions similar to luteinising hormone, so that the corpus luteum no longer degenerates and instead continues to secrete progesterone and oestrogens. This prevents degeneration of the endometrium and therefore, there is no menstruation. It is the rising levels of hCG which indicates biochemical confirmation of pregnancy and can be detected in blood or urine from around 12 days post fertilisation. Other hormones produced by syncytiotrophoblast cells are the placental hormones human placental lactogen, prolactin and relaxin, giving the placenta its endocrine function.

Embryogenesis

This is the stage of embryo development from approximately the second week until week nine, when it officially becomes a fetus. Early stages of embryogenesis see two main events:

1) The formation of the three main germ layers from which all tissues develop

2) The formation of the extra-embryonic membranes which lie outside and protect the developing embryo (and fetus)

Formation of primary germ layers: Gastrulation

Up to this point, the **inner cell mass** has developed two key layers, and for this reason is known as the **bilaminar embryonic disc**. These two layers are known as the outer **ectoderm** and the inner **endoderm.** During **gastrulation**, the bilaminar embryonic disc undergoes significant changes and becomes **trilaminar** (three-layered). The third layer, the **mesoderm**, forms by migration of cells from the ectoderm towards a central 'line'

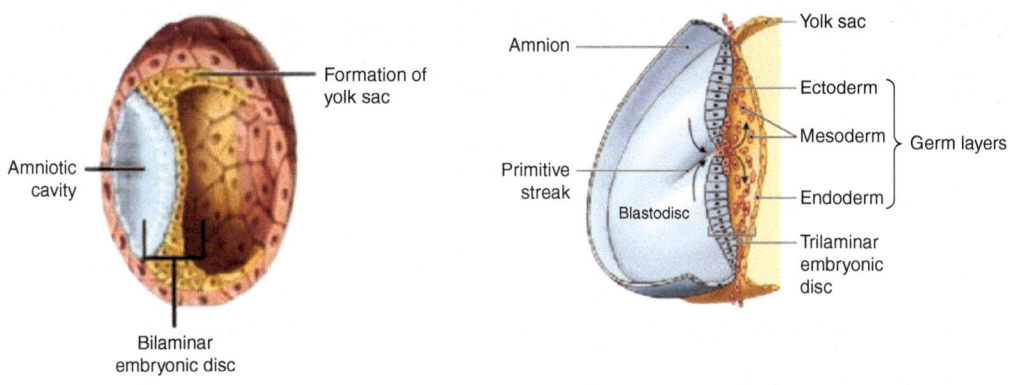

Figure 2.4.6 Gastrulation/bilaminar to trilaminar disc

called the **primitive streak**. Cells from the surface migrate between the two existing layers (see Figure 2.4.6). These three layers are called **germ layers**:

1. Ectoderm – superficial cells which did not migrate to the interior
2. Endoderm – cells facing the yolk sac
3. Mesoderm – loosely organised migrating cells between the endoderm and ectoderm

It is the body of this disc which eventually forms the fetus; it first begins to separate from other cells and bulges into the amniotic cavity forming first a head fold and, by four weeks, a tail fold (see Figure 2.4.7). Further development, folding and growth, forms an embryo with internal organs.

All the tissues and organs of the body develop from the three embryonic germ layers. Broadly speaking, the endoderm layer forms the epithelial linings of organs such as the gastrointestinal tract and endocrine system; the mesoderm forms muscle, bones, gonads and blood; and the ectoderm forms nerve, hair, eyes and epidermis of skin. Table 2.4.1 shows the main body structures produced from the three primary germ layers.

Formation of extra-embryonic membranes

The other cells of the original blastocyst form the **extra-embryonic membranes**. All lie outside and protect the growing embryo.

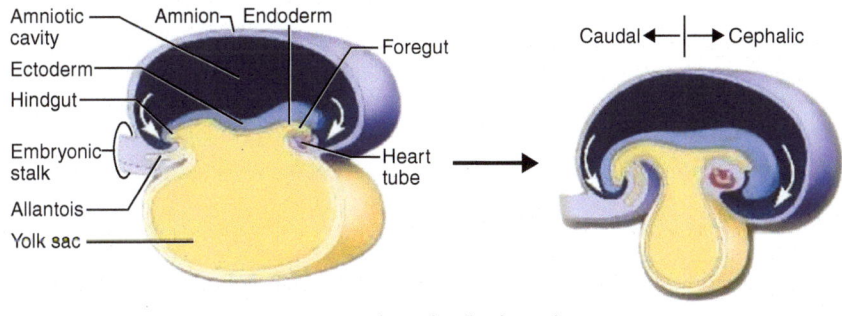

Longitudinal sections

Figure 2.4.7 Embryogenesis week 3–4 head fold formation

Table 2.4.1 Main body structures produced from three germ layers

Endoderm	Mesoderm	Ectoderm
Endocrine – thymus, thyroid gland, pancreas	Muscle tissue, heart	Nervous tissue
Epithelium – liver, bladder, gallbladder	Cartilage, bone, connective tissue	Skin epidermis, hair follicles, nails, skin glands, mammary glands, sebaceous glands
Epithelium – gastrointestinal tract	Blood, bone marrow, lymph	Teeth enamel, eye lens, internal and external ear
Epithelium – respiratory tract, auditory tubes, tympanic cavity	Dermis of skin	Mucus epithelium – oral cavity, nasal cavity, salivary glands, anal canal
Epithelium – reproductive tract	Kidneys and ureters, spleen	Epithelium – pituitary gland, pineal gland, adrenal medulla
Gamete stem cells, distal reproductive ducts	Gonads, adjacent reproductive ducts	

They are the yolk sac, the amnion, the allantois and the chorion (see Figure 2.4.8).

We saw earlier the creation of the **yolk sac** from the inner layer of cells of the blastocyst. This is the primary source of nutrients for the developing embryo, but its main function is as a site of blood formation. The thin, protective membrane of the **amnion** is first formed when ectoderm cells, and then mesoderm cells, line the inside surface of the amniotic cavity which surrounds the developing embryo. The **amniotic fluid** which fills the cavity buffers the embryo from external forces.

The **allantois** is formed (around the same time as the head fold) by an extension of endoderm cells, surrounded by mesoderm, towards the trophoblast cells. It is a small, vascular sac which also serves as a site of blood formation. At around four weeks, the overall area of allantois plus surrounding mesoderm cells connecting the embryo body to the trophoblast are termed the body stalk. Constriction of this stalk (and similarly the stalk to the yolk sac) means both connections become narrower and more pronounced (Figure 2.4.8). The **body stalk** later forms the umbilical cord, including some vessels of the allantois.

The **chorion** is derived from the mesoderm cells, which spread outwards from the

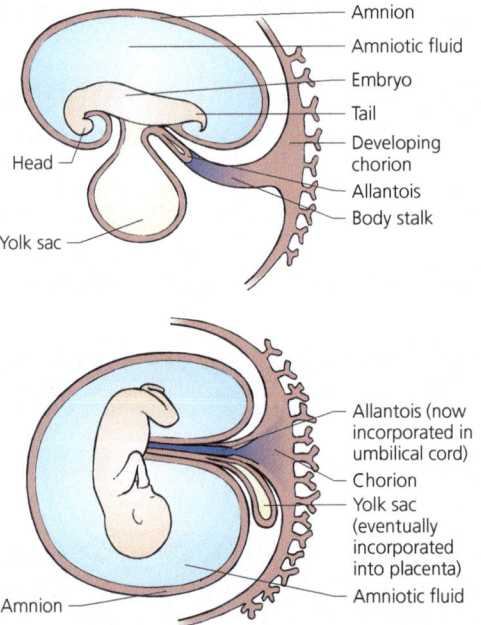

Figure 2.4.8 Extra-embryonic membranes
Source: Figure 19.8, p.532, Clancy and McVicar (2009)

Amnion
Amniotic fluid
Embryo
Tail
Developing chorion
Allantois
Body stalk
Head
Yolk sac

Allantois (now incorporated in umbilical cord)
Chorion
Yolk sac (eventually incorporated into placenta)
Amniotic fluid
Amnion

allantois and line the inner surface of the trophoblast. The mesoderm extends along all of the trophoblastic villi, forming chorionic villi which have contact with maternal tissues. The further enlarging and branching of these villi are significant in placental development, which is fully described in Chapter 2.5.

Late embryogenesis

By four weeks of development, the embryo is already distinct, having a certain orientation and shape, with head, eye, limb buds and heart all recognisable. From the first few cells it is now around 5 mm in size. The extra-embryonic membranes are also differentiated.

By the end of embryogenesis (8 weeks) the fundamental organs are formed and the embryo measures around 1.6 cm. Table 2.4.2 outlines some of the milestones of organ development in this period. The embryo moves further away from the site of the placenta, but remains connected by the umbilical cord, which has formed by the fusion of the body stalk

Table 2.4.2 Milestones of organogenesis during the embryonic period

2.4

Week	Key milestones of organogenesis
Week 3	Starting development of the brain, heart, blood cells, circulatory system, spinal cord and digestive system
Week 4	Starting development of bones, facial structures and limbs Heart begins to beat
Week 5	Starting development of eyes, nose, kidneys, lungs Heart valves formed
Week 6	Starting development of hands, feet and digits
Week 7	Starting development of hair follicles, nipples, eyelids and gonads Urine formed in kidneys, evidence of brain waves
Week 8	Facial features more distinct, internal organs now developed, brain signals muscle movement, beginning formation of external sex organs

and the yolk sac stalk. From nine weeks, development and growth continue in the fetal period (Chapter 2.5).

The placenta and developing fetus

Ginny Mounce

LEARNING OUTCOMES

▶ Describe the key stages of placental development

▶ Understand the core functions of the placenta, and the mechanisms by which these occur

▶ Describe the role of the placenta as an immunological barrier

▶ Explain key stages of fetal development from nine weeks to term

▶ Describe the structure and key landmarks of the fetal skull at term

This chapter describes the development of the placenta and fetus from the implantation of the fertilised ovum in the womb until birth. Although they are separate, but connected units, as the products of conception, the placenta and fetus are often referred to as the 'fetoplacental unit'. The placenta is a temporary organ of pregnancy, forming an interface between mother and fetus. The fetus is utterly dependent on this organ while *in utero*, as it is via the placenta that oxygen, nutrients and other vital substances needed by the fetus are obtained, in exchange for its carbon dioxide and other waste products. The placenta is much more than a passive receptacle, however, as it also produces hormones which promote an ideal environment for fetal growth and development.

Placental development

The initial development of the embryo into a blastocyst with an outer trophoblast (which will form the placenta and chorionic membrane) and an inner cell mass (which will form the fetus and amniotic membrane) was outlined in Chapter 2.4. We pick up the story of the developing placenta here after the blastocyst has implanted into the uterine wall.

DOI: 10.4324/9781003227571-10

Pre-lacunar stage

At implantation, nutrients required by the inner cell mass simply diffuse across from surrounding trophoblast cells. However, as the distances between cells and the demands of the embryo increase, this is not sustainable for long. The development of a more efficient and rapid system to deliver nutrients – the placenta – begins with the formation of chorionic blood vessels.

Lacunar stage

As early as days 8–9 after implantation the embryonic trophoblast cells extend towards and around the capillaries of the uterine endometrium. The uterine capillary walls begin to break down, causing blood to pool into spaces called **lacunae**. The trophoblastic 'finger like' extensions become known as **chorionic villi**.

The inner uterine endometrium is vascularised by coiled blood vessels called spiral arteries and veins. These are most prolific in the luteal phase of the reproductive cycle, ensuring an optimal environment for the embryo. The action of chorionic villi remodels the endometrial capillaries in two main ways:

▶ The lumen becomes wider
▶ The muscle wall becomes less elastic and restrictive

These changes maximise the flow of maternal blood into the lacunae. In some cases these vascular changes may be compromised – a scenario that is implicated in the development of pre-eclampsia.

Primary, secondary and tertiary villus stages

These first extensions of chorionic villi are **primary villi**, containing only cytotrophoblastic cells. As they reach further into the interior of the endometrium they grow larger, branch and become more complex. After two weeks, the mesoderm from the inner surface of cytotrophoblast grows into the villi, meaning the core contains trophoblast and mesoderm, forming looser connective tissue. These are **secondary villi**. Increasingly, they erode larger blood vessels, resulting in greater flow of maternal blood through the lacunae. As they develop further, embryonic blood vessels arising from the mesenchymal cells of the connective tissue core form in each chorionic villus. These are the **tertiary villi** as they contain trophoblast, mesoderm and a network of capillaries. The branching tertiary villi provide a large surface area that aids diffusion.

Note that all the chorionic villi are surrounded by (bathed in) maternal blood of the lacunae. As the vasculature develops in each villus they connect to the vessels serving the embryo, arising from the allantois. By week 3, when the fetal heart beats, blood starts to flow through these vessels (see Figure 2.5.1). This all means that the blood vessels of the fetus and mother are brought very close together, allowing for exchange of nutrients and gases. Importantly, the two circulations do not join and there is usually no mixing of blood because they are separated by layers of trophoblast (the placental membrane). This is the placental barrier. Placental circulation and functioning are described later.

By week 4 extra-embryonic membranes have formed (see Chapter 2.4). The early embryo, amnion and yolk sac are suspended in a fluid-filled chamber. The body stalk which contains the embryonic blood vessels, connects the embryo and chorion, while the yolk stalk connects the yolk sac and embryo endoderm. Both stalks become constricted and narrower, and by week 5 when the chorion enlarges and bulges into the uterine cavity; they fuse forming the umbilical stalk.

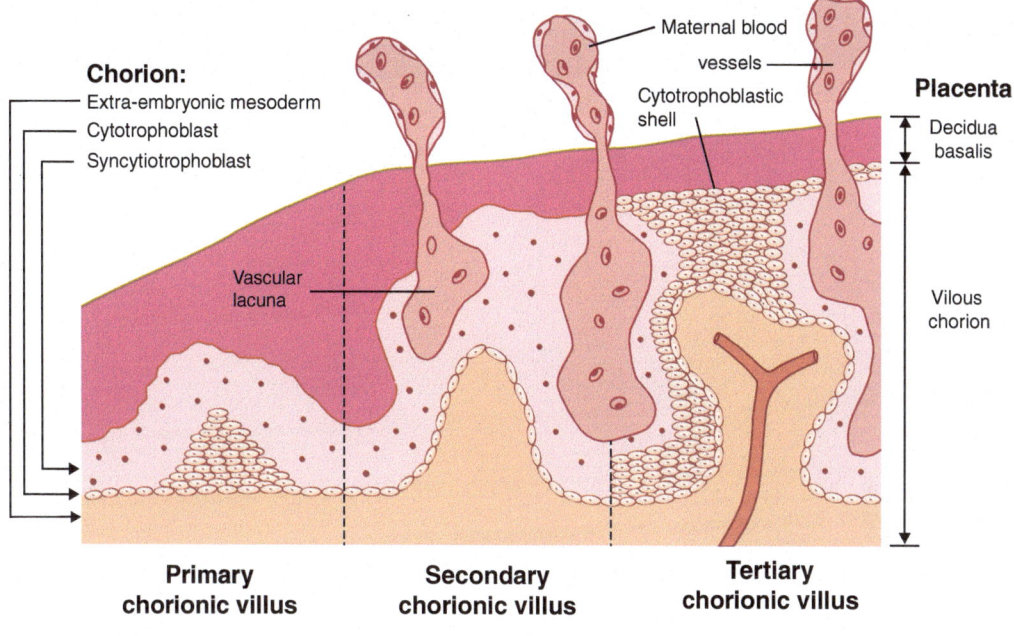

Chorion:
- Extra-embryonic mesoderm
- Cytotrophoblast
- Syncytiotrophoblast

Vascular lacuna

Maternal blood vessels

Cytotrophoblastic shell

Placenta 2.5

Decidua basalis

Vilous chorion

Primary chorionic villus

Secondary chorionic villus

Tertiary chorionic villus

Figure 2.5.1 Primary, secondary and tertiary chorionic villi

The endometrium into which the chorion expands and modifies is known as the **decidua**. It includes all but the basal layer of uterine endometrium. When the placenta is expelled after birth it separates at the basal layer.

Three regions of the decidua are named according to their location relative to the site of implantation. See Figure 2.5.2 and observe that while the chorion encloses the entire embryo and amnion, only the parts with chorionic villi remain involved in nutrient and gaseous exchange and form the functioning placenta. The chorionic villi develop most in the region called the **decidua basalis**, which is between the implanted embryo and the myometrium, and are most concentrated near the umbilical stalk or placental region. It is the decidua basalis which forms the maternal plate of the mature placenta. The region of endometrium located between the chorion and uterine cavity is called the **decidua capsularis**. This thinner portion has no associated chorionic villi. As the fetus enlarges, the smooth decidua capsularis stretches more and more. Eventually, it fuses with the **decidua parietalis** which is the remaining endometrial region of the uterus, and then there is no longer a uterine cavity. The decidua capsularis itself degenerates at around week 27.

The placenta is formed from both maternal and embryonic tissues; the chorion of the embryo and decidua basalis from the mother. As the fetus grows it moves further away from the placenta, but remains connected by the umbilical cord, itself developed from the umbilical stalk. The umbilical cord contains the blood vessels of placental circulation (Figure 2.5.3) plus the allantois and yolk stalk. By the end of the first trimester of pregnancy the placenta is developed and fully functional (see Figure 2.5.3).

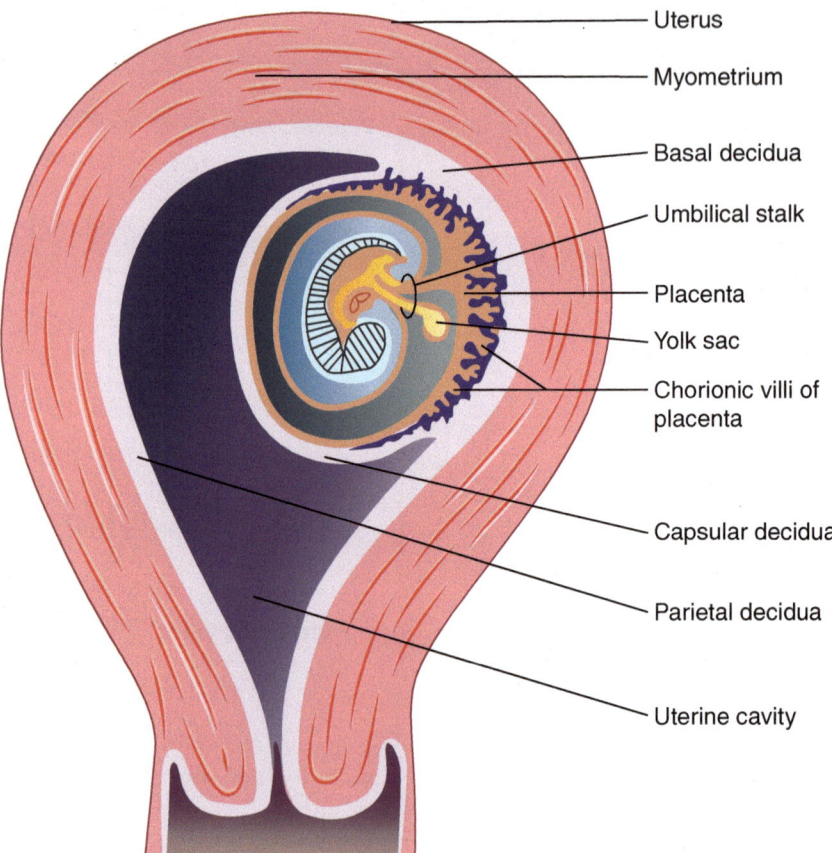

Uterus

Myometrium

Basal decidua

Umbilical stalk

Placenta

Yolk sac

Chorionic villi of placenta

Capsular decidua

Parietal decidua

Uterine cavity

Figure 2.5.2 Week 5 early placental development

Mature placenta

The mature placenta is a discoid-shaped organ, 22 cm diameter and 2.5 cm deep at the centre. It weighs approximately 500 g. The placenta is the site of exchange of gases, nutrients and waste products for fetus and mother. It is considered an endocrine organ.

The placenta has two sides: 1) the chorionic plate which faces the fetus and contains the umbilical cord; and 2) the basal plate which is formed of the decidua. In between the plates are the **intervillous spaces**, the pools of maternal blood or lacunae described earlier. It is worth stating again that while they are in extremely close

proximity (separated by only epithelial cells), the maternal and fetal circulations do not join together and there is no mixing of blood.

Placental circulation

From around eight weeks of gestation, maternal blood pools in the intervillous space around the chorionic villi. Maternal blood is pumped into the intervillous space under pressure from the arterial system, and blood drains away into the venous system. This creates a concentration gradient, so that oxygen and nutrients in maternal blood diffuse across cell membranes into the fetal blood vessels,

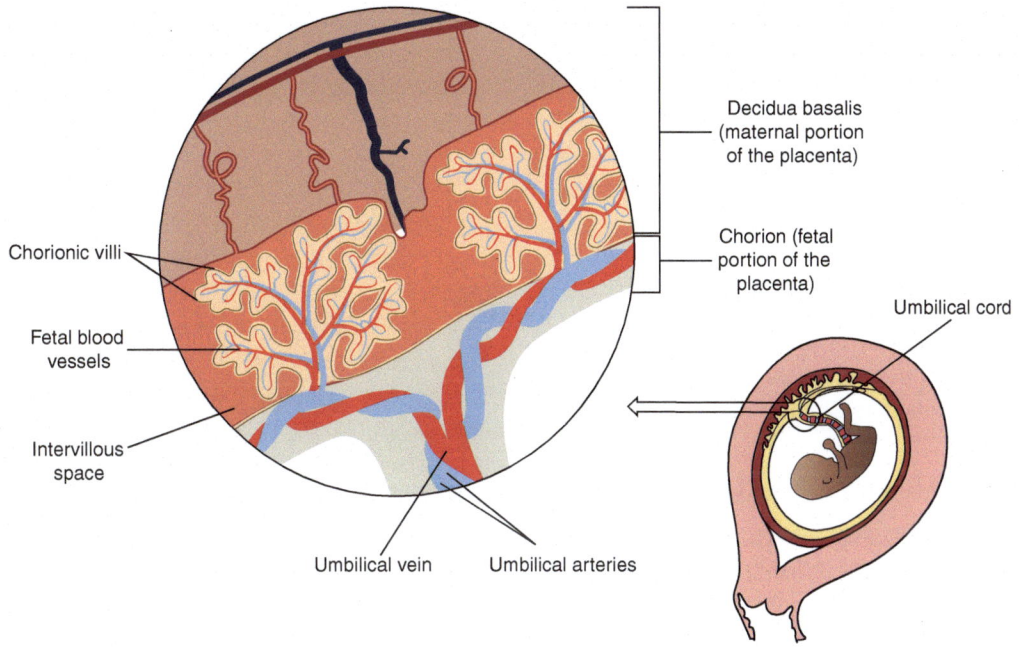

Chorionic villi

Fetal blood vessels

Intervillous space

Decidua basalis (maternal portion of the placenta)

Chorion (fetal portion of the placenta)

Umbilical cord

Umbilical vein   Umbilical arteries

Figure 2.5.3 The placental barrier

and waste products and carbon dioxide in the fetal vessels diffuse across in the opposite direction. The fetal blood vessels connect to the fetus by the **umbilical cord**.

Umbilical cord

The umbilical cord contains two paired umbilical arteries which carry blood from the fetus to the placental barrier, and the single umbilical vein that returns blood to the fetus. It also contains remnants of the allantois. All are enclosed in a gelatinous substance known as Wharton's jelly and are covered by an outer sheath of smooth amnion. Usually, an umbilical cord is 50–60 cm long and 1 cm diameter. When an umbilical cord is cut (Figure 2.5.4) it is easy to see the two arteries and one vein in cross section, and a common way to remember this is 'AVA', noting that it is the vein which carries oxygenated blood to the fetus (unlike veins in adult circulation).

Fetal blood is carried to the capillaries of chorionic villi via the umbilical arteries of the umbilical cord. This blood is deoxygenated, containing carbon dioxide

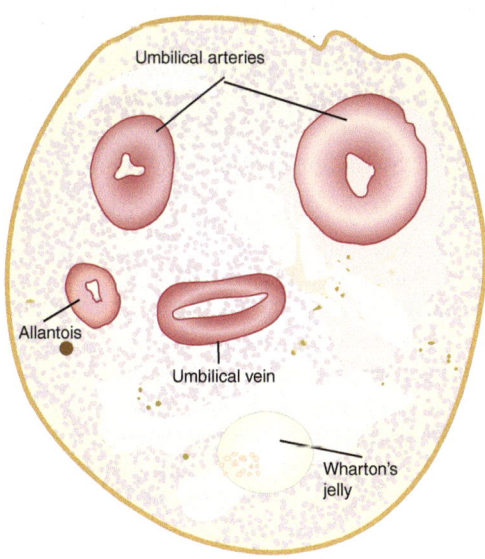

Umbilical arteries

Allantois

Umbilical vein

Wharton's jelly

Figure 2.5.4 Umbilical cord cross section

and other wastes which diffuse across into the pools of maternal blood. In exchange, the oxygen and nutrients in the pools surrounding the villi are taken up and returned to the fetus by the umbilical vein.

Fetal circulation

Oxygenated blood and nutrients in the umbilical vein enter the fetus and travel either to the liver or directly to the fetal heart via the ductus venosus and inferior vena cava (see Chapter 5.2).

Functions of the placenta

The placenta has several important functions that support the growing fetus; oxygenation, nutrition, excretion, hormone production (endocrine), protection and immunity.

Oxygenation

The fetus relies totally on the placenta for respiratory gas exchange, i.e. for all its oxygen and does not use lungs to breathe.

Oxygen needed by the fetus diffuses from the higher area of concentration in maternal blood in the intervillous space to the lower concentration found in the fetal blood vessels in the chorionic villi and is then carried to the fetus via the umbilical vein. There are a number of mechanisms that maximise oxygen transport to the fetus:

- ▶ The numerous intervillous spaces slow down the passage of maternal blood at the placenta, giving more time for the diffusion of oxygen across the trophoblast layers into the fetal circulation.
- ▶ Fetal red blood cells contain fetal haemoglobin, which has a higher affinity for oxygen than adult haemoglobin. Gas exchange takes place at the placental barrier, but when equilibrium is reached (the PO_2 becomes the same) the fetal haemoglobin saturation will be much greater than that for adult haemoglobin.

That is, each fetal haemoglobin carries more molecules of oxygen. This same quality means that when the oxygenated fetal blood reaches the peripheral fetal tissues it gives up a larger amount of oxygen during gas exchange to achieve the PO_2 equilibrium.

The respiratory function of the placenta extends to the diffusion of carbon dioxide in exchange for oxygen at the placental barrier. Other molecules which are present during the process of respiration are hydrogen ions, bicarbonate ions and lactic acid. These are exchanged freely via diffusion and maintain the optimal acid-base balance.

Nutrition

Exchange of compounds across the placental membrane is by passive transport (such as the simple diffusion of oxygen and carbon dioxide described above), active transport (such as carrier-mediated transport or ion channels) or vesicular transport (such as exocytosis).

The main nutrient the fetus relies on from the mother is glucose. This is transferred by protein-mediated facilitated diffusion via a glucose transporter (GLUT). Glucose provides energy and is the substrate for glycogen, itself synthesised and stored by the placenta. The placenta also synthesises proteins, fatty acids and cholesterol for the fetus. The placental cholesterol is a precursor for steroid hormones, oestrogen and progesterone (see endocrine function below). Amino acids are actively transported across the placenta, while free fatty acids and glycerol cross by simple or facilitated diffusion. The placenta also has nutrient demands, and extracts glucose, amino acids and oxygen for its own requirements.

Excretion

The placenta also functions like a kidney, meaning it removes waste products that are not needed by the fetus. Ammonia, converted to uric acid and urea, passes passively across into the maternal circulation for excretion. Other waste metabolites that are eliminated include creatinine and bilirubin. Water passes freely between circulations via osmosis. Micronutrients and electrolytes, such as calcium and potassium, are exchanged via active transport or ion pumps, but others move across via diffusion. All of this maintains the correct chemical balance between fetus and mother.

Endocrine function

The syncytiotrophoblast cells of the placenta synthesise several pregnancy hormones that are released into the maternal circulation. In Chapter 2.4 we described how, soon after implantation of the embryo, the chorionic cells (later of the placenta) secrete hCG, which rescues the corpus luteum in the ovary from degeneration, meaning it continues to produce oestrogens and progesterone. However, oestrogens are produced by the chorion from the first month of pregnancy and progesterone by week 6. Both are steroid hormones derived from cholesterol, synthesised from fatty acids stored by the placenta.

By the first trimester onwards, the placenta has completely taken over the function of **oestrogen** and **progesterone** production from the corpus luteum, supplying all the amounts of these hormones required to maintain the pregnancy. By the fourth month, secretion of hCG is vastly reduced. Oestrogens and progesterone maintain the endometrium during pregnancy, prepare mammary glands for lactation and play a part in stimulating labour and birth.

Another hormone initially produced by the corpus luteum and later also by the placenta is **relaxin**. This peptide hormone increases flexibility of the symphysis pubis and other pelvic ligaments, and helps to dilate the cervix during labour. It also has an inhibitory effect on uterine smooth muscle contractions, delaying early onset of labour.

The two other main peptide hormones produced by the chorion are **human placental lactogen (hPL)** and **corticotrophin releasing hormone (CRH)**. Maximum hPL levels are reached and maintained around 32 weeks of pregnancy. This hormone has a role, along with several other hormones such as prolactin, in activating mammary glands for lactation. It also stimulates maternal protein synthesis for growth and regulates some aspects of metabolism, for example decreasing glucose uptake by the mother so making more available to the fetus.

In non-pregnant people, CRH is a hormone of the hypothalamus involved in stress responses, but in pregnancy it is produced from around 12 weeks from the placenta until the end of pregnancy when its levels increase greatly. It is thought to be the 'clock' for the timing of birth as higher levels are associated with premature delivery (and vice versa). Additionally, it increases secretions of cortisol, a steroid that matures fetal lungs, and surfactant production. Other regulatory molecules produced by the placenta are placental growth factor, vascular endothelial growth factor, cytokines and chemokines.

Protection and immunity

The placenta is a physical barrier. This means it is protective since it can prevent harmful molecules and foreign bodies (xenobiotics), including most bacteria and viruses, from crossing into the fetal circulation. However, the majority of drugs readily cross the placenta and may be harmful. Some bacteria (e.g. listeria, and those causing syphilis), protozoa (e.g. toxoplasma) and various viruses (HIV, cytomegalovirus, rubella, Zika, polio and varicella) are able to cross. The membrane is also selective, allowing some proteins but not others to pass. The placenta produces enzymes which destroy some xenobiotics, while other placental enzymes act to modify any maternal molecules, such as sex hormones, into forms which would otherwise be harmful to the fetus.

The fetus remains vulnerable to any toxic substances and pathogens that cross the placental barrier as it is unable to produce antibodies. This is most critical early in pregnancy when the placenta is undeveloped or when poorly functioning. From around 13 weeks the fetus acquires passive immunity from the mother when her IgG antibodies cross the barrier, via pinocytosis. This means that any historic immunity the mother has acquired, either by a response to previous infection or vaccination, will be passed to the fetus. IgG antibodies are the dominant source of immunity for the fetus. Exposure to a pathogen will produce IgM antibodies by the mother, but these molecules are too large to pass across the barrier. This means that the fetus has little protection against any new pathogen or infection the mother encounters during pregnancy. After birth, IgA antibodies are transferred to the baby via breastmilk.

The placenta as an immunological barrier

Since the fetus is genetically dissimilar to its mother, it could be subject to immunological recognition and attack, but the placenta provides an immunological barrier that prevents the mother's body from rejecting her own fetus.
This is achieved in the following ways:

▶ The placental barrier is comprised of syncytiotrophoblasts, which are fused multinucleated cells or syncytium. As this has no extracellular spaces it limits the migration of immune cells between fetus and mother, something which a normal epithelial barrier does not prevent.

▶ The IgG antibodies which pass through the placenta do not generally target fetal cells. The placenta secretes special peptides which help mask the presence of fetal cells and produces suppressor cells to inhibit the effects of interleukin-2 cytokine, which has a role in recognising foreign bodies.

▶ The major histocompatibility complex molecules on the surfaces of trophoblast cells are altered in ways that appear to prevent their destruction by maternal T-cells and natural killer cells.

This higher immunological tolerance for the fetus in pregnancy is thought to increase the severity of some infections, such as influenza and malaria, in pregnancy.

Fetal development

The ninth week of pregnancy marks the start of the period of fetal development. During the previous embryological period, the three germ layers of the embryo differentiate into three germ layers, from which all body tissues and organs develop (see Chapter 2.4). As the placenta establishes an oxygen and nutrient supply, and acts to maintain a hospitable environment, the fetus starts to develop and grow.

Fetal growth

The fetal period is one of continual growth and differentiation. The tissues, immature structures and organs formed during the embryonic period fully develop during the 30 remaining weeks.

The fetus is surrounded by amnion and by 12 weeks (the beginning of the second trimester) of pregnancy, the mesoderm of the outer amnion and inner chorion fuse forming the **amniochorionic membrane** or amniotic sac. The amniotic fluid which fills the sac is initially filtrate of maternal blood and later excreted urine from the fetus. **Amniotic fluid** functions as a protective cushion from shock for the fetus, regulates fetal temperature and protects the fetal skin from damage by contact with surrounding tissues. Fragments of shed fetal epithelial cells, which are found in the amniotic fluid, can be collected during pregnancy in a process called **amniocentesis**, and examined to ascertain fetal karyotype, for example, presence of trisomy 21.

From 12 weeks onwards the fetus grows rapidly in terms of both function, size and weight. During this period, also known as organogenesis, the organ systems of the fetus are fully developed. At the start of the second trimester, the fetus weighs around 14 g, which increases to around 0.6 kg by the end of the second trimester.

Although the rate of growth slows, the final three months of pregnancy sees the fetus gain a further 2.6 kg, meaning that at the end of the third trimester (9 months) the fetus weighs around 3.2 kg. The major changes and growth are illustrated in Table 2.5.1.

Table 2.5.1 Development timeline

Age	Image	Key development points
9–12 weeks/ month 3 9 weeks		Head dominant, but growth in body length and limbs accelerates Brain continues to enlarge Ears low set Retina of eye present Facial features crudely present Lungs begin to develop, fetus inhales/exhales amniotic fluid Blood cell formation begins in bone marrow Skin epidermis and dermis obvious
13–16 weeks/ month 4		Sensory organs differentiated, eyes blinking and sucking of lips visible Growth of body now outpacing head Most bones now distinct, joint cavities apparent Kidneys develop usual structure Intestines collect meconium Crown to rump length at 16 weeks is c. 140 mm
17–20 weeks/ month 5	16 weeks	Vernix caseosa covers body, lanugo (silk-like hair) covers skin Limbs reach near final proportions Fetal movements can usually be felt Crown to rump length at 20 weeks is c. 190 mm
21–30 weeks/ months 6 and 7	 28 weeks	Period of substantial increase in weight Body well-proportioned Myelination of spinal cord Limb bones begin to ossify Fingernails and toenails complete Crown to rump length at 30 weeks is c. 280 mm
30–38 weeks/ months 8 and 9	 38 weeks	Fat accumulates Firm grasp Circumference of head and abdomen roughly equal Crown to rump length at 38 weeks is c. 360 mm Weight c. 3.2 kg

Source: Figure 19.4, p.526, Clancy and McVicar (2009)

The growing uterus

As pregnancy proceeds, the uterus expands to accommodate the growth of the fetus. By the second trimester, it occupies the entire pelvic cavity, and extends higher into the abdominal cavity. A non-pregnant uterus is only 7.5 cm long and weighs 30–40 g, but at term is 30 cm in length weighing just over 1 kg. This growth is by expansion of existing smooth muscle fibres, called hypertrophy. Eventually, the uterus fills most of the abdominal cavity, nearly reaching the xiphoid process of the sternum, pushing many maternal organs out of position. The intestines, liver, stomach and diaphragm are pushed upwards, the thoracic cavity widens, and ureters and urinary bladder are compressed in the pelvic cavity. In total, including fetus, fluid and placenta, the uterus can weigh 6 or 7 kg.

Fetal skull

This section describes the fetal skull, whose features are significant in relation to the requirements of physiological childbirth.

The fetal skull is an ovoid shaped structure made up of 22 interlocking bones. Its two main parts are the **cranium**, which encloses and protects the brain housed in the cranial cavity, and the **face/jaw**. Compared to the rest of the fetal skeleton, the skull is large, although it has a relatively small face and jaw in contrast with the **vault** (posterior, lateral and superior) area of cranium. The skull bones are thin, but

these thicken after birth. The bones of the vault are compressible (see below) while those of the cranial base and face are fixed. Fetal facial bones are undeveloped and dramatic changes in facial shape occur for around two years after birth. Also, at this time, there is rapid brain growth and expansion of the top part of the skull. This is most significant for the first two years but continues until early adulthood.

Fetal skull development

The periosteum contains special cells called **osteoblasts**. They are responsible for the formation of fetal skull bones by a process called **intramembranous ossification**, where bone is directly laid down on connective tissue. During embryogenesis, the fetal skull is entirely membranous, but ossification spreads outwards from specific sites on the vault area as bones form. The centres of ossification are marked by rounded projections; the **occipital protuberance**, **parietal eminences** and **frontal bosses**.

At birth, the skull remains membranous in places; these are the gaps between bones known as **sutures**. Where sutures meet, they form larger soft areas of membrane called **fontanelles** (Figure 2.5.5). All these features of the fetal skull are landmarks for midwives in the process of physiological birth (see Chapter 4.3).

Structures of the fetal skull

Cranial bones and sutures

There are fourteen facial bones. The largest, the mandible or lower jawbone, is attached to the cranium by ligaments and is the only moveable bone of the skull. The cranium is the region of the skull of most interest, consisting of eight bones locked together by joints called sutures (as described above). These are the **frontal bone**, two **parietal bones**, two **temporal bones**, the

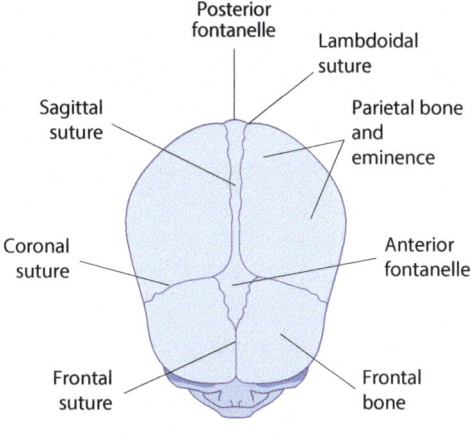

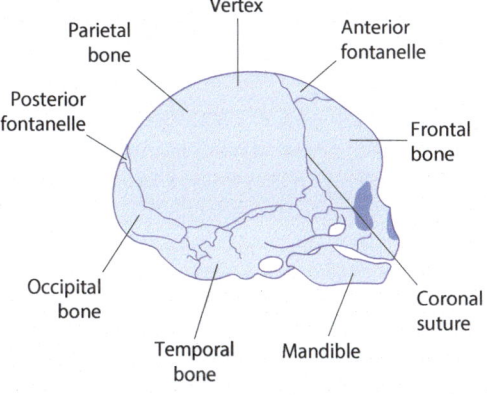

Figure 2.5.5 Landmarks and structures of the fetal skull

floor and roof of the two eye sockets. As a frontal suture unites the two sides of the frontal bone shortly after birth it is commonly described as a single bone. The two parietal bones are on either side behind the frontal bone, forming the sides and roof of the cranium. They are fused in the middle by the **sagittal suture** and meet the frontal bone at the **coronal** (named for crown) **suture**. The two temporal bones lie on each side below the parietal bones along the squamous suture, forming part of the base and sides of the cranium. Of greater significance is the large occipital bone which makes up the back of the skull and base of the cranium. It joins the parietal bones along the **lambdoid suture** (named for the Greek letter lambda, λ). A large circular opening at the base of the skull is the **foramen magnum** where the spinal cord and nerves enter the brain.

The bones of the vault are flat, and their dimensions correlate with those of the maternal pelvis (see Chapter 4.3 and Figure 2.5.6). During labour, under pressure of uterine contractions, the shape of the skull is modified as it passes through the maternal pelvis. This is due to the dense,

occipital bone or occiput, the sphenoid bone and ethmoid bone. These last two are of less interest to midwives as they are not included in the vault region. The sphenoid bone is a complex, bat-shaped keystone at the base and partly sides the cranium, while the ethmoid is a sponge-like bone in front of the sphenoid bone forming a mass either side of the nasal cavity. Hollow spaces inside the cranium, paranasal sinuses, help to resonate sound for voice and lighten the weight of the skull. Cranial bones are joined to the facial bones and base of the skull by sutures.

The frontal bone forms the anterior part of the cranium (the forehead) and cranial

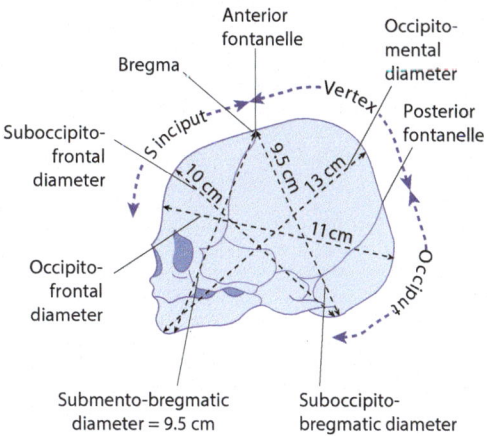

Figure 2.5.6 Approximate diameters of the fetal skull

fibrous connective tissue of the sutures and fontanelles between bones that allows for slight movement and flexibility, sometimes including overlapping of the thin sheets of bone. The alterations in skull shape during labour can reduce the size of the presenting part by around 1 cm, causing other skull parts to elongate in compensation. This phenomenon, resulting in a more oblong or flattened shape of the fetal skull, is called **moulding**, and resolves within a few days of birth. Sometimes areas of **caput** or swelling are also present in areas where circulation has been restricted. Excessive moulding strains the underlying dura matter and internal structures of the brain, which can be damaging. The flexibility of bone plates also accommodates the rapid brain growth and development after the baby is born.

Fontanelles

As described, the fontanelles ('soft spots') are membrane-filled spaces between bones where sutures meet. They will eventually be replaced by bone, by the same intramembranous ossification process as the rest of the skull and sutures. When this ossification is completed is dependent on location. It is known as the 'closure' of the fontanelle.

Two of the six fontanelles of the skull are particularly significant. The **anterior fontanelle** is the largest. It is diamond shaped, approximately 2.6 cm in size, found at the fore of the vault where the frontal and two parietal bones meet, at the junction of the frontal, sagittal and coronal sutures. It usually closes 18–24 months after birth and becomes known as the bregma.

The **posterior fontanelle** is smaller, approximately 0.6 cm in size, and triangular. It lies between the two parietal bones and the occiput at the rear of the skull and closes by 2–3 months after birth.

Regions of fetal skull

Midwives and obstetricians use the named regions of the fetal skull to identify the position of the fetal head during pregnancy or in labour (see Figure 2.5.6). The **vertex** is bounded by the anterior fontanelle at the front, posterior fontanelle to the rear and parietal eminences laterally. The **occiput** is the region of occipital bone from the posterior fontanelle to the base of the skull. The **brow** or sinciput is the region of frontal bone from the anterior fontanelle to the orbital ridges. The face region is the area below this to the chin.

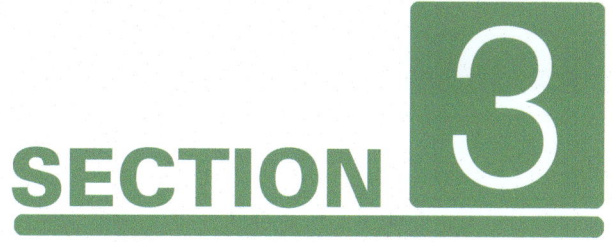

SECTION 3

Maternal Changes and Adaptations to Pregnancy

Jane Carpenter, Giada Giusmin, Louise Hunter and Claire Smith

With our new-found knowledge of the incredible complexity of the reproductive systems, female reproductive cycle, fertilisation, embryology and fetal development we now move on to consider the implications of being pregnant and maintaining the pregnancy on the maternal body. Indeed, pregnancy affects each and every body system, and each and every body system must change and adapt throughout pregnancy in order to enable and support the growing fetus. Therefore, in this section, we will take each of those main systems and consider how they function outside of pregnancy, as well as exploring the changes and adaptations which occur as a result of pregnancy.

DOI: 10.4324/9781003227571-11

The blood and cardiovascular system

Giada Giusmin

LEARNING OUTCOMES

▶ Describe the structure and function of the blood and cardiovascular system
▶ Describe the maintenance of haemostasis
▶ Explain the ABO blood groups and their significance
▶ Understand the key anatomical and physiological changes to the blood and cardiovascular system during pregnancy, and apply these to practice

Overview of blood

Blood is a fluid, connective tissue which transports oxygen, nutrients, waste, hormones and antibodies around the body.

It constitutes 6.5% of female body weight, approximately 4.5–5 litres in a 70 kg woman. Reference values for males are slightly higher. Blood is composed of two parts which separate when spun in a centrifuge: a liquid portion **(plasma)**, and a cellular portion containing **red blood cells**, **white blood cells** and **platelets** (see Figure 3.1.1).

Plasma

Plasma is 55% of the total blood volume and is mostly made of water (90%). It also contains:

▶ **Proteins**: Albumin is the most important and is responsible for maintaining the pressure inside blood vessels and avoiding fluid moving into the tissues and causing oedema (swelling).

DOI: 10.4324/9781003227571-12

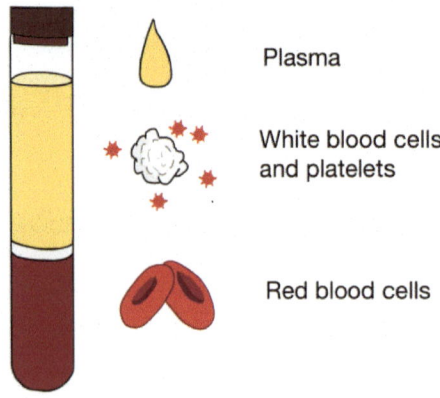

Figure 3.1.1 Blood composition

- ▶ **Electrolytes**, such as sodium and potassium, which are essential to cell function.
- ▶ **Nutrients**, such as glucose and vitamins, are essential for metabolic function.
- ▶ **Hormones**: These chemical messengers secreted by the endocrine glands into the bloodstream target specific receptors around the body.
- ▶ **Antibodies**, or immunoglobulins, are proteins that neutralise foreign microorganisms.

- ▶ **Clotting factors**, also technically proteins. Fibrinogen is the most numerous. Plasma without clotting factors is called **serum**.
- ▶ **Waste products** like carbon dioxide, which are transported to the lungs for excretion, or urea and creatinine, which are transported from the liver to the kidneys.

The cellular component of blood

The cellular component of blood comprises red blood cells **(erythrocytes)**, white blood cells **(leukocytes)** and platelets **(thrombocytes)**.

The vast majority of these cells are produced in red bone marrow from pluripotent stem cells through a process called **haematopoiesis**. Through haematopoiesis, pluripotent stem cells develop into one of the three types of blood cells (see Figure 3.1.2). Until approximately the age of seven years, red bone marrow is found in every bone. With time, the majority of red bone marrow changes into yellow, which is unable to support haematopoiesis, leaving only the end of long bones, flat and irregular bones

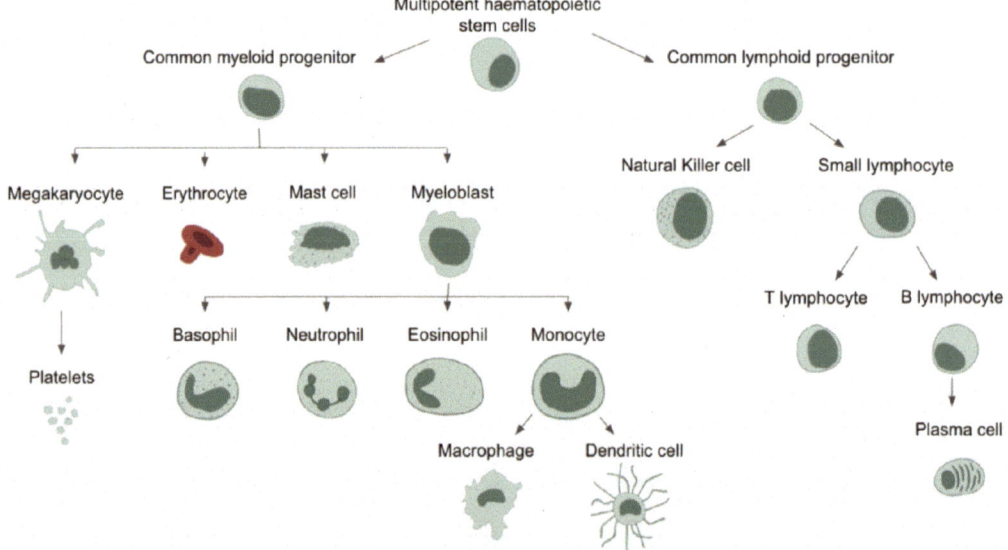

Figure 3.1.2 Blood cells' origins

able to host this process. Some lymphocytes (one of the five types of white blood cells) are produced in lymphoid organs.

Red blood cells (erythrocytes)

Erythrocytes are the most abundant blood cell. Their function is to circulate in the body and transport gases, especially oxygen. Erythrocytes are small biconcave cells (doughnut shape) without a nucleus or mitochondria (see Figure 3.1.3). Their shape and the lack of a nucleus are particularly useful as these increase the area for gas exchange, and the space for **haemoglobin**, an important protein used to transport oxygen. Erythrocytes are also particularly flexible and can squeeze through small blood vessels.

As erythrocytes are non-nucleated cells, they cannot replicate and have a lifespan of about three months. For this reason, the bone

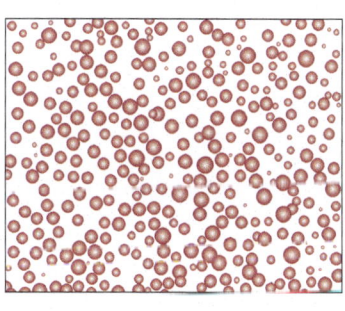

(a)

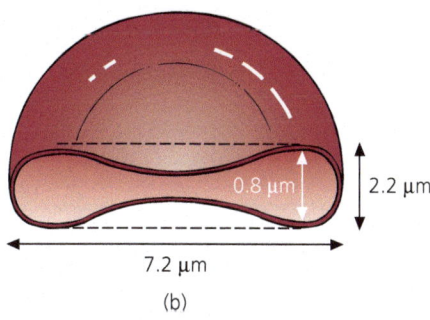

(b)

Figure 3.1.3 The structure of an erythrocyte. (a) viewed in a standard blood smear and (b) in cross-section
Source: Figure 11.6(a) and 11.6(b), p.278, Clancy and McVicar (2009)

marrow needs to constantly produce more, at the same rate as they are destroyed, to maintain a stable number. It takes about one week for their precursors to become erythrocytes, and this whole process is known as **erythropoiesis**. It is controlled by a hormone called **erythropoietin**, which is released by the kidneys and works under a negative feedback loop. It is released when body cells are deprived of oxygen (haemorrhage, anaemia, high altitude etc.) to stimulate the production of erythrocytes and attempt to reinstate adequate oxygen levels to the tissues.

In addition to erythropoietin, folic acid and vitamin B12 play a crucial role in the production of erythrocytes. A deficiency of these vitamins directly affects the development of erythrocytes and causes the death of their precursors, effectively leading to anaemia.

At the end of their life, erythrocytes are destroyed by macrophages in the spleen, liver and bone marrow; this process is called **haemolysis**. The iron atoms will be utilised again by the bone marrow to make more haemoglobin. Bilirubin, a pigment released during haemolysis, is transported back to the liver, and then excreted in bile.

Haemoglobin

Haemoglobin is a large molecule made of four *haem* units and four *globin* chains (see Figure 3.1.4). Each haem unit contains an atom of iron that can attach to an oxygen molecule, which means that each haemoglobin molecule can carry up to four oxygen molecules.

Once a haemoglobin molecule has all four oxygen molecules bound, it becomes saturated. This leads to changes in the colour of the blood, giving blood its red colour. Blood that has a lower oxygen level will appear more bluish in colour.

White blood cells (leukocytes)

White blood cells are essential to ensure optimal functioning of the immune system.

3.1

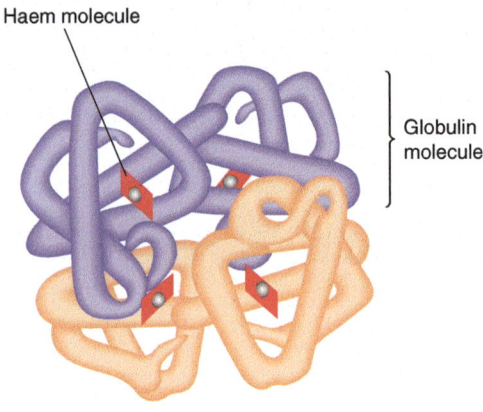

Haem molecule

Globulin molecule

Figure 3.1.4 Haemoglobin molecule

White blood cells are larger in size than their red counterparts but make up only about 1% of the total blood volume. Unlike erythrocytes, which are contained in the bloodstream, leukocytes can move from tissues to the bloodstream and back by squeezing through capillary walls, a process called **diapedesis** (further explained in Chapter 3.8).

White blood cells contain a nucleus, and some also contain granules in the cytoplasm. This allows the differentiation between two key groups of white blood cells, **granulocytes** (neutrophils, eosinophils and basophils) and **agranulocytes** (lymphocytes and monocytes) – see Table 3.1.1 and Figure 3.1.5.

Table 3.1.1 White blood cells

Leukocytes	Blood cell	Percentage	Function
Granulocytes	Neutrophils	60–65%	Important in the fight against bacterial and fungal infections, neutrophils are summoned to infected areas via chemical signals (discussed further in Chapter 3.8), where they can reach high numbers very rapidly. Small in size but highly mobile, they engulf bacteria and debris and destroy them by phagocytosis (Figure 3.1.5).
	Eosinophils	2–4%	These are mostly deployed against parasite infections. They engulf and destroy smaller invaders via phagocytosis, and surround larger parasitic worms, releasing toxic chemicals to destroy them.
	Basophils	1%	Least common leukocyte but important as they release histamine. Histamine is needed in the inflammatory response to make the capillaries leaky and attract other leukocytes (see Chapter 3.8).
Agranulocytes	Lymphocytes	20–35%	Circulate mostly in the lymphatic tissue like lymph nodes and spleen but are also found in the blood. Lymphocytes derive from a different stem cell compared to other leukocytes, and then develop into two different types of lymphocytes, B and T, which are of vital importance in the adaptive immune defences.
	Monocytes	3–8%	**Monocytes** are the largest type of leukocytes. These divide into **macrophages**, which roam in the tissues, and **dendritic cells**, which roam in the bloodstream. Macrophages are extremely important leukocytes as they link innate and adaptive immune defences. Macrophages are phagocytic, like neutrophils, but are much larger, more powerful and long-lasting.

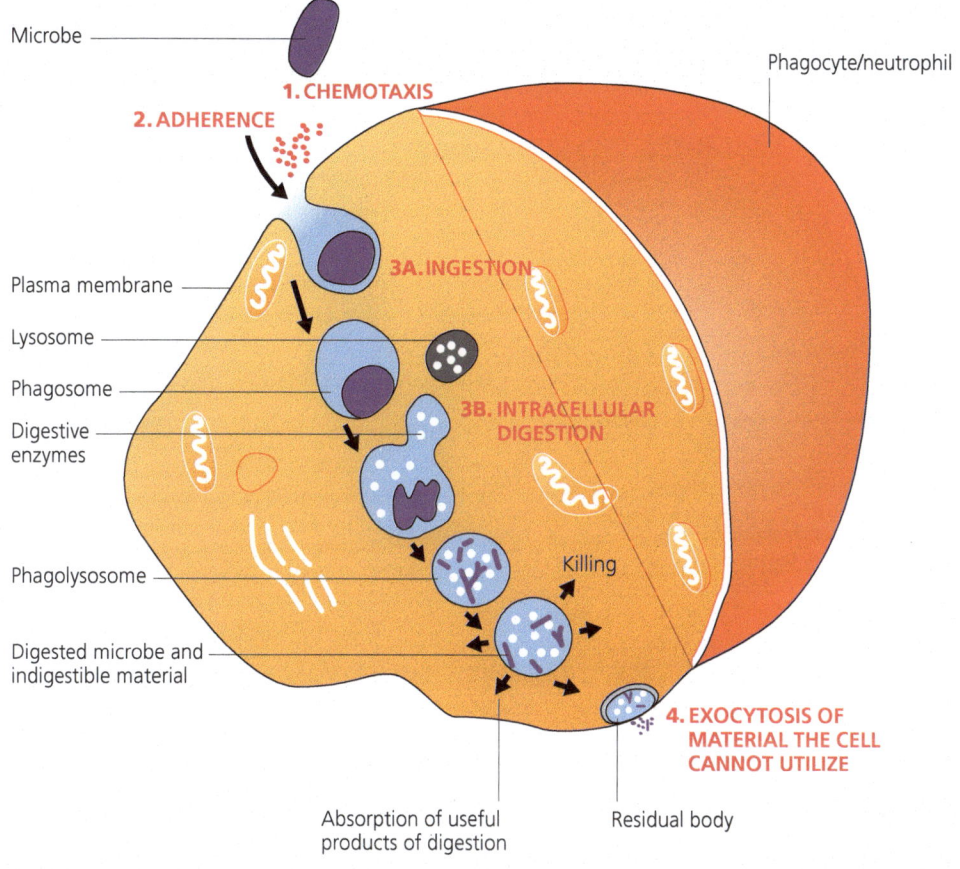

Figure 3.1.6 Neutrophil showing phagocytosis process
Source: Figure13.10(a), p.378, Clancy and McVicar (2009)

Platelets

Platelets are cell fragments (not technically cells) that originate from megakaryocytes breaking into thousands of irregularly shaped pieces. Platelets have no nucleus but contain granules in their cytoplasm that promote haemostasis (arrest of bleeding from damaged blood vessels) by blood clotting.

It is not known how platelet production is regulated, apart from that the hormone thrombopoietin is responsible for accelerating the production of platelets from megakaryocytes.

Platelets live for just over a week and are mostly stored in the spleen, ready in case of emergency. Also in the spleen, platelets are destroyed by macrophages if they have not been used for haemostasis.

Maintenance of haemostasis

When a blood vessel is damaged, causing blood loss, platelets play a major role in repairing the damage and restoring haemostasis – the maintenance of stable blood volume in the body. This process is outlined below and in Figure 3.1.6.

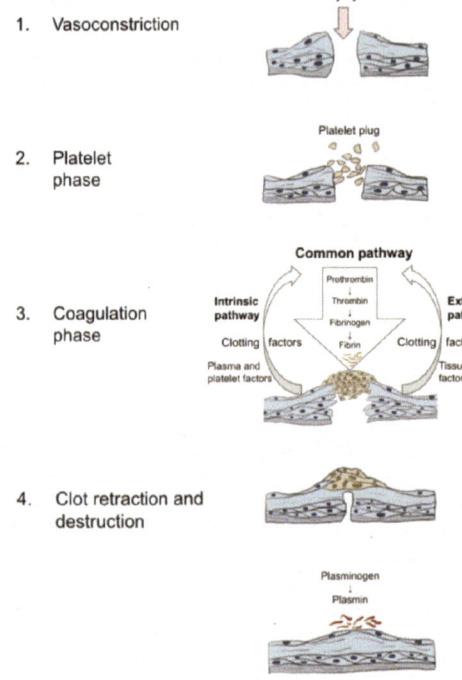

1. Vasoconstriction

2. Platelet phase

3. Coagulation phase

4. Clot retraction and destruction

Figure 3.1.6 Haemostasis

Vasoconstriction

Once a blood vessel has been damaged, vascular spasm occurs – the smooth muscle in the vessel walls contracts, narrowing the lumen (the space in the vessel) and slowing blood flow.

Platelet phase

Platelets roll along vessel walls and adhere to any broken edges. Once they have adhered, the platelets are 'activated' by chemicals released from the injury site, and by contact with the extracellular collagen (the collagen outside the blood vessel). The platelets change shape from smooth discs to become spiked and secrete chemicals such as adenosine diphosphate (ADP) and Von Willebrand factor. These help platelets adhere to each other and to the damaged vessel wall. Serotonin, prostaglandins and phospholipids maintain vasoconstriction,

attract further platelets to the site (a positive feedback loop) and **help activate clotting factors**.

Activated platelets then **aggregate** – interconnect with each other and the endothelial lining of the damaged vessel – forming a **weak platelet plug** to cover the break. Platelet aggregation is aided by **fibrinogen**, which forms bridges between adjacent platelets.

Coagulation phase

This phase is complex, and a detailed explanation is outside the scope of this book; therefore, only some of its steps are described here.

Coagulation involves **clotting factors** acting in a **cascade**. There are twelve clotting factors, numbered I to XIII (number VI is redundant). They are secreted primarily by platelets and the liver (which requires vitamin K to produce many of them). They are usually inactive but become activated when blood vessel damage occurs.

Activation happens via three pathways. The **extrinsic pathway** is triggered when clotting factors encounter substances outside the blood vessel. The **intrinsic pathway** is triggered when clotting factors encounter substances inside the blood vessel. The **common pathway** is formed when the extrinsic and intrinsic pathways merge.

In the common pathway, **factor X** is activated to become the enzyme **prothrombinase**. This converts **factor II**, the inactive enzyme **prothrombin** into the active enzyme **thrombin**. Thrombin then converts **factor I**, the soluble plasma protein **fibrinogen**, into insoluble **fibrin** protein strands. These insoluble fibrin molecules join to form a mesh around the platelet plug, which is further stabilised by **factor XIII** (fibrin-stabilising factor). This lays the foundation of the final blood clot, which is much more stable and resistant than the initial platelet plug.

Clot retraction and destruction

Very shortly after the final blood clot has been completed, platelets contract and cause the clot to start expelling serum. This will bring the injured sides of the blood vessel closer together and allow the endothelium to start regenerating.

The breakdown of the clot happens as **plasminogen** is activated into **plasmin**, an enzyme which breaks down the fibrin in the clot.

Overall, haemostasis is a very quick process, a platelet plug can be formed in only 6 minutes, but also a very accurate one. It relies on numerous mechanisms that activate or suppress the function of clotting factors to ensure clots are not formed where not needed (e.g. deep vein thrombosis, DVT) and bleeding is not left uncontrolled (e.g. in hereditary haemophilia).

Blood groups

Erythrocytes or red blood cells (RBCs) carry different proteins (called **antigens**) on their plasma membrane. These antigens determine an individual's blood group. They are also recognised as foreign when transferred from one individual to another. Therefore, if an individual receives a blood transfusion from a donor with a different blood group, their immune system will be prompted to mount an attack on the foreign antigens present in the donor's blood. They will produce antibodies which will attach themselves to the foreign antigens and cause **agglutination** (the formation of clumps or clots which then block small blood vessels in organs such as the kidneys), **haemolysis** (the destruction of RBCs) and death.

If an individual is transfused with the same blood group, however, the immune system will not recognise the erythrocytes as foreign, as they will have the same antigens as the ones it is usually exposed to and therefore, will not attack them with antibodies. Despite blood transfusions presently being a common life-saving procedure, the existence of different blood groups was only discovered in 1901.

In the human species, there are about 30 different types of RBC antigens. The commonly known ones are the **ABO** and **Rhesus factor**, because of their potentially catastrophic transfusion reactions from blood incompatibility. However, as other antigens could also cause harmful reactions during blood transfusions, a sample containing blood of the recipient must be crossmatched with the intended transfusion unit prior to administration to the patient to ensure compatibility.

ABO blood groups

The four main blood groups are A, B, AB and O. An individual's blood group is genetically determined. As shown in Table 3.1.2, people with blood group A have erythrocytes carrying A antigens and will develop naturally occurring anti B antibodies in early childhood. People with blood group B have erythrocytes carrying B antigens and will develop naturally occurring anti-A antibodies in early childhood. People with blood group AB have A and B antigens and therefore, will not develop antibodies against either, making blood group AB the 'universal recipient'.

Conversely, people with blood group O have no antigens displayed, making them 'universal donors', as the absence of antigens on their RBCs will mean no immune response occurs in the recipient. On the other hand, people with blood group O can only receive the blood of the same blood group as they will have anti-A and

Table 3.1.2 ABO blood group system

Blood Group	A	B	AB	O
Red blood cell type Antigen	A antigen	B antigen	A and B antigens	None
Antibodies	Anti-B	Anti-A	None	Anti-A and Anti-B
Who can they donate blood to?	A and AB	B and AB	AB	A, B, AB and O
Who can they receive blood from?	A and O	B and O	A, B, AB and O	O

anti-B antibodies. Table 3.1.2 shows in more detail all the different combinations in terms of ABO blood groups and the safety of transfusions.

In addition to the antigens discussed above, there is another antigen of vital importance in midwifery and during blood transfusions, the Rh system (formerly known as the Rhesus system). This will be discussed in detail in Chapter 3.8.

Overview of the cardiovascular system

The cardiovascular system is composed of the heart, the blood vessels and the blood. Its function is to distribute oxygen and nutrients around the body and to collect waste products via the blood. It is essential to remember that the cardiovascular system is closely linked to all the other body systems: in fact, whenever the cardiovascular system fails to perform its function, tissues and organs will be depleted of oxygen and nutrients and will eventually die.

The heart: structure and function

The heart is a hollow cone-shaped muscular organ positioned in the thoracic cavity, with the apex obliquely pointing towards the left side of the body. Around the heart, on either side, there are the lungs, posteriorly the oesophagus and trachea, and anteriorly the sternum and ribs.

The heart is surrounded by a double-layered, fluid-filled sac called the **pericardium**. The function of the pericardium is to protect and anchor the heart, as well as to allow its smooth movement during each beat. The heart is also lined on the inside by a smooth membrane, called the **endocardium**, which covers all the chambers and valves.

The cardiac muscle, also called the **myocardium**, is composed of **myocytes** (see Chapter 1.2 for more information on these specialised cells). Myocytes are stimulated by targeted electrical signals produced by conducting fibres. The electrical signals are insulated by a fibrous

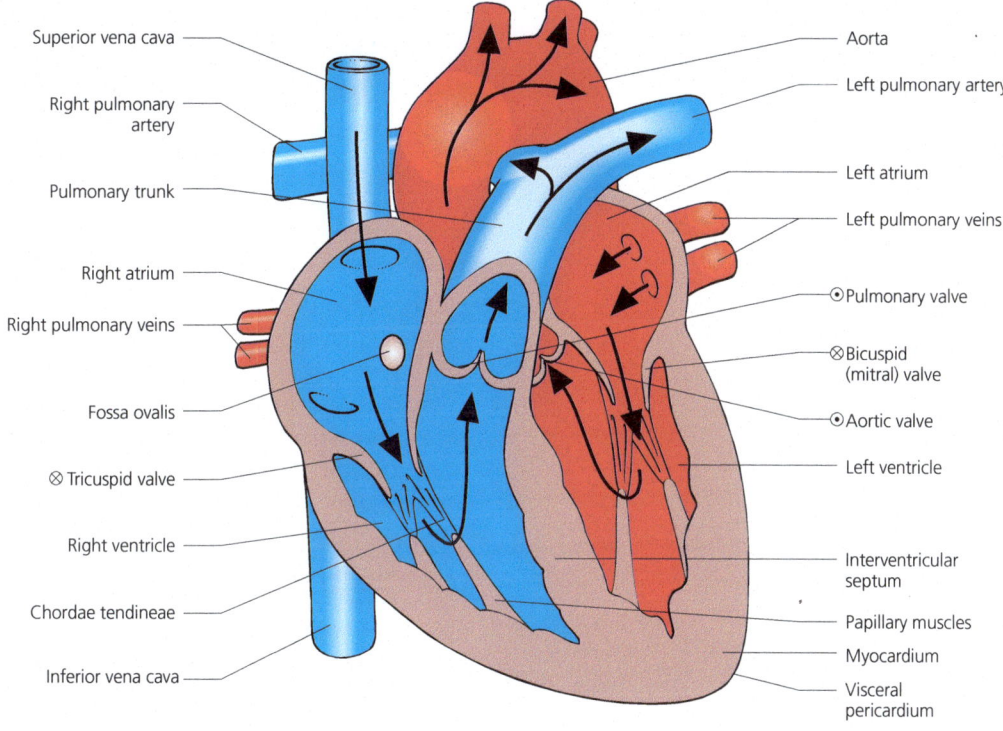

Superior vena cava

Right pulmonary artery

Pulmonary trunk

Right atrium

Right pulmonary veins

Fossa ovalis

⊗ Tricuspid valve

Right ventricle

Chordae tendineae

Inferior vena cava

Aorta

Left pulmonary artery

Left atrium

Left pulmonary veins

⊙ Pulmonary valve

⊗ Bicuspid (mitral) valve

⊙ Aortic valve

Left ventricle

Interventricular septum

Papillary muscles

Myocardium

Visceral pericardium

3.1

Figure 3.1.7 Frontal section of the heart
Source: Figure 12.4, p.308, Clancy and McVicar (2009)

skeleton: a rigid connective tissue structure between the atria and ventricles.

The heart is divided into **four chambers**: **two atria** and **two ventricles**, and into **two sides**: **right** and **left** (Figure 3.1.7). The atria are considered the receiving chambers, as they do not have pumping activity, whereas the ventricles are considered the discharging chambers, and are the true pumps. The atria are positioned above the ventricles.

A system of **valves** ensures blood only enters the heart via the atria and then is moved into the ventricles, in a unidirectional flow. **Atrioventricular valves** open when the pressure in the ventricles is low, moving blood from the atria, where the pressure is higher, to the ventricles. When the pressure is higher in the ventricles, the valves close to prevent blood from flowing back into the atria. The right atrioventricular valve has

three flaps; hence, it is called the **tricuspid valve**. The atrioventricular valve on the left has two flaps and is called the **bicuspid or mitral valve.** Two **semilunar valves** are located just outside the ventricles, one at the base of the pulmonary artery (pulmonary valve) and the other at the base of the aorta (aortic valve). Both valves are made of three cusps and they both open when the ventricles contract to push the blood out, then close back when the ventricles are relaxed and filling. This means that due to their different functions, atrioventricular and semilunar valves open and close at different times.

The left and right sides of the heart are separated by the septum, made of myocardium lined by the endocardium. Each side pumps blood into different, but consecutive, circulation systems (see Figure 3.1.8). The right side of the heart

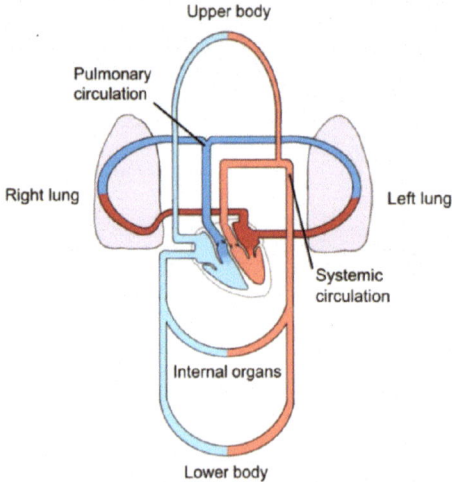

Figure 3.1.8 Pulmonary and systemic circulation

distributes blood to the lungs to allow gas exchange; this is called the **pulmonary circulation**. The left side of the heart, after receiving oxygenated blood coming from the lungs, pumps blood to the rest of the body; this is called the **systemic circulation**.

Blood vessels: arteries, veins and capillaries

Blood vessels make up the vascular system, and together with the heart, these comprise the cardiovascular system. As an analogy, the vascular system could be described as a road network. It starts from motorways (larger blood vessels), from which smaller roads stem, going all the way down to countryside lanes.

Arteries, as a general rule, carry blood away from the heart. These branch out into smaller and smaller vessels, arterioles, until they become capillaries. The capillaries are where the exchange of gases, as well as nutrients and waste products, occurs. From the capillaries, the opposite network can be seen as these come together in larger and larger vessels, venules, which then drain into veins. Veins, as a general rule, carry

blood back to the heart. An exception to this rule can be seen in the fetus' umbilical cord (see Chapter 5.1).

Anatomical structure of blood vessels

There are three layers of tissue that compose blood vessels (see Figure 3.1.9):

▶ **Tunica intima** or **endothelium**, is the inner layer. It is composed of only one cell layer, and in the case of capillaries, this is the only layer thus making them very permeable. The endothelium rests on a layer of basement membrane.
▶ **Tunica media** is the middle layer. This contains a varying amount of elastic tissue and smooth muscle. As the smooth muscle is controlled by the sympathetic nervous system, this layer can change the diameter of the blood vessels.
▶ **Tunica adventitia** (or externa), which is made of fibrous tissue. It is the outer layer of the blood vessels and functions as a structural support.

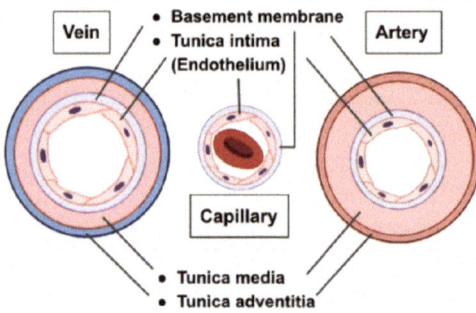

Figure 3.1.9 The structure of arteries, veins and capillaries
Source: Figure 12.4, p.308, Clancy and McVicar (2009)

Arteries

Compared to veins, arterial walls are much thicker, especially at the level of the tunica media. This allows arteries to stretch when the blood is pumped by the heart into the systemic circulation and then to return to a normal diameter without compromising their structure. For this reason, the tunica media of the arteries has more elastic tissue than smooth muscle. Conversely, when the arteries branch out into arterioles, the composition of the tunica media changes, with gradually more smooth muscle than elastic tissue. This allows the arterioles to be under the control of the sympathetic nervous system and change their diameter, which influences systemic blood pressure.

In the human body, the **aorta** is the largest artery, and its shape resembles a hairpin bend. It goes up from the left ventricle before descending through the thorax down to the abdominal cavity (see Figure 3.1.10). From the aorta, arteries to the organs branch out at different levels, for example, coronary arteries branch out from the first portion of the aorta (ascending). Arteries supplying the head and upper limbs stem from the aortic arch (the curved portion of the aorta). The lungs and the diaphragm receive oxygenated blood from the thoracic aorta. Arteries from the abdominal section of the aorta supply the digestive tract, kidneys, ovaries and lower limbs.

Veins

Compared to the respective artery, veins have a larger diameter, their tunica media is thinner and the tunica adventitia is thicker. Veins return blood to the heart and need to ensure the same amount of blood that has been pumped out by the heart is brought back to it. However, as blood pressure in the venous circulation is not sufficient on its own to push blood against gravity, larger veins have valves to prevent back flow. Valves are half-moon-shaped folds of tunica intima and connective tissue. Skeletal muscle activity also promotes venous return – the contraction and retraction of skeletal muscles exerts pressure on neighbouring veins, squeezing blood back towards the heart.

There are two major veins in the human body, these are the **superior** and the **inferior venae cavae**. The superior vena cava receives deoxygenated blood from the veins of the upper body (head and upper limbs). The inferior vena cava, which is the largest vein, returns blood from the lower body. It has one valve at the level of the right atrium, where, together with the superior vena cava, these return the deoxygenated blood to be re-oxygenated by the pulmonary circulation (see Figure 3.1.11).

3.1

APPLICATION TO PRACTICE

Left lateral position in pregnancy

Left lateral position, especially in the second half of pregnancy, is a recommendation that has been supported by numerous studies over the last century. The gravid uterus in a supine position can cause aortocaval compression, reduced venous return due to an occlusion of the abdominal aorta and inferior vena cava (IVC). This causes systemic hypotension in the mother which may result in fetal compromise. Both right and left lateral positions help relieve the pressure on abdominal aorta and IVC by the gravid uterus and restore adequate cardiac output. However, the left lateral position seems to be more beneficial than the right lateral at the level of the renal veins joining the IVC, showing increased blood flow (see Figure 3.1.12).

It is important to note that, despite their size and importance in the pulmonary and systemic circulation, arteries and veins are only conducting vessels. It is the capillaries, the narrow countryside roads of our road

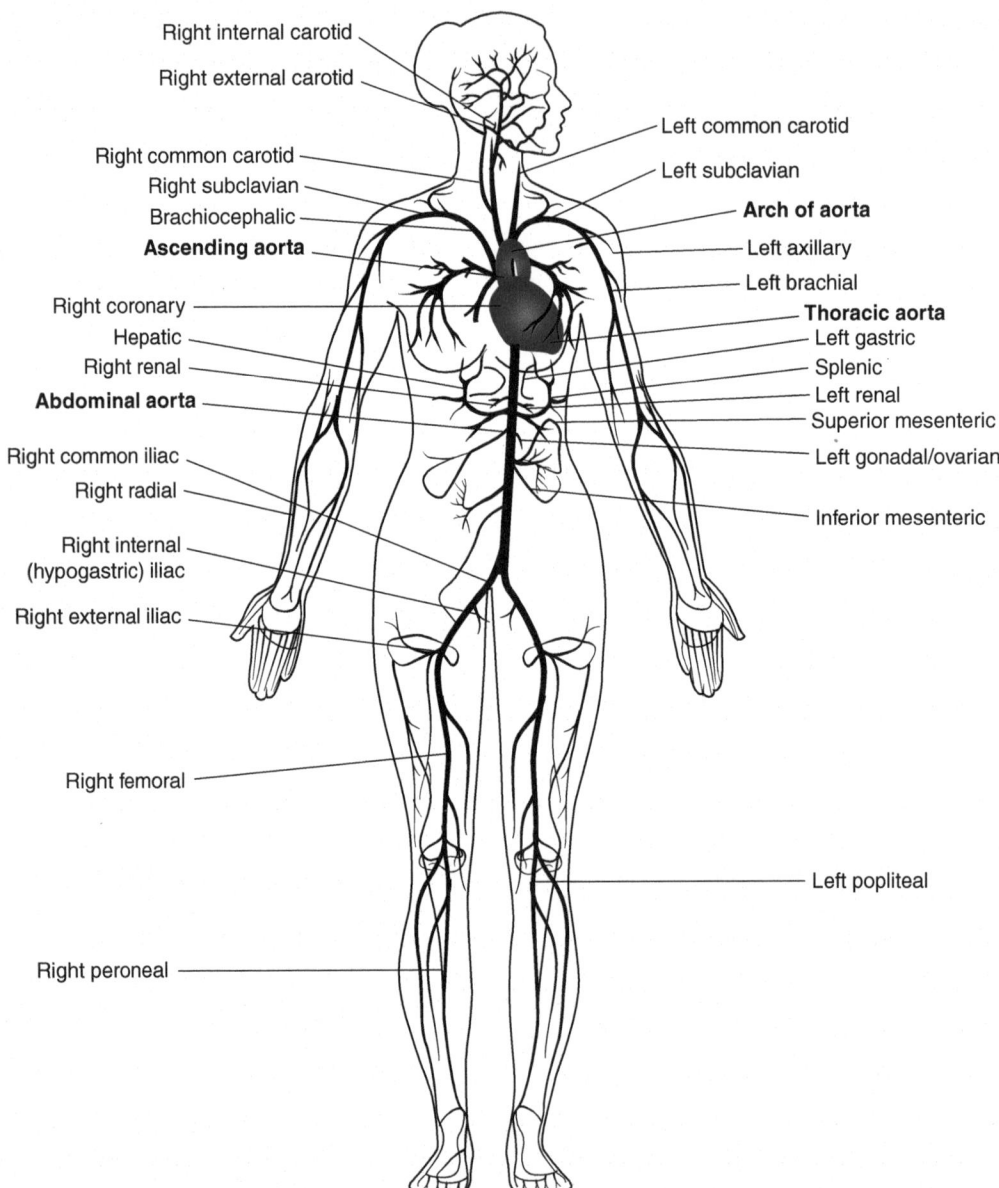

Figure 3.1.10 Major arteries in the body

network analogy, which allow the blood to reach the individual cells, the individual houses.

Capillaries

The capillaries are the smallest blood vessels and are composed of a single layer of endothelial cells lying on a basement membrane (see Figure 3.1.9). This arrangement facilitates gaseous exchange, as well as the passage of nutrients and waste products, between the blood vessels and the tissue cells. The movement of oxygenated blood from the

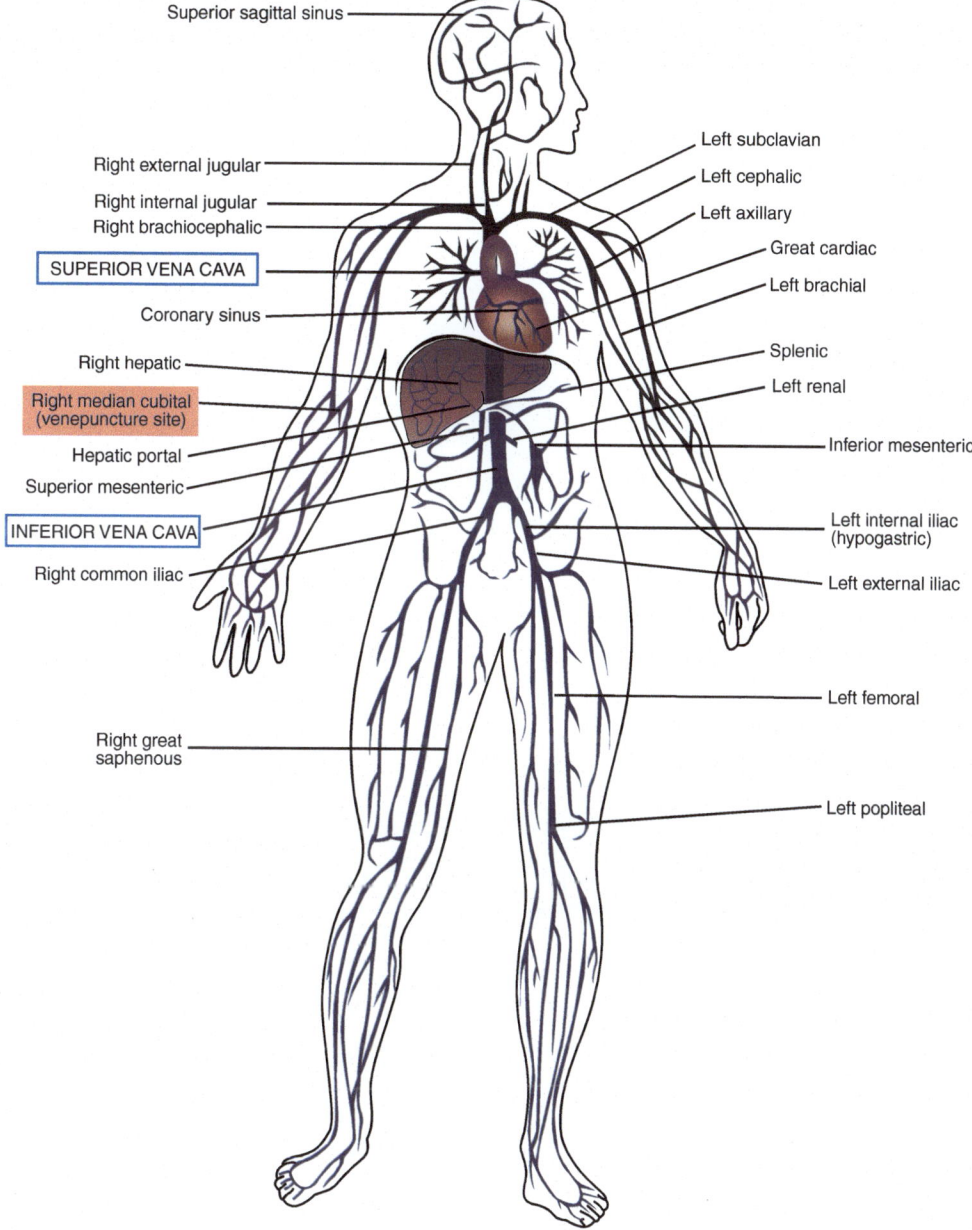

Superior sagittal sinus

Right external jugular

Right internal jugular

Right brachiocephalic

SUPERIOR VENA CAVA

Coronary sinus

Right hepatic

Right median cubital (venepuncture site)

Hepatic portal

Superior mesenteric

INFERIOR VENA CAVA

Right common iliac

Right great saphenous

Left subclavian

Left cephalic

Left axillary

Great cardiac

Left brachial

Splenic

Left renal

Inferior mesenteric

Left internal iliac (hypogastric)

Left external iliac

Left femoral

Left popliteal

Figure 3.1.11 Major veins in the body

arteriole, through the network of capillaries and back with deoxygenated blood and waste products to the venule, is called **microcirculation**. The vast majority of the body cells (skin is an exception) lie near a capillary. Body cells are surrounded by interstitial fluid (also called tissue fluid), which is where gases, nutrients and wastes move between cells and capillaries, see Figure 3.1.13.

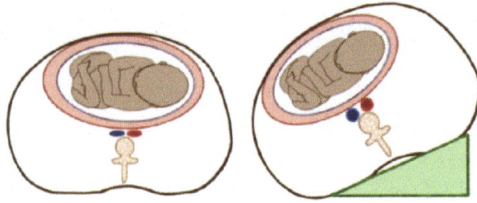

Figure 3.1.12 Supine hypotension and use of a lateral position to relieve this

Physiology of heart and blood circulation

Deoxygenated blood reaches the heart via the superior and the inferior venae cavae which enter the heart at the level of the right atrium. From the right atrium, blood flows into the right ventricle before being pumped out through the pulmonary trunk and reaching the lungs via the left and right pulmonary arteries. Here the deoxygenated blood offloads CO_2 and picks up O_2 (see Chapter 3.2). The pulmonary arteries are the only arteries to carry deoxygenated blood. Similarly, once the blood has become oxygenated in the lungs, it is carried back to the heart via the pulmonary veins. The blood now enters the left side of the heart via the left atrium, and flows into the left ventricle before being pumped out to the rest of the body via the aorta; then, the cycle starts all over again.

Vasculature of the heart

Despite the heart pumping blood 24/7, the blood contained in the heart does not actually oxygenate the myocardial cells. In fact, the myocardium receives oxygenated blood via the coronary arteries, which are generated directly from the ascending part of the aorta. When the myocardial cells have been oxygenated, the blood is returned via the cardiac veins, which drain into the coronary sinus and then reach the right atrium.

If the heart does not receive a sufficient supply of oxygenated blood, some areas might die, and this results in a myocardial infarction, also known as a heart attack.

Conduction system

The cardiac conduction system refers to the electrical supply of the heart. The heart has an **intrinsic conduction system**, consisting of specialised neuromuscular cells that cannot be found anywhere else in the body (see Figure 3.1.14). This enables the production of electrical impulses which travel from the atria to the ventricles, causing the heart to contract and beat. Although the cardiac conduction system is situated entirely within the heart, it can be modified by **extrinsic factors** such as the nervous system, hormones and

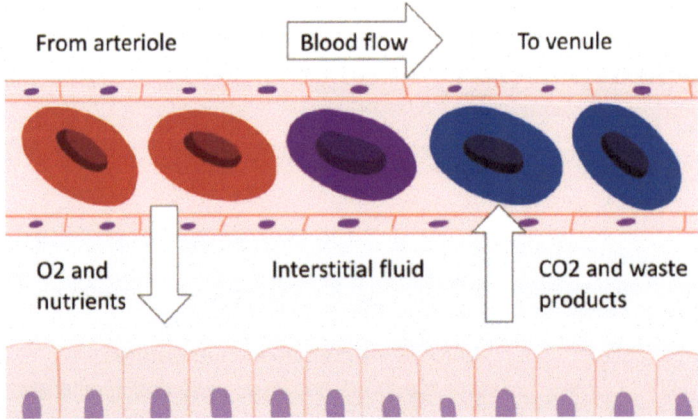

Figure 3.1.13 Gas and nutrient exchange at capillary level

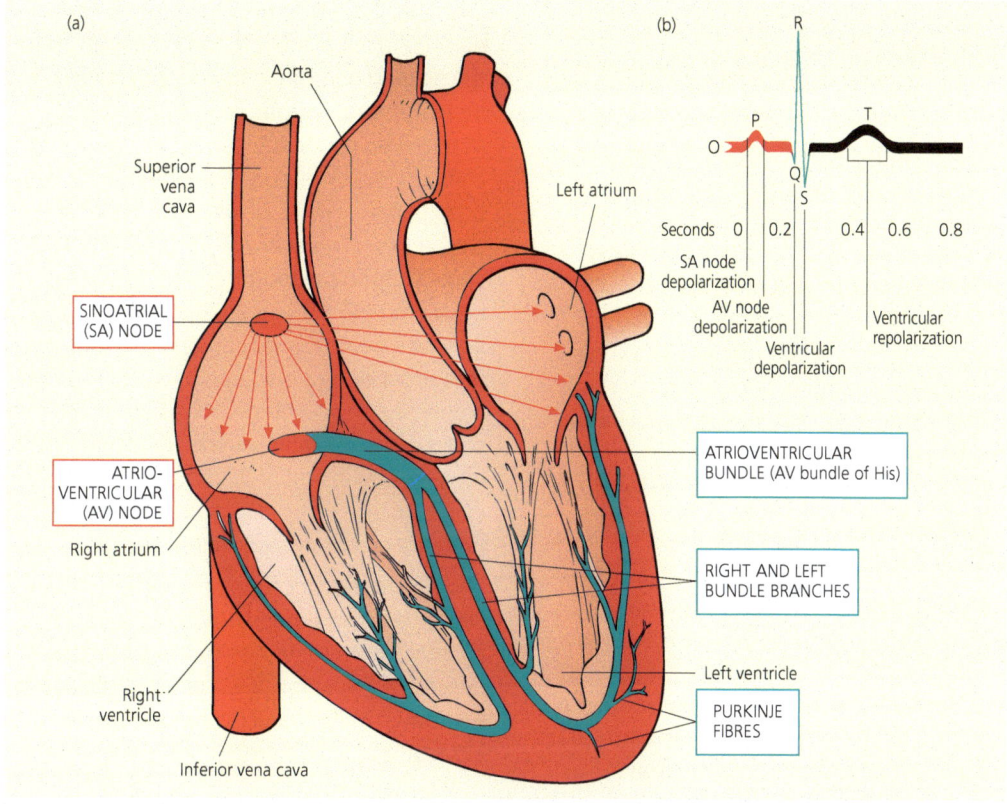

Figure 3.1.14 (a) Conduction in the heart and (b) corresponding electrocardiogram
Source: Figure 12.8, p.315, Clancy and McVicar (2009)

electrolytes. The heart is supplied with nervous fibres from the autonomic nervous system (see Chapter 3.3), which can affect the heart rate by increasing or lowering it. Hormones such as adrenaline and electrolyte imbalances (particularly involving potassium) can also affect heart rate. Additional factors such as age also have an impact: the fetal heart rate can reach 160 bpm during a rest phase, and it gradually decreases throughout an individual's life to 60–80 bpm in adults.

There are three main components of the intrinsic conduction system: the **sinoatrial node**, the **atrioventricular node** and the **bundle**. The sinoatrial (SA) node is positioned in the right atrium close to the superior vena cava's entrance (see

Figure 3.1.14). The cells of the SA node discharge regular electrical impulses (depolarisation) because they are unstable and as soon as they have repolarised, they are unstable again and depolarise, and so on. Their action causes the atria to contract, and because this rhythm is faster than any other part of the heart, the SA node is also known as the heart's pacemaker. The SA node is connected to the atrioventricular (AV) node, and this is the only electrical pathway between the atria and the ventricles.

The AV node is located in the atrial septum close to the AV valves, and its function is to transmit the impulses from the atria to the ventricles. Because there is a 0.1-second delay between the impulse going from the atria to the ventricles, this allows the atria to complete the contraction before the ventricles start theirs.

The atrioventricular (AV) bundle, or bundle of His, stems from the AV node and splits into the right and left bundle branches in the ventricular septum. These branches then split even further into smaller fibres called Purkinje fibres. The AV bundle function is to transmit the impulses from the AV node to the apex of the heart where the ventricular contraction starts. Sympathetic and parasympathetic nerves supply the SA and AV nodes and can increase or decrease the heart rate.

Cardiac output and blood pressure

Cardiac output is defined as the amount of blood pumped by the heart within one minute. To calculate it, we need to multiply the **stroke volume**, the amount of blood pumped by the heart during each individual ventricular contraction, by the **heart rate**.

The stroke volume depends on the amount of blood physically present inside the ventricles just before they contract. Consequently, this depends on the venous return to the heart via the venae cavae (superior and inferior). The heart can adjust to a reduced or increased venous return, within physiological limits, in order to eject the same amount of blood as it receives. However, excessive or insufficient venous return, such as during a sudden haemorrhage, can lead the heart to reduce the stroke volume and the cardiac output and then deteriorate. Hormones, such as adrenaline, and sympathetic nervous system activity, will cause an increase in heart rate and, therefore, cardiac output.

Blood pressure (BP) is, literally, the pressure of the blood against the blood vessel walls and is reported in millimetres of mercury (mmHg). As a parameter, it is generally presented as two numbers, for example, 120/80 mmHg, where the first number is the systolic blood pressure, and the second number is the diastolic blood pressure. The **systolic blood pressure** is determined by the left ventricle contracting and pushing oxygenated blood into the body and therefore, is the maximal force on the vessels (usually around 120 mmHg). The **diastolic pressure** reflects the blood pressure whilst the heart is at rest in between beats (usually around 80 mmHg). It is important for blood pressure to remain within the normal range. High blood pressure could damage blood vessels, leading to their rupture. Low blood pressure could result in inadequate blood flow to vital organs, potentially causing permanent damage.

The tunica media of the smaller arteries and arterioles is mostly made of smooth muscle which responds to the sympathetic nerves of the autonomic nervous system. As shown in Figure 3.1.15(b), when the sympathetic nerves reduce the diameter of the blood vessels (also known as vasoconstriction), this increases the pressure inside and the systemic blood pressure. On the other hand, when there is a signal for the blood pressure to be lowered, the sympathetic output will be reduced, leading to blood vessels widening their diameter (vasodilation).

There are various factors that determine how much resistance blood encounters in the blood vessels (peripheral resistance), for example sex and age, however, there are two main pathways:

▶ Short-term control, mostly influenced by the nervous system
▶ Long-term control, mostly influenced by the renal system. This topic will be discussed in Chapter 3.6.

The short-term control of blood pressure is regulated by the cardiovascular centre (CVC), located in the brain. The CVC works together with other areas in the brain, plus

3.1

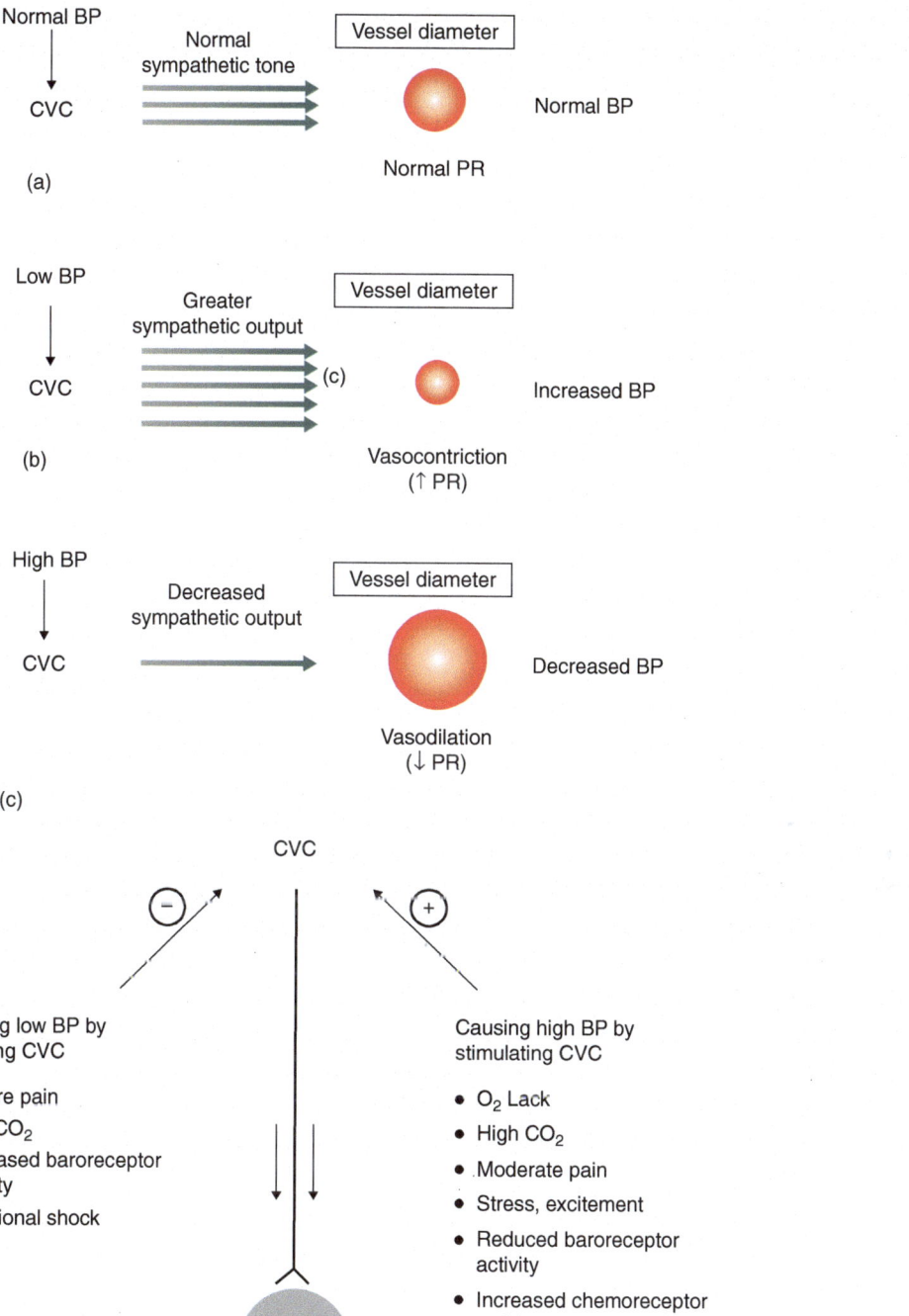

Figure 3.1.15 Blood pressure and vessel diameter (CVC – Cardiovascular Centre, BP – Blood Pressure, PR – Peripheral resistance)

baroreceptors and chemoreceptors, to control blood pressure and heart rate via sympathetic and parasympathetic nerves. Baroreceptors are special nerve cells which can detect changes in pressure and signal the CVC to increase or slow down the heart rate. The chemoreceptors are also special nerve cells, but these detect changes in the chemical composition of the blood, like raised carbon dioxide and lowered oxygen levels. When this happens, the chemoreceptors send signals to the CVC, which in turn amplifies the sympathetic impulses to increase blood pressure and heart rate. In order to restore adequate levels of oxygen to the tissues, the CVC will also stimulate the respiratory centre to increase respiratory activity and have more oxygen available.

Other factors that can influence the CVC to adjust blood pressure and heart rate are emotional states like pain, stress, shock or fear, but also body temperature or exercise.

Changes and adaptations during pregnancy

The cardiovascular system is possibly the most influenced by physiological changes

in pregnancy, as these affect not only the heart and blood vessels but also the blood.

Haematological changes during pregnancy

Many changes to the cardiovascular system happen from early pregnancy. The total blood volume increases between 30% and 50% (approx. 1.5 litres) and is more marked in the case of multiple pregnancies, even up to 70%. However, looking at the specific components, the plasma volume increases by 50% but the RBC volume only increases by around 20–30%. This 'mismatch' results in an apparent reduction of haemoglobin concentration **(haemodilution)** and what is known as **physiologic anaemia of pregnancy**. The increase in blood volume starts as early as six to eight weeks gestation and plateaus towards the end of the third trimester (see Figure 3.1.16). It is thought that the increase in blood volume is stimulated by oestrogen and progesterone, which stimulate vasodilation and nitric oxide (which is a strong vasodilator) production. In addition to this, oestrogen and progesterone act on the kidneys, increasing

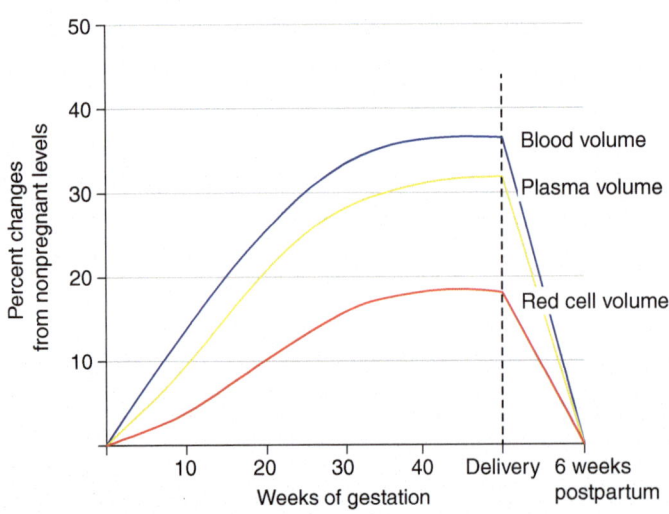

Figure 3.1.16 Increases in blood volume during pregnancy

water and sodium retention by stimulating the renin-angiotensin-aldosterone system.

There are a number of advantages to the increased blood volume during pregnancy. There is a growing demand for blood flow to the breasts, skin, kidneys and uterus for placental perfusion. Also, due to the peripheral vasodilation occurring in pregnancy, the increased blood volume ensures that blood pressure is maintained within a stable range. It is also protective at birth as it reduces the impact of blood loss for the mother.

In a full blood count (FBC) test result, the physiological changes in pregnancy will translate into:

▶ A lower RBC count than pre-pregnancy due to the haemodilution.
▶ A lower haemoglobin (Hb) level, as it is also influenced by haemodilution. Pre-pregnancy levels are around 12–15 g/dl, whereas in pregnancy it can drop to 10.5–11 g/dl, especially in the second trimester.
▶ Stable mean cell volume (MCV), however, if there is iron deficiency this could be decreased.
▶ Slight drop in platelet level, with a normal platelet count between 150–400 × 10^9/L, despite an increase in production. This drop is also due to the haemodilution.
▶ Increased white cell count (WCC), with the normal range being between 6–16 × 10^9/L. This is mostly due to an increased neutrophil count, and it increases until the peak is reached at the beginning of the third trimester. The WCC count increases further during labour and birth.

Another aspect to consider when discussing haematological changes is haemostasis. Pregnancy is known to be a state of induced **hypercoagulability** or **pro-coagulatory**, caused by increased levels of some coagulation factors (like VII and VIII) and plasma fibrinogen, as well as reduced

fibrinolytic activity. Although designed to ensure the mother is protected from the risk of haemorrhage once the placenta has separated after birth, hypercoagulability puts women at a higher risk of thrombosis. This risk is further heightened by reduced venous return from the lower limbs. Regarding the routine coagulation blood tests, these remain unchanged during pregnancy.

Cardiovascular changes during pregnancy

There are a number of changes to the heart that occur throughout pregnancy. Anatomically, its volume increases by about 12%, it is moved upwards by the diaphragm and rotated forward. Additionally, the left ventricular wall increases in thickness to sustain the increased blood volume. These changes lead to the alteration of some heart sounds, like systolic or diastolic murmurs, which are considered benign.

Cardiac output increases by 30–50% from early pregnancy to accommodate the increased blood volume. This significant change occurs in response to the stroke volume and heart rate both increasing, rather than to supply the uterus, which has not enlarged in early pregnancy yet. The stroke volume is increased by about 10% and the heart rate by about 10–20%; however, the heart rate should remain within the normal range.

Blood pressure in pregnancy tends to be slightly lower than in the non-pregnant state. This is due to the relaxing effect of progesterone on the vascular tone in the peripheral vessels and to the formation of new blood vessels. Overall, systolic blood pressure changes minimally, however, diastolic blood pressure drops more significantly in the first and second trimesters before it returns to a pre-pregnancy state in the third trimester. Postural changes can also affect blood

3.1

pressure, with pregnant mothers having their blood pressure when sitting up to 10% higher than when lying down.

Briefly returning to peripheral vessels, resistance decreases by 35–40%, which, combined with reduced venous return due to gravity and the pregnant uterus, causes lower limb oedema.

During pregnancy, some organs particularly benefit from the increased blood flow; these are the uterus, kidneys, breasts and skin. The uterus is the key target of the increased blood flow in pregnancy, as the uterus, placenta and fetus are responsible for the majority of the increased oxygen consumption. The kidneys receive a greater blood flow from early pregnancy, which tails towards the end. Increased blood flow to the breasts and skin is responsible for an increased temperature, especially of the hands and feet.

Anaemia in pregnancy and haemoglobinopathies

Anaemia in pregnancy

Anaemia is described as an insufficient number of RBCs or haemoglobin concentration, which results in a lower level of oxygen being carried to the body organs and tissues. It has two main causes: excessive blood loss or breakdown of RBCs, or insufficient or defective production of RBCs. In pregnancy, a deficiency in iron or folate can adversely affect RBC production.

Due to the increase in plasma volume and RBC volume in pregnancy, extra iron is required. This increased iron requirement (3.0–7.5 mg a day at the end of pregnancy) can be met only if there is sufficient absorption of iron from the diet and by utilising body iron stores. However, some mothers become pregnant with insufficient iron stores and considering that the iron

obtained from the diet is insufficient to meet the requirements of pregnancy alone, iron supplementation may be required. This is particularly important as a very low Hb level in the mother can cause her increased cardiovascular stress and a higher risk of haemorrhage, and fetal growth restriction or even death in the unborn baby. In order to test for iron-deficiency anaemia, serum ferritin is a reliable parameter to assess the status of the iron stores in the body, even before anaemia becomes obvious, showing low haemoglobin levels. If the serum ferritin is low, then iron supplementation should be sufficient to treat the anaemia. In particular circumstances, intravenous iron or a blood transfusion might be required to correct the anaemia.

Folates and vitamin B12 are essential for erythropoiesis and their deficiency slows down the production of RBCs leading to anaemia. In pregnancy, there is an increased requirement of folates and vitamin B12; therefore, anaemia could be caused by folate deficiency rather than iron deficiency and further blood tests are required to confirm this. In this case, iron supplementation is not going to be beneficial and vitamin B12 injections and a high dose of folic acid might be more appropriate.

Haemoglobinopathies

The term haemoglobinopathies describes a range of inherited disorders that affect the quantity or the structure of haemoglobin, resulting in a reduction of the RBCs' ability to carry oxygen. The most common haemoglobinopathies encountered in midwifery are sickle-cell disease and thalassaemia. Sickle-cell disease is most prevalent in people of Black African or Asian descent and causes RBCs to have an abnormal shape. This leads to RBCs having a shorter life, causing anaemia, and blocking

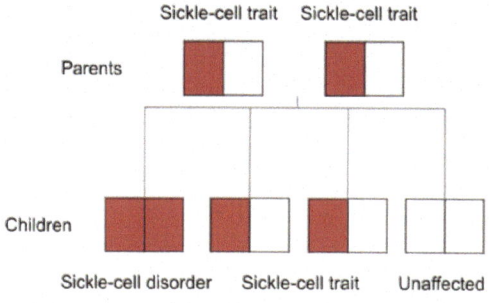

Figure 3.1.17 Sickle-cell disease inheritance

the blood flow in the capillaries, causing clots and severe pain (sickle-cell crisis).

Thalassaemia is more prevalent in people of Mediterranean or Asian descent and causes abnormal production of haemoglobin. There are four types of thalassaemia, which have different clinical significance. These range from being asymptomatic, to anaemia, and to severe complications for the individual and for the unborn baby, like Bart's hydrops fetalis.

Both sickle-cell disease and thalassaemia are recessive conditions. Parents carrying a faulty gene are considered carriers, also called 'trait' If both parents are carriers, then the offspring has a one in four chance of getting the disease (see Figure 3.1.17). Very rarely these genetic conditions present *de novo* when neither of the parents has

the mutation and it is only present in the affected individual. Routine antenatal screening in the UK offers the possibility to detect high-risk couples and offer specific counselling and genetic testing.

Further reading

Dean L. The Rh blood group. In *Blood groups and red cell antigens* [Internet]. Bethesda (MD): National Center for Biotechnology Information (US), 2005. www.ncbi.nlm.nih.gov/books/NBK2269/.

Humphries A., Thompson J. et al. The effect of positioning on maternal anatomy and hemodynamics during late pregnancy. *Clin. Anat.* [Internet] 2020, 33(6):943–9. https://onlinelibrary.wiley.com/doi/10.1002/ca.23614.

Public Health England. Understanding haemoglobinopathies [Internet]. 2018. www.gov.uk/government/publications/handbook-for-sickle-cell-and-thalassaemia-screening/understanding-haemoglobinopathies.

Sanghavi M., Rutherford J. Cardiovascular physiology of pregnancy. *Circulation* [Internet] 2014, 130(12):1003–8. www.ahajournals.org/doi/10.1161/circulationaha.114.009029#d3e409.

3.1

The respiratory system

Giada Giusmin

LEARNING OUTCOMES

▶ Describe the structure and function of the respiratory system

▶ Describe the processes of inspiration, expiration and gas exchange

▶ Understand the differences between aerobic and anaerobic cellular respiration, including the role of Krebs cycle in aerobic respiration

▶ Understand the anatomical and physiological changes to the respiratory system during pregnancy, and apply these to practice

Overview of the respiratory system

Overall, the main function of the respiratory system is to allow the entrance of oxygen into the body and to expel carbon dioxide as a waste product of respiration. In the previous chapter, when looking at the blood and cardiovascular system, we explored how oxygen, carbon dioxide and other nutrients are exchanged at the level of the capillaries. In this chapter, all the processes before and after this exchange are further explained.

Description of the key structures of the respiratory system

As shown in Figure 3.2.1, the respiratory tract comprises the nose, nasal cavity, pharynx, larynx, trachea and lungs with bronchi and alveoli.

The nose and the nasal cavity

Starting from the only structure in contact with the exterior, the nose is made of bone and cartilage. The internal part of the nose, the nasal cavity, is divided into two nostrils by the nasal septum. The nasal cavity is where the olfactory receptors

DOI: 10.4324/9781003227571-13

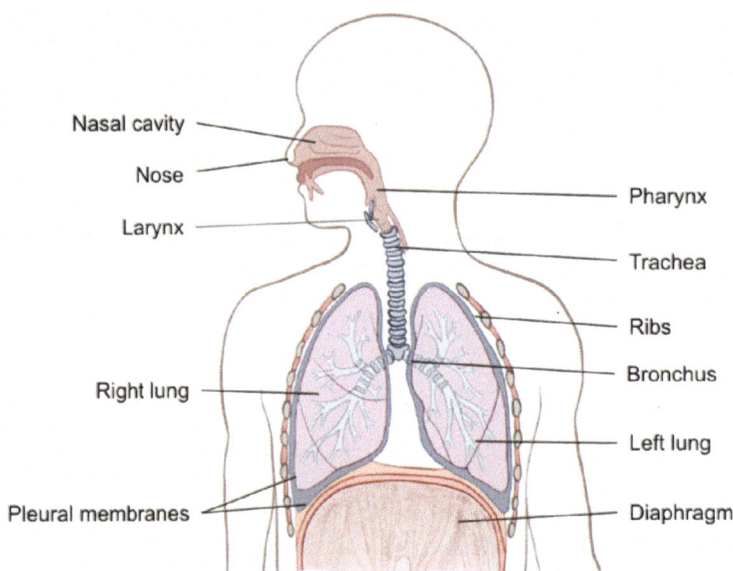

Figure 3.2.1 Anatomy of the respiratory tract

(sense of smell) are located. The oral cavity is found below it, and is divided by the palate. The nasal cavity is also surrounded by paranasal sinuses within the bone structure of the head. These are important for producing mucus, which drains into the nasal cavity, and to lessen the weight of the bone structure. The nasal cavity is covered by respiratory mucosa, which also produces mucus important for protecting the respiratory tract from foreign microorganisms and for humidifying the entering air. Cilia are present in the nasal mucosa, and their action allows the mucus to move towards the throat and be swallowed.

The pharynx

Following the movement of air from the external environment, after the nasal cavity, the pharynx is the next structure found. Commonly referred to as the throat, it is a muscular, funnel-shaped communal passageway for food as well as air. The pharynx can be divided into three sections,

the nasopharynx, the oropharynx and the laryngopharynx. The tonsils, lymphatic organs important for the immune system, are located in the pharynx. These become swollen during infections and can be palpable.

The larynx

The larynx is where food and air find their way into the different passageways. It is a hollow tube with a cartilaginous skeleton, ligaments and muscles. One of the nine laryngeal cartilages is the epiglottis. The epiglottis is a leaf-shaped flap that usually rests upright, allowing air to move towards the lower respiratory tract. The epiglottis closes when we swallow food or liquids to direct these into the oesophagus and the stomach. If, by accident, food or fluids enter the larynx, the cough reflex stops these from continuing down the wrong route.

The larynx is also where the vocal cords are located, for this reason, it is also called the voice box. The vocal cords are folds of mucous membranes that vibrate when the air passes through from the lungs, which is what allows us to speak.

The trachea

The trachea connects the larynx to the lungs and is approximately 10 cm long, running alongside the oesophagus (food and fluid passageway). The trachea is mainly rigid because of C-shaped hyaline cartilage, which allows the airway to be kept open and prevents its collapse. Nevertheless, the trachea also has a flexible side that allows the oesophagus to expand towards the front when we swallow a large chunk of food. Internally, the trachea is covered by ciliated mucosa that, together with the production of mucus, push debris trapped in the mucus upwards, away from the lungs.

The bronchi

The bronchi are the two passageways (right and left) that originate from the division of the trachea and separately enter the side of each lung. At this level, the bronchi are labelled as **main bronchi**, this is because further branching out of the bronchi occurs inside the lungs leading to the alveoli. The main bronchi are made of cartilage and tissue, and in the smaller the branches less cartilage is present.

The lungs and the respiratory zone

The lungs are positioned in the thoracic cavity. They have an elongated triangular shape, with the apex at the top at the clavicle level and the base lying on the diaphragm. Each lung is covered by the pulmonary pleura, which allows smooth movement against the parietal pleura that lines the inside of the thoracic cavity. Both pleaurae produce fluid that allows the lungs to move without friction inside the thoracic cavity during breathing.

Within the lungs, the bronchi branch out and become smaller and smaller (like in a tree) until they become bronchioles, the narrowest passageways. Further down, the bronchioles become terminal just before reaching the respiratory zone. The respiratory zone includes the respiratory bronchioles, the alveolar ducts and sacs, and the alveoli – these are the only places where gas exchange happens, whereas all the other parts are only for conduction (see Figure 3.2.2).

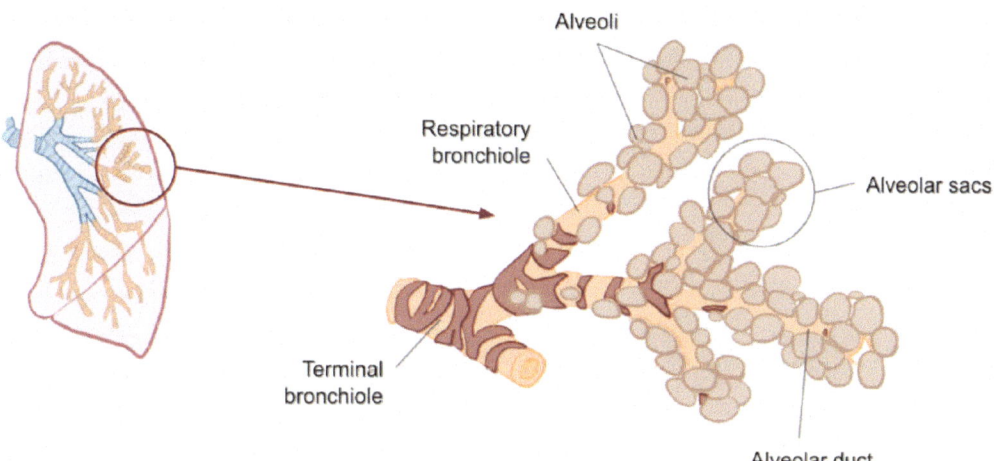

Figure 3.2.2 Focus on the structures between terminal bronchioles and alveoli

The lungs, in order to reoxygenate the circulating blood, need their own supply to function. The oxygenated blood comes from the bronchial arteries, which are generated from the aorta, whereas the deoxygenated blood is returned by the bronchial and pulmonary veins.

The alveoli

The alveoli are clustered together and resemble bunches of grapes. There are about 700 million alveoli, and these constitute the volume of the lungs. The alveolar walls are made of a single layer of cells and are surrounded by pulmonary capillaries. The capillary and alveolar walls are fused together at the level of the basement membrane, which creates the respiratory membrane, also called the air-blood barrier. As shown in Figure 3.2.3, gas exchange occurs by diffusion through the respiratory membrane as blood and air flow next to the other. During this process, the oxygen goes from the alveoli into the blood, and the carbon dioxide goes in the opposite direction.

Among the cells that are part of the alveolar walls are cells that produce surfactant. Surfactant is a mix of lipids and proteins which lower surface tension, thereby preventing alveolar walls from sticking together when they touch.

Physiology of respiration

After this overview of the anatomy of the respiratory system, the focus will now be on the physiology of respiration, how the human body actually acquires the necessary oxygen and expels carbon dioxide. There are four separate phases that together constitute the process called respiration. These four phases are:

▶ Pulmonary ventilation, also known as breathing, is the process in which the air enters and exits the lungs to ensure oxygenated air reaches the lungs.
▶ External respiration occurs when the pulmonary blood exchanges gases with the alveoli. Oxygen from the external environment is transferred to the blood and carbon dioxide is unloaded from it.

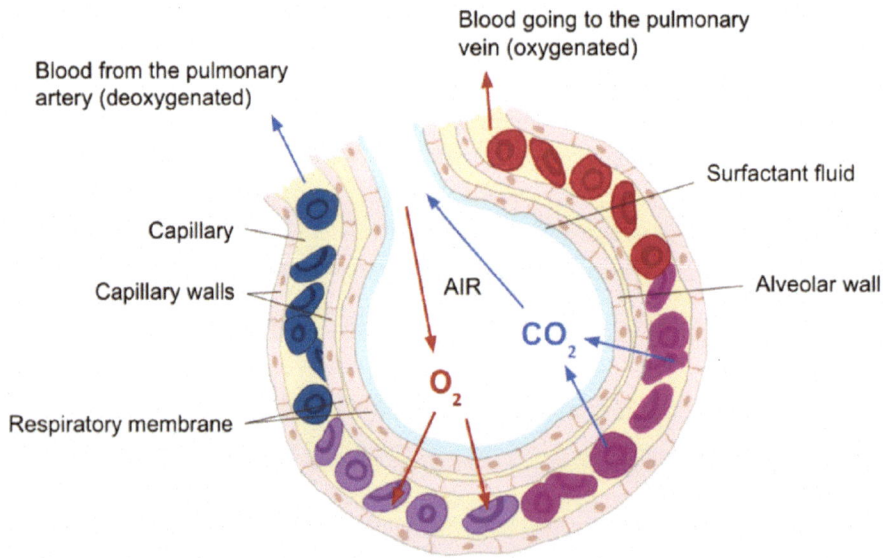

Blood going to the pulmonary vein (oxygenated)

Blood from the pulmonary artery (deoxygenated)

Surfactant fluid

Capillary

Capillary walls

AIR

Alveolar wall

CO_2

O_2

Respiratory membrane

Figure 3.2.3 Gas exchange at the level of the alveoli

▶ Respiratory gas transport is the part of the process in which oxygen and carbon dioxide are transported via the bloodstream from the tissue cells around the body to the lungs and vice versa.

▶ Internal respiration is the gas exchange at the level of the tissue cells. This occurs when oxygen and carbon dioxide are exchanged between the capillaries and the nearby tissue cells.

In the next section, some of these processes are discussed in further detail, starting with pulmonary ventilation or breathing.

Pulmonary ventilation

Volume changes within the thoracic cavity cause the mechanical process called breathing. The tendency is for a flow of gases to occur in order to even out the pressure, which previously changed because of the volume changes. These volume changes are different according to which one of the two phases of breathing, inspiration and expiration, occurs.

Inspiration and expiration

During inspiration, the thoracic cavity expands due to the diaphragm and the external intercostal muscles contracting. This leads to the lungs expanding too, as they adhere to the internal thoracic walls thanks to the pleural membranes. As the lungs are larger, the volume within the lungs (intrapulmonary volume) also increases, resulting in the gases within the lungs now needing to fill a greater space. The drop in gas pressure in the lungs, compared to the external atmospheric pressure, creates a vacuum that forces air to enter the lungs. Air carries on entering the lungs until the pressure inside the lungs is the same as the external atmospheric pressure.

3.2

Expiration is the second half of the breathing process and is mostly a passive event due to the lungs' elasticity. At the end of inspiration, the muscles that initially contacted, now return to their relaxed state and the lungs recoil. At this stage, both the thoracic and the lung volumes drop, causing the gases in the lungs to be more compressed. Now, the pressure inside the lungs increases to a level higher than the atmospheric pressure, which forces the gases to flow out to even the pressure with the external environment. Both inspiration and expiration are shown in Figure 3.2.4.

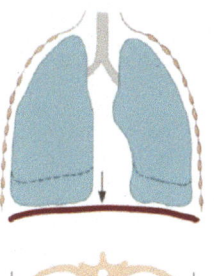
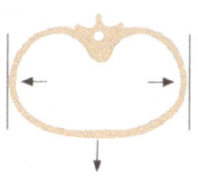

(a) Inspiration

The thoracic cavity expands as the external intercostal muscles and the diaphragm contract. The lungs expand as well, which allows for air to enter the lungs (inspiration).

(b) Expiration

Air exits the lungs (expiration) as the external intercostal muscles and the diaphragm relax back to their original state. The lungs and the thoracic cavity reduce their volumes and air is forced out.

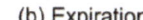
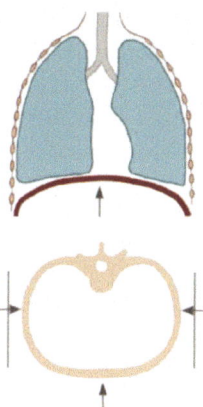

Figure 3.2.4 Inspiration and expiration shown from the front and across the thoracic cavity

Gas exchange in the alveoli of the lungs

As previously mentioned, gas exchange between blood and alveoli occurs during the external respiration phase. The deoxygenated blood (darker in colour) coming from the body reaches the lungs where it becomes oxygenated (brighter in colour) before being pumped out by the heart to supply all body tissues. In the lungs, gas exchange occurs by simple diffusion, which means that the diffusing substance, in this case, oxygen and carbon dioxide, are forced to move toward the area of lower concentration. The deoxygenated blood coming from the body through the pulmonary capillaries acquires oxygen from the air in the alveoli, where there is a greater concentration of oxygen. At the same time, the carbon dioxide, which is in greater concentration in the pulmonary capillaries, leaves these to move to the alveoli, where the concentration is lower.

Oxygen and carbon dioxide are transported in different ways in the blood. Oxygen mostly binds to haemoglobin molecules, whereas a small part is transported dissolved in the plasma. Carbon dioxide, on the other hand, is mostly transported in plasma as bicarbonate ions after the carbon dioxide molecules are converted to bicarbonate ions within the red blood cells. Bicarbonate ions are important for maintaining a stable blood pH with their buffering activity (refer to Chapter 1.3). In addition to this, a small amount of carbon dioxide is also transported by haemoglobin, but it does not hinder the transport of oxygen.

Internal respiration

Internal respiration occurs when the oxygenated blood coming from the lungs reaches the tissue cells in order to offload the oxygen and pick up carbon dioxide. Before reaching the tissue cells, the blood coming from the lungs has a higher concentration of oxygen and a lower concentration of carbon dioxide. Therefore, when it reaches the tissues, gas exchange occurs by simple diffusion through the capillary wall, in the opposite direction to external respiration. For more information, see Chapter 3.2 regarding gas exchange at the capillary level.

However, simple diffusion is not the only mechanism for facilitating gas exchange. The heat caused by cell metabolism and the carbon dioxide within the cell also lower the affinity of haemoglobin for oxygen, encouraging its entry into the cell. Furthermore, the carbon dioxide, combined with the water present in the blood, forms carbonic acid, which breaks down into hydrogen and bicarbonate ions (which impact on the blood pH); these further encourage the haemoglobin to offload oxygen to the tissue cells. At this stage, the haemoglobin picks up the carbon dioxide and this deoxygenated blood makes its way to the lungs before the whole cycle starts again.

Control of respiration

The muscles involved in inspiration and expiration, mentioned in the previous section, are controlled by the phrenic and intercostal nerves receiving impulses from the brain. In particular, the phrenic nerve originates from cervical nerves 3–5, whereas the intercostal nerves originate from the thoracic nerves 1–12, see further information in Chapter 3.3. In the brain, the breathing control centres are mainly found in the pons and medulla. In the medulla, the ventral respiratory group (VRG) houses both the neurons that control inspiration and expiration. Via the phrenic and intercostal nerves, the inspiratory neurons release stimuli to the diaphragm and external intercostal muscles to inhale (see Figure 3.2.5). Stimuli from expiratory neurons bring the stimulation of the diaphragm and

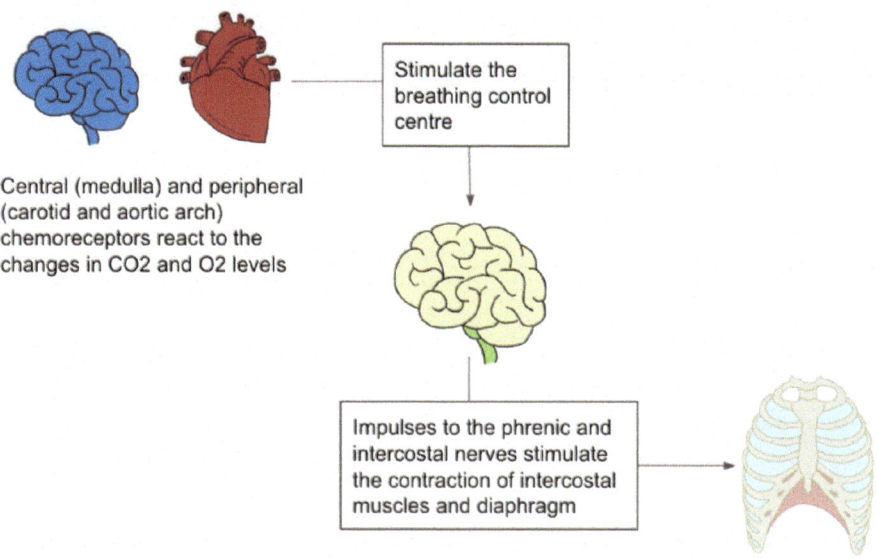

3.2

Stimulate the breathing control centre

Central (medulla) and peripheral (carotid and aortic arch) chemoreceptors react to the changes in CO2 and O2 levels

Impulses to the phrenic and intercostal nerves stimulate the contraction of intercostal muscles and diaphragm

Figure 3.2.5 Neural control of respiration

external intercostal muscles to an end, enabling exhalation. The VRG is responsible for maintaining a regular breathing rhythm. The dorsal respiratory group (DRG) is also found in the medulla. The DRG is responsible for combining the information from the peripheral receptors and relies on this information to the VRG to adjust breathing rhythms. The pons respiratory centres help to coordinate the breathing rhythms, by liaising with the VRG during various activities, such as running or singing.

Apart from the neural control of respiration, there are more factors that can affect the rate and depth of respiration. For example, during yoga or hypnobirthing, individuals can voluntarily control their breathing patterns. However, this conscious control is limited as the respiratory centres will retake control of respiration whenever the oxygen supply in the blood becomes low, preventing the individual from dying. Additionally, other factors can have an impact on the rate and depth of respiration, such as physical (i.e. coughing) and emotional (i.e. fear) factors. Chemical factors, such as the level of oxygen

and carbon dioxide in the blood, have a principal role in modifying breathing patterns. Excessive carbon dioxide in the blood and a lower pH level represent the most significant stimuli to ensure that the rate and depth of respiration are increased. These changes in the chemical composition of the blood are picked up by chemoreceptors (respond to chemical changes), which are located in different areas of the body. When the level of carbon dioxide increases in the blood, messages are sent to the respiratory centre in the brain to breathe more often.

Respiration at the cellular level

In Chapter 1.1, we introduced the cell and its structures, now we discuss a process called cellular respiration, which can be considered the final stage of respiration. Now that oxygen has been brought into the tissues via the processes described above, this oxygen can be used at the cellular level to produce energy, via **cellular respiration**. Glucose is broken down to produce energy, which is essential to enable our bodies to

127

function (for example, muscles to contract). Energy comes in the form of **adenosine triphosphate (ATP)**, a molecule that is often referred to as the 'energy currency', as it is a form of energy readily expendable by body cells. ATP is made of a base plus a sugar unit, which together is called adenosine, attached to three phosphate groups (see Figure 3.2.6).

ATP is synthesised in the mitochondria (see Chapter 1.1), and it is necessary to run most processes in living beings. **Aerobic**

respiration (in the presence of oxygen) can be summarised as follows:

Glucose + Oxygen → Carbon dioxide + Water + ATP

Glucose reaches the cells where it meets oxygen and these react, producing carbon dioxide, water and ATP.

Below, the process is described in more detail, albeit some aspects are omitted/shortened to ease understanding. The process starts in the digestive tract, where nutrients, like glucose, are absorbed. These nutrients reach the tissue cells carried in the blood. Once in the cell, three steps occur (Figure 3.2.7):

1. In the cells, in particular in the cytoplasm, these nutrients are either combined into bigger molecules or broken down into smaller parts. In the case of glucose, this is broken down in a process called glycolysis (glyco = glucose, lysis = break up). Here, one molecule of glucose is converted into two molecules of pyruvic

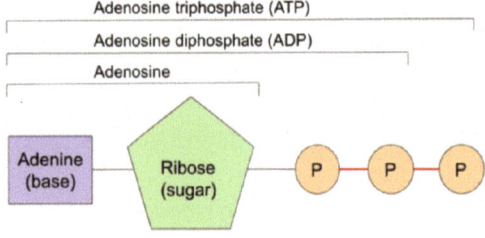

Figure 3.2.6 ATP composition

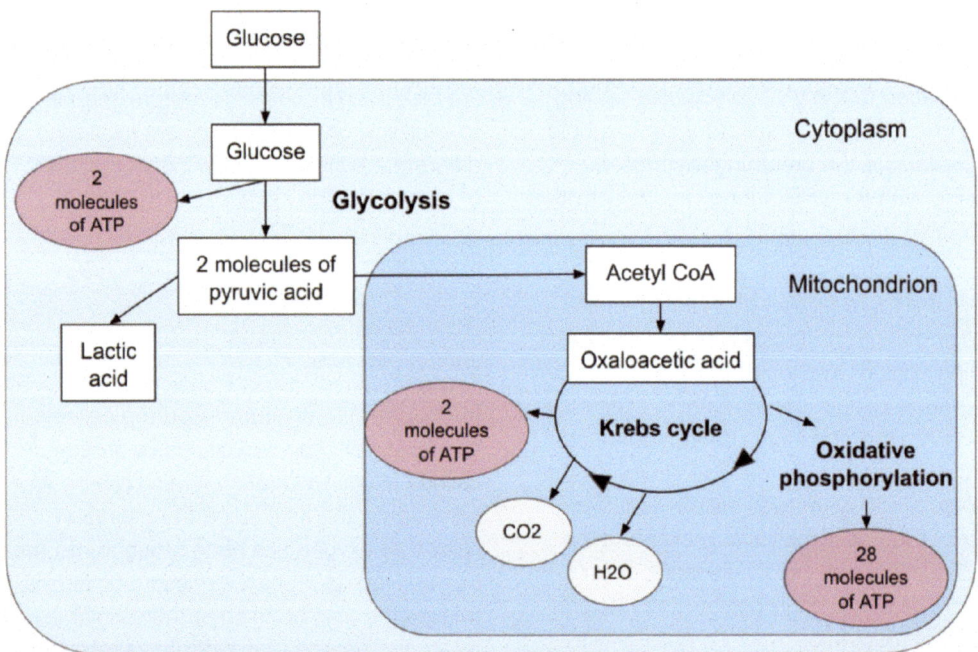

Figure 3.2.7 Cellular respiration

acid, and this produces two net ATP molecules (actually produces 4 ATP but uses 2 to run). Glycolysis occurs whether or not oxygen is available, so it is considered an **anaerobic process**.

2. The next stage takes place in the mitochondria where, in the presence of a sufficient amount of oxygen (**aerobic pathway**), most of the pyruvic acid molecules become Acetyl CoA before entering Kreb's cycle (also known as the citric acid cycle). This produces another two ATP molecules, carbon dioxide and water.

3. However, the majority of the ATP molecules (34, for a total of 38 ATP molecules) derive from a third process called oxidative phosphorylation. Oxidative phosphorylation can only happen if oxygen is available.

It is worth noting that the whole process also costs energy to run, so it is suggested that the actual number of ATP molecules produced from glucose is 29–30 ATP, depending on the efficiency of the cell.

In the event of oxygen not being readily available, ATP can still be produced from the glycolysis of a glucose molecule, as this process is anaerobic (Step 1), but in much less quantity. In this case, the pyruvic acid is converted into lactic acid via an anaerobic process **(anaerobic pathway)** and therefore, is prevented from entering Krebs cycle and oxidative phosphorylation. The excessive amount of lactic acid in the tissues is what causes the feeling of sore muscles after excessive physical exercise. An excessive amount of lactic acid due to prolonged anaerobic metabolism can also lead to acid-base issues.

Changes and adaptations during pregnancy

Changes to the respiratory system in pregnancy occur on an anatomical and physiological basis, in order to sustain the growing fetus. These changes, especially the physiological ones, occur as early as six weeks due to hormonal and biochemical changes.

Anatomical changes to the respiratory system

3.2

In pregnancy, due to the increase of oestrogen and progesterone, the mucosa in the nasal cavity becomes more oedematous, which is accompanied by increased secretion of mucus. This can lead to more frequent episodes of nosebleeds (epistaxis) and nasal congestion.

The growing uterus is the main reason for anatomical changes in the thorax during pregnancy. The diaphragm becomes displaced upwards (about 4–5 cm), reducing chest height, but the thoracic transverse diameter increases (about 2 cm) to compensate. In addition to this, the area between the lower part of the sternum and the ribs on either side, known as the **subcostal angle**, widens from 68.3° to 103.5° (see Figure 3.2.8).

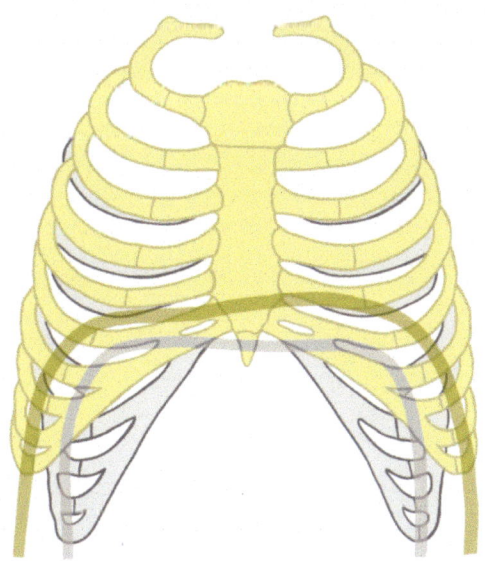

Figure 3.2.8 Anatomical changes during pregnancy (Grey outline – outside of pregnancy, yellow outline – change as a result of pregnancy)

Physiological changes to the respiratory system

During pregnancy, the hormones progesterone, oestrogen and prostaglandins contribute to some physiological changes in the respiratory system. Firstly, progesterone increases the sensitivity of the medulla oblongata to carbon dioxide, causing this to be expelled more easily and lowering its concentration in the arterial blood. Progesterone, with its relaxant effect, also induces a **bronchodilator** effect (up to 50%) due to its action on the airway's smooth muscle, making the flow in the airways greater. Oestrogen mostly acts as a mediator for progesterone, increasing the number and sensitivity of those receptors. Prostaglandins, according to their type, on one hand, increase the resistance of the bronchial smooth muscle (bronchoconstriction), and on the other, act similarly to progesterone, having a bronchodilator effect.

Changes to respiratory parameters

In pregnancy, the overall ventilation increases not because of a higher respiratory rate, but because the breaths are deeper. Interestingly, no difference in function can be observed in the case of twin pregnancy. As shown in Table 3.2.1 and Figure 3.2.9, expiratory reserve volume (ERV) and residual volume (RV) are reduced due to anatomical changes. Similarly, the functional residual capacity (FRC) decreases, but the total lung capacity (TLC) remains unchanged thanks to an increase in tidal volume (TV) and inspiratory capacity (IC). In addition to this, oxygen consumption is increased by 20% to meet the pregnancy requirements, which, combined with increased minute ventilation, leads to a lower arterial carbon dioxide concentration. The blood pH remains stable, despite these respiratory changes, due to renal system compensation.

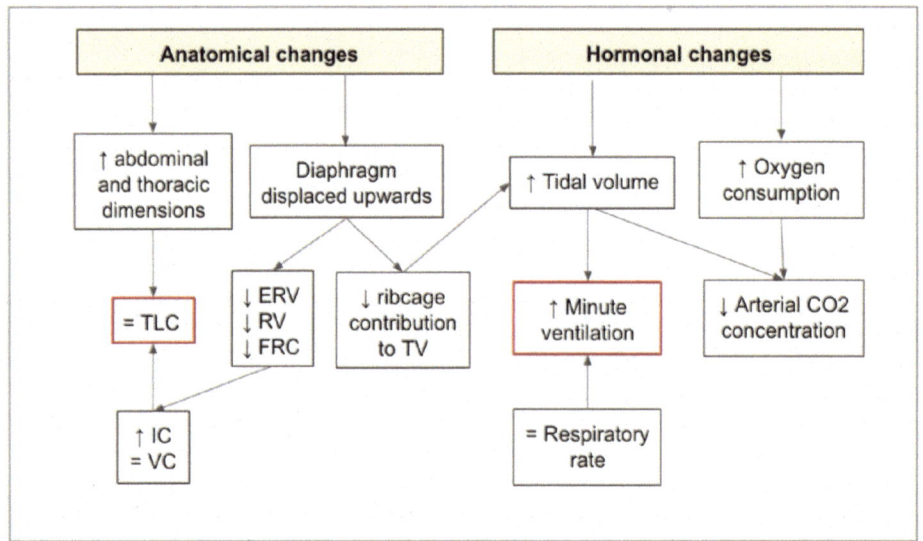

Figure 3.2.9 Summary of changes to the respiratory system during pregnancy (TLC – Total lung capacity, ERV – Expiratory reserve volume, RV – residual volume, FRC – Functional residual capacity, TV – Tidal volume, IC – Inspiratory capacity, VC – Vital capacity)

Table 3.2.1 Respiratory parameters in a healthy woman and their changes in pregnancy

3.2

	Parameter	Description	Normal value for a healthy female	Change in pregnancy
Respiratory volumes	Tidal volume (TV)	The amount of air entering and exiting the lungs in one normal breath	500 ml	40% increase (approx. 200 ml)
	Inspiratory reserve volume (IRV)	The maximum volume of air that can be inspired above the TV value during the deepest inspiration with extra effort	1900 ml (higher for males)	Stable
	Expiratory reserve volume (ERV)	The maximum volume of air that can be voluntarily expired after a normal breath with extra effort	700 ml	8–40% reduction
	Residual volume (RV)	The amount of air that is left in the lungs after forceful expiration	1100 ml (higher for males)	7–22% reduction
Respiratory capacities	Total lung capacity (TLC)	The amount of air present in the lungs after maximum inspiration. It is the sum of TV, IRV, ERV and RV	4200 ml (higher for males)	Stable
	Vital capacity (VC)	The total amount of air expelled after maximal inspiration. It is the sum of TV, IRV and ERV	3100 ml (higher for males)	Stable
	Inspiratory capacity (IC)	The total amount of air that can be inhaled after a normal expiration. This is the sum of TV and IRV	2400 ml (higher for males)	10% increase
	Functional residual capacity (FRC)	The amount of air left in the lungs after a normal expiration. It is the sum of ERV and RV	1800 ml (higher for males)	10–25% reduction
Other parameters	Respiratory rate (RR)	Number of breaths in one minute	12 resp./minute	Slight increase to 15 resp./minute but still within normal parameters
	Minute ventilation	The amount of air that is inhaled and exhaled in one minute (TV × respiratory rate). Of this, approximately 150 ml remain stuck in the dead space and do not take part in gas exchange	500 ml × 12 resp./minute = 6000 ml a minute	40% increase
	Alveolar ventilation	The amount of air entering the alveoli in one minute. This is calculated as (TV – dead space) × respiratory rate	(500 ml – 150 ml) × 12 resp./minute = 4200 ml a minute	50% increase

CHAPTER CHALLENGE

The most common respiratory disorder in pregnancy is asthma. Although around a third of women with the condition report improved symptoms during pregnancy, asthma is associated with poorer pregnancy outcomes and maternal morbidity.

Read Popa M., Peltecu G. et al. Asthma in pregnancy. Review of current literature and recommendations. *Maedica (Bucur)* [Internet] 2021, 16(1):80–7. www.ncbi.nlm.nih.gov/pmc/articles/PMC8224723/ and answer the following questions:

▶ Describe the symptoms of asthma.

▶ Why might symptoms improve in pregnancy? Why might they get worse?

▶ What complications and adverse outcomes have been linked with asthma in pregnancy?

▶ What advice could you give to women in your care around managing asthma in pregnancy and childbirth?

Further reading

LoMauro A., Aliverti A. Respiratory physiology of pregnancy. *Breathe* [Internet] 2015: 11:297–301. www.ncbi.nlm.nih.gov/pmc/articles/PMC4818213/.

CHAPTER 3.3

The nervous system

Jane Carpenter

LEARNING OUTCOMES

▶ Understand the structure and function of the nervous system
▶ Describe the unique structures of the neuron, and the three different types of neuron
▶ Explain how neuron structure and function enable communication between neurons via the action potential
▶ Explain the structure and function of the central nervous system and peripheral nervous system
▶ Describe key changes to the nervous system which occur in pregnancy, and apply these to practice

The nervous system can be thought of as the master command and communication system of the human body. It receives, integrates and then reacts to information. Think of when you remove your hand from a hot plate before you have even registered it was a hot plate – this is the nervous system at work!

This chapter will first consider the normal structure and function of the nervous system, before considering how the nervous system responds, acts and changes during pregnancy.

Nervous system overview

Organisation and functions of the nervous system

Structurally, the nervous system is split into two separate parts for ease of learning: the **central nervous system (CNS)**, which consists of the brain and spinal cord, and the **peripheral nervous system (PNS)**, which is any part of the nervous system extending outside of the CNS (Figure 3.3.1).

The PNS is then further split, functionally, into the **sensory (afferent) division** and the **motor (efferent) division**. The sensory division is concerned with transmitting information from sensory receptors throughout the body to the CNS. The motor division transmits information away from the CNS to muscles or glands, which can then effect a response. The motor division

DOI: 10.4324/9781003227571-14

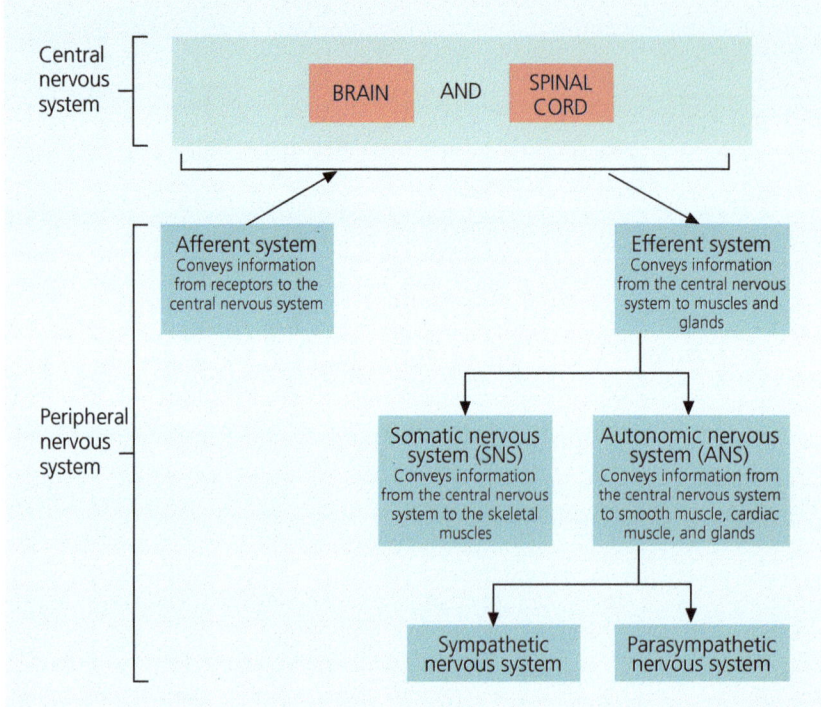

Figure 3.3.1 Overview of the central and peripheral nervous systems
Source: Figure 8.3(a), p.165, Clancy and McVicar (2009)

is split into the somatic nervous system and the autonomic system, and these will be further explored below.

Neurons and neuroglia

The nervous system performs its function via the function of highly specialised cells called **neurons**, supported by specialist support cells – **neuroglia**.

The structure of the neuron

The neuron has a highly specialised cell structure, which enables it to carry out its function. Neurons carry nerve impulses from one part of the body to another – and this is how messages are communicated around the body. Due to their specialisation, neurons do not usually undergo further mitotic division. However, they are also built

to last, and can survive for a long time, in some cases even a lifetime.

In order to carry out their function, neurons have a specific structure which varies slightly depending on their particular function. Neurons which extend from the CNS to tissues elsewhere in the body are referred to as **efferent neurons** or **motor neurons**. Key structures of motor neurons are described and shown in Table 3.3.1 and Figure 3.3.2. Neurons which carry impulses from sensory receptors in the tissues back to the CNS are referred to as **afferent neurons** or **sensory neurons**. Key structures of sensory neurons are described and shown in Table 3.3.2 and Figure 3.3.2. A third type of neuron, known as an **interneuron**, is found exclusively within the CNS. Interneurons form connections between the motor and sensory neurons in the CNS.

Table 3.3.1 Key structures of the motor neuron and their functions

Cell structure	Description
Cell body	Located at one end of the neuron is the cell body. This contains a nucleus, smooth and rough endoplasmic reticulum, mitochondria and other cellular components to enable normal cellular function.
Axon	Each neuron has a maximum of one axon. In some cases, the axon may be very short, or rarely, absent. However, axons are often extraordinarily long – stretching a metre or more! Bundles of axons are called tracts in the CNS, and nerves in the PNS. The axon, if triggered, generates a nerve impulse and transmits it **away from the cell body** down its length to the axon terminal within the target tissue.
Dendrite	Extending from the cell body are fine, branching processes, called dendrites. Via these processes, the neuron receives electrical impulses from other nerve cells in the vicinity.

Table 3.3.2 Key structures of the sensory neuron and their functions

Cell structure	Description
Cell body	Located in an 'off-shoot' from the fibre. This off-shoot is usually located close to where the fibre enters the CNS. This leads to many cell bodies being located at the same point, giving rise to a distended area known as the **dorsal root ganglion**.
Axon	The elongated fibre of the cell that extends from the cell body to the CNS.
Dendron	The elongated fibre of the cell that extends from the sensory receptor to the cell body.

Source: Table 8.6, p.200, Clancy and McVicar (2009)

3.3

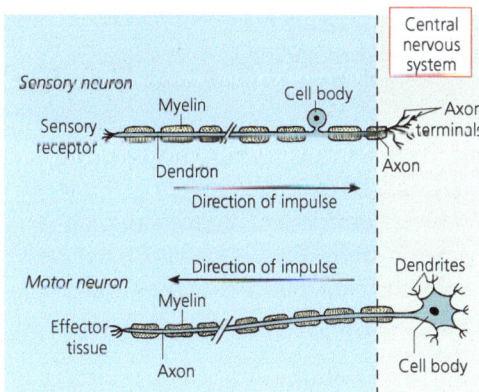

Figure 3.3.2 The sensory and motor neuron
Source: Figure 8.2, p.163, Clancy and McVicar (2009)

Structures common to sensory and motor neurons

Myelin is a fatty substance which often, although not always, covers the axon or dendron of neurons (Figure 3.3.2). This fatty substance functions to insulate the neuron to aid the passage of the electrical impulse down the fibre. Myelin is secreted by **Schwann cells**, which are non-neural cells closely association with neurons. Gaps in the myelin, known as **nodes of Ranvier**, are important as myelin is not a perfect insulator – therefore the electrical current must periodically be regenerated (see communication between neurons, below, for further detail on conduction of the nerve impulse).

The **synapse** is the junction between the nerve cells. It is a gap, rather than a physical structure, as the cells do not normally actually touch. However, this gap is extremely small (c. 20 nm wide) and is where communication occurs between the **presynaptic** cell (giving the signal) and the **postsynaptic** cell (receiving the signal). The synapse is important in determining whether the impulse is transmitted forwards or not. Most synapses are chemical, where the process is mediated by a chemical known as a neurotransmitter. However, some can be electrical, where the charge of one cell is influenced by the charge of an adjacent cell.

INTERRUPTER

Using the appropriate table in your workbook (or create your own), draw an image of a motor and sensory neuron, and then in your own words describe the key components of the structure. Explain how the key structural components help each neuron type to undertake their function.

Communication between neurons – the action potential

Neurons are 'excitable' cells – this means they can conduct an electrical signal along the axon, known as the **action potential**. They do this via the use of a concentration gradient, or a difference in ion concentration, between the inside and outside of the neuron.

Most of the time this concentration gradient is stable or 'resting'; but it is **polarised**, meaning that the inside of the neuron has a different potential to the outside. The **resting potential** of a neuron sits at about −70 mV. Although this is stable, there is nonetheless a constant flow of sodium and potassium ions in and out of the neuron.

When a neuron is 'triggered', sodium channels along the membrane open, allowing sodium ions to rush into the cell. This changes the membrane potential from its resting potential of −70 mV to + 40 mV. This is known as **depolarisation**. This depolarisation flows down the axon in a wave – the action potential. After depolarisation has occurred, the cell begins to pump out sodium ions via a sodium/potassium pump. This active process pumps three sodium ions out, and two potassium ions back in. This continues until **hyperpolarisation** occurs at a potential of −90 mV before the resting potential then restores. During hyperpolarisation, known as the **refractory period**, the cell cannot generate another action potential.

In order for an action potential to be triggered, a **threshold** of −55 mV must be reached. If the stimulus does not reach the threshold, an action potential will not occur. If it does meet the threshold an action potential will follow. The size of the stimulus does not affect the strength of the impulse, but instead causes *more* impulses.

Figure 3.3.3 provides a diagrammatic representation of the action potential.

The synapse

The impulse created by the action potential, as described above, flows down the axon, eventually reaching the **axon terminal**. Here, it reaches the **synapse**, a junction or gap, through which the impulse must travel, either chemically or electrically, to transfer from the presynaptic neuron to the postsynaptic neuron, or to an effector cell.

Chemical synapses are much more common than electrical synapses. These synapses allow the release of neurotransmitters from the axon terminal or the presynaptic neuron, via **synaptic vesicles**. The neurotransmitter is released from the vesicles and empties into the **synaptic cleft**. Neurotransmitters diffuse across the cleft and bind to receptors on the postsynaptic membrane. This can either cause the postsynaptic neuron to be excited (and so the impulse continues) or inhibited. This process is shown in Figure 3.3.4.

Less common **electrical synapses** work via channel proteins, connecting one neuron to the next and allowing direct transfer of ions from one neuron to the next. This is a much simpler way of transferring information, whereas chemical synapses allow for more complex transmission of information.

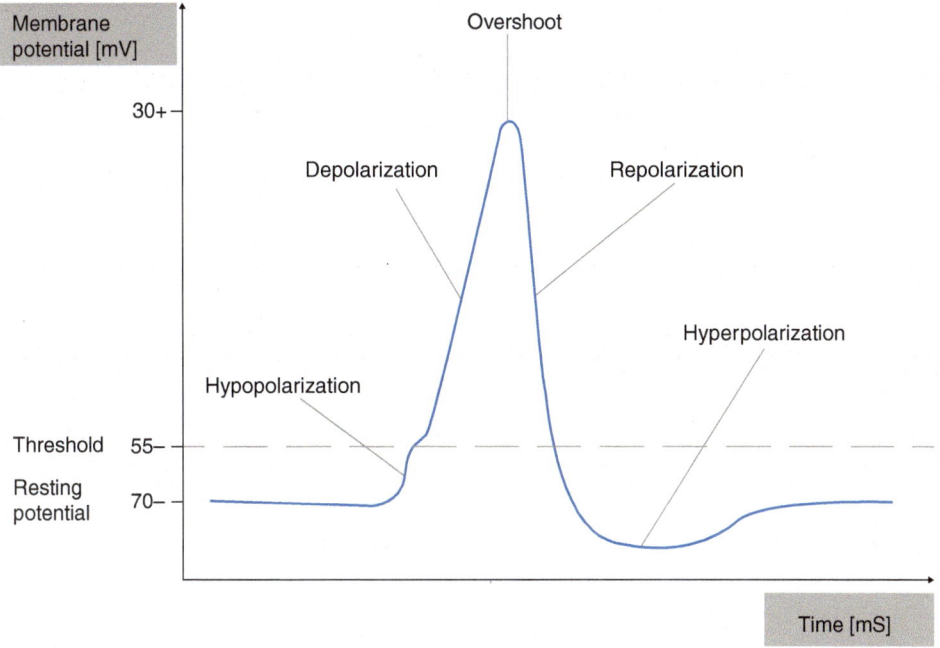

Figure 3.3.3 The action potential

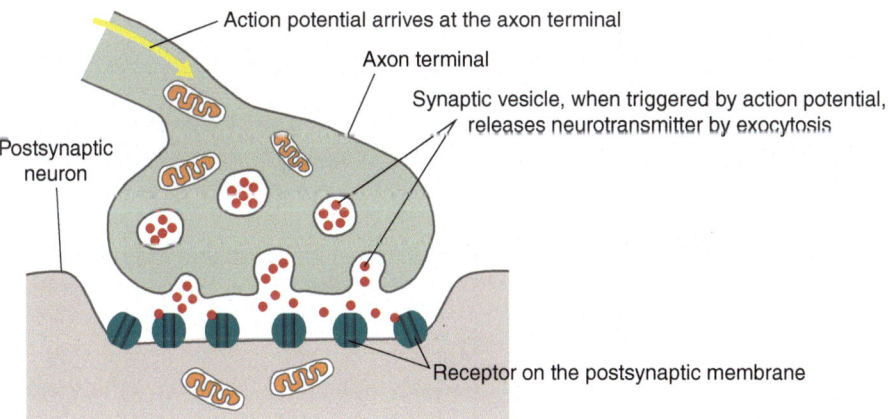

Figure 3.3.4 Close up of an axon terminal where it meets the dendrite of another neuron

Figure 3.3.4 shows a close up of an axon terminal where it meets the dendrite of another neuron.

Neuroglia

Neuroglia serve to support, protect and insulate neurons. Although neurons receive much focus as the way in which communication in the nervous system occurs, neuroglia are crucial for the smooth function of those neurons and hence, the nervous system.

Some neuroglia have projections which attach to neurons and anchor them in place, providing structure and support. Others are phagocytes, and as such protect the neurons of the CNS. Still others produce the myelin which insulates neurons throughout the CNS and PNS.

APPLICATION TO PRACTICE

To understand the crucial role of the neuroglia, we can consider the disease **multiple sclerosis (MS)**. MS gradually destroys the myelin sheath, provided by glial cells, around the neurons of the CNS. Instead, the myelin becomes hardened, or may eventually be destroyed altogether. Those neurons no longer function well, or at all. Initially, the signal may be able to pass along an alternative route which may take longer but will reach its intended destination. However, over time, areas of damage can become too large leading to permanent loss of function.

Symptoms of MS include pain, numbness in the limbs and extremities, and speech difficulties. Symptoms become progressively worse over time as damage to myelin and hence neuron function becomes irreparable. Currently, there is no cure for MS, although there are several treatments, which help with symptoms and slow the effect of the disease.

Central nervous system (CNS)

The brain – key structures and function

The brain is a highly complex organ at the centre of the nervous system. There is still much to be understood about how the brain functions. Here, we will consider some of the main anatomical structures and overarching functions of the brain, allowing a basic understanding of this fascinating

organ – as is required for the profession of midwifery.

Figure 3.3.5a shows a side view of the brain, annotating the **forebrain**, **midbrain** and **hindbrain**. Note that in this diagram, the midbrain is not actually visible. Figure 3.3.5b shows a cross section through the brain, and here you can clearly see the three regions of the brain. The midbrain and hindbrain together are called the **brainstem**.

The forebrain

The forebrain consists of the **cerebrum** and the **diencephalon**. The cerebrum is the highly convoluted structure which is perhaps what we think of first when we picture the human brain. It is divided into two hemispheres, the right and left, and these are connected by the corpus callosum. This is an important brain structure, as it allows communication between the hemispheres. Each hemisphere consists of the outer cerebral cortex, which comprises of grey matter and inner cerebral nuclei.

The hemispheres' outer cerebral cortex has various complex processing functions; four 'lobes' on each hemisphere are generally associated with different functions. The **frontal lobes** are considered to be most associated with development of intelligence and conscious thought, and function to plan, carry out and evaluate actions. The **parietal lobes** are associated with sensory reception and perception such as language and face recognition. The **occipital lobes** consist of the visual cortex, and as such are involved in visual processing. Finally, the **temporal lobes** are associated with spatial reasoning and auditory processes.

The cerebral nuclei are also known as white matter. This white colour comes from myelinated axons of nerve cells – demonstrating a key function of this area in conveyancing information from one

3.3

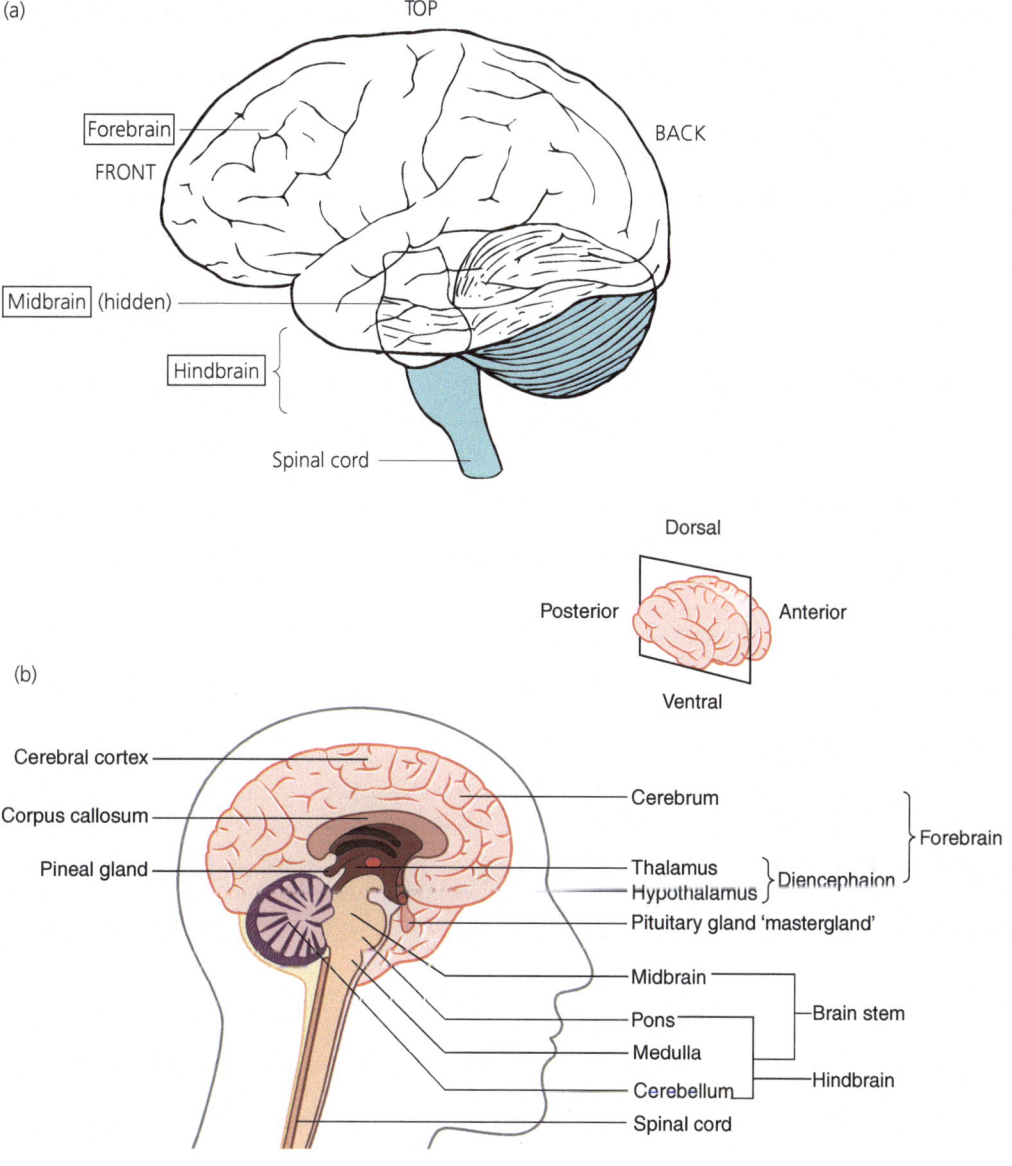

Figure 3.3.5 a) Side view of the brain, b) cross section through the centre of the brain

part of the brain to another. However, also within this region of the brain are the **basal ganglia**, involved in control of movement, and the **limbic system**. The limbic system has a role in memory, behaviour and emotion.

APPLICATION TO PRACTICE

The limbic system has received some attention in recent years. It may play an important role in activating the effects of aromatherapy, which can be used by women during labour, as the nerves

139

activated by this method pass directly to the limbic system. Additionally, the limbic system potentially has a key role to play in inhibiting or supporting behaviour change due to its role in 'holding' emotions. When a part of the limbic system known as the **amygdala** is activated, the focus is on survival – running towards safety or away from danger. This is clearly a good thing! However, at the same time, it reduces our ability to think clearly and creatively. Therefore, if the amygdala is activated inappropriately, such as in response to a suggested behaviour change, we are more likely to perceive this as a danger, and less likely to be able to think clearly or creatively about it. Thus, if the public health role of the midwife is to support behaviour change, the midwife must explore how to work *with* the limbic system. If a woman perceives danger, or feels uncertain, this may trigger the limbic system. This will not support clear decision making! Ask yourself – how could midwives create dialogue around behaviour change without triggering this response in the limbic system?

'**Diencephalon**' actually means 'through brain'; and this reflects the fact that the key function of this section of the forebrain is communication of information from the cerebrum to the rest of the nervous system. The two main regions of the diencephalon are the **thalamus** and **hypothalamus**, although there are other regions such as the **epithalamus** and **subthalamus**. The thalamus is concerned with sensory perception, motor function regulation and sleep cycle regulation. The hypothalamus, although small, serves as the control centre for many autonomic functions via the release of hormones, and is also responsible for homeostatic regulation. The epithalamus contains the **pineal gland**, and its main function is the regulation of sleep and wake cycles. Melatonin, released by the pineal gland, is thought to play an important role in this. The subthalamus is closely interconnected with the basal ganglia in the cerebrum, and as such is strongly linked to motor control and movement.

The brainstem

The brainstem connects the spinal cord with the cerebrum.

The midbrain lies deep within the brain and is not visible externally. It consists of two component parts, the **tectum** and **tegmentum**. The midbrain aids in the processing of auditory and visual information including eye movements, and is involved in motor function.

The hindbrain is made up of the **cerebellum**, **pons** and **medulla oblongata**. The cerebellum, 'little brain', is located behind and below the rest of the brain and bears a resemblance to the cerebrum. It functions to relay information between muscles and the cerebral cortex, and thereby aids in fine movement coordination, maintaining balance and equilibrium. The pons assists in the control of autonomic functions, as well as states of sleep and arousal, and relays information to and from the higher centres of the brain. The medulla oblongata sits at the top of the spinal cord, and links this to the rest of the brain. It is also involved in regulation of autonomic functions such as breathing, cardiac function, vasodilation and reflexes like vomiting, coughing, sneezing and swallowing.

The spinal cord

The spinal cord is situated within the vertebrae of the spine. Each vertebra has a 'spinal foramen', and it is through this that the cord passes. The spinal cord functions to carry sensory information from around the body to the brain and carry motor activity from the brain to the tissues via the PNS.

Information passes from the PNS into the spinal cord, and vice versa, at intervals along the cord. Nerve 'roots' leave the cord at intervals to form spinal nerves. At each vertebral joint there is a pair of dorsal (posterior) and ventral (anterior) roots. Sensory neurons, transmitting information from the body into the cord, form the dorsal root whereas motor neurons, sending signals out to the body tissues from the

CNS, form the ventral root. Cell bodies of sensory neurons are located in the same area of the dorsal root, forming the dorsal root ganglion. Cell bodies of motor neurons are located within the cord itself. Figure 3.3.6 shows these spinal nerve roots in relation to the vertebrae. Located at the end of the spinal cord is the **cauda equina** (Latin for horse's tail, due to its appearance), which is the result of the collection of roots of various nerves which enter or exit the vertebral column below this point. As the

3.3

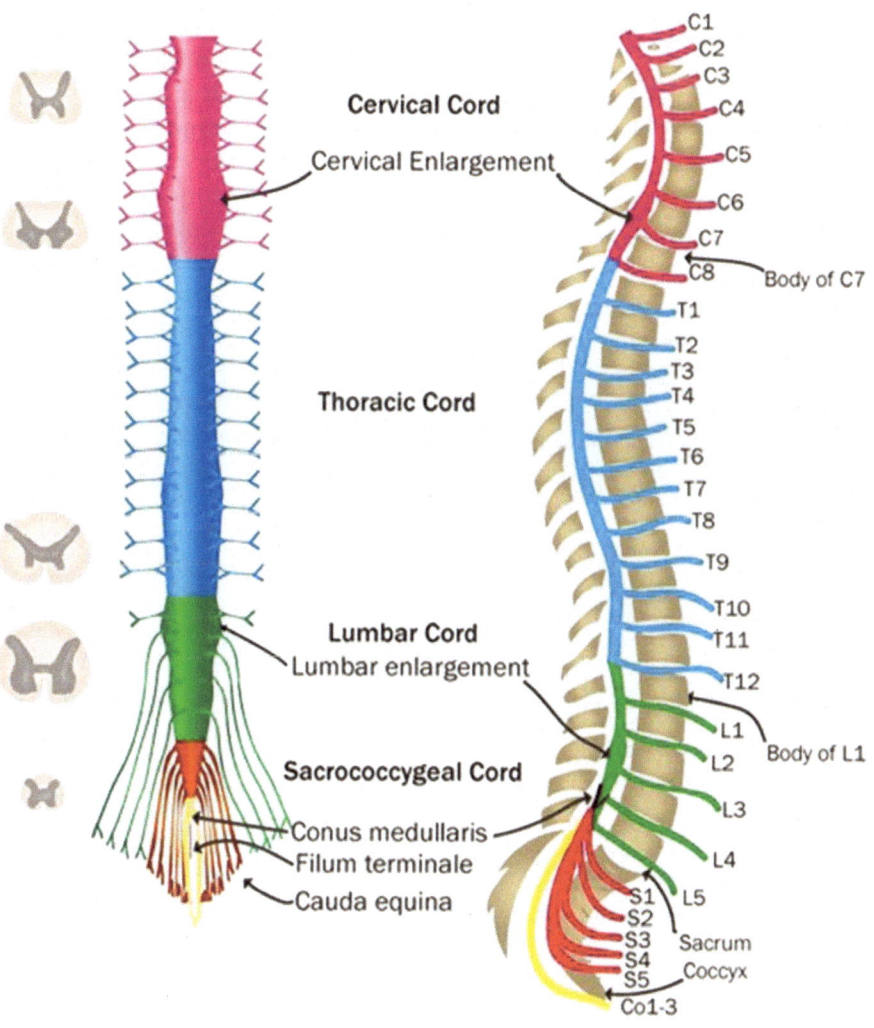

Figure 3.3.6 Spinal nerve root relation to vertebra

cord itself ends here, all nerves extending below this point must enter or exit the cord here, creating this 'horse's tail' effect (Figure 3.3.6).

Protective membranes and cerebrospinal fluid

Surrounding both the brain and spinal cord are three membranes (the **meninges**). The **dura mater** is the outermost layer and is a tough protective collagen-based layer. The **arachnoid mater** is the middle layer. Between this delicate membrane and the dura mater is the narrow subdural space, and the larger subarachnoid space exists between this and the third membrane, the **pia mater**. The pia mater covers the surface of the brain and spinal cord and therefore, is rich in blood vessels which supply the neural tissue.

The subarachnoid space, and various other spaces within the brain, contain the cerebrospinal fluid. This 'transcellular' fluid is secreted by the pia mater. It functions to provide a stable, protective environment for the brain and spinal cord, and is the fluid in which the brain is suspended within the skull. This prevents friction and damage from the bony skull, and enables an element of 'shock absorption' from sudden head movements.

The cells which secrete the cerebrospinal fluid also form the 'blood-brain barrier'. This critically important barrier ensures that toxic blood components, blood cells and pathogens are unable to transfer into the CNS and regulates transfer of other molecules. This ensures that the neuronal environment can be tightly regulated, as neurons are susceptible to any changes in their intra or extracellular environment. Although the blood-brain barrier is largely successful in its tight regulation, it is not perfect, and certain drugs and other molecules can cross this barrier. The mechanisms for this are not always clear.

Peripheral nervous system (PNS)

Somatic nervous system

The key function of the somatic nervous system is to control conscious, or voluntary, actions.

Afferent nerves, comprised of sensory neurons, send sensory information received via sensory receptors to the brain and spinal cord. One way by which sensory receptors are classified is by the type of stimulus that generates a response in the receptor. **Chemoreceptors** detect chemical stimuli, for example, chemicals that lead to the sense of smell. **Mechanoreceptors** detect movement or pressure changes, including sound and balance. **Thermoreceptors** detect temperatures above or below normal body temperature. **Photoreceptors** detect changes in light. Pain is detected through **nociceptors**, which may detect chemical (detecting tissue damage from chemicals), but sometimes mechanical, stimuli.

Once a receptor has detected a stimulus, this will be sent via sensory neurons in afferent nerves into the CNS. The CNS must then determine what, if any, response is required. If a response is required, efferent nerves, comprised of motor neurons, will send information from the brain back to the somatic nervous system, to cause voluntary movement via the musculoskeletal system in response.

Reflex activity

It was stated above that the somatic nervous system controls voluntary actions. The use of 'voluntary' is often taken to assume that we are in control of the somatic nervous system – and often we are. However, on occasion it will act without conscious control – via a reflex arc.

A reflex action is performed in response to a dangerous stimulus, for example standing

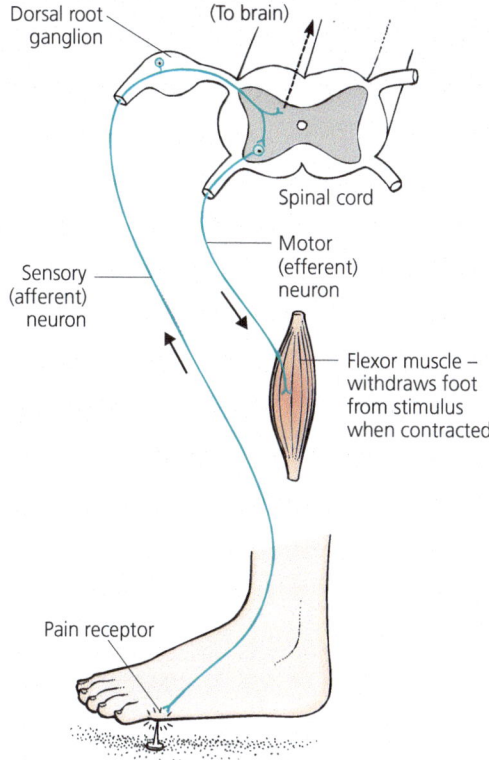

Dorsal root ganglion

(To brain)

Spinal cord

Motor (efferent) neuron

Sensory (afferent) neuron

Flexor muscle – withdraws foot from stimulus when contracted

Pain receptor

Figure 3.3.7 A reflex arc
Source: Figure 8.25, p.194, Clancy and McVicar (2009)

3.3

on a sharp object (Figure 3.3.7). In this case, the PNS and CNS act together to respond to the stimulus, but without requiring input from the brain. There are five key stages to a simple reflex arc:

1. Receptor (e.g. pain receptor) receives a signal
2. Sensory neuron transmits the signal to the spinal cord
3. Interneuron in the spinal cord connects input from the sensory neuron to output via the motor neuron
4. Motor neuron transmits the output signal to the effector
5. Effector tissue turns the signal into action, usually a muscle

This is how the body can respond so quickly to such episodes – have you ever removed your hand from a hot surface before realising it was hot? This is a reflex arc in action. The brain will then receive the information *after* the nervous system has already caused removal of the hand, at which point you realise your hand was burning! There will usually also be other actions in response – other muscles may then need to move to stabilise the body for example – but these actions kick in later, after the initial quick action caused by the reflex arc.

Gate control theory of pain

Pain, and how pain is experienced in the body, is highly complex – and in the most part, therefore, is well outside the scope of this book. However, it is useful to explore the gate control theory of pain, as this is pertinent to understanding certain pain-relieving processes often used during labour. This theory is also complex, however, and so a simplified version of the gate control theory of pain is presented here.

At the heart of the gate control theory of pain is the idea of a gate, located where sensory neurons enter into the spinal cord and would then transmit their signal to the interneuron. Only so much information can enter through this gate at once, and the gate lets through certain pain signals. When the gate is open, therefore, if a pain receptor is triggered the pain signal will travel via sensory neurons to the gate. It can pass through the open gate and up to the brain. If the gate is closed, or blocked by another stimulus, the pain signal cannot travel through the gate, and so does not reach the brain. Therefore, pain is not perceived (Figure 3.3.8).

If someone experiences a painful stimulus, the application of a non-painful (soothing) stimulus can help activate the gate control mechanism, shut the gate, and thereby reduce the pain.

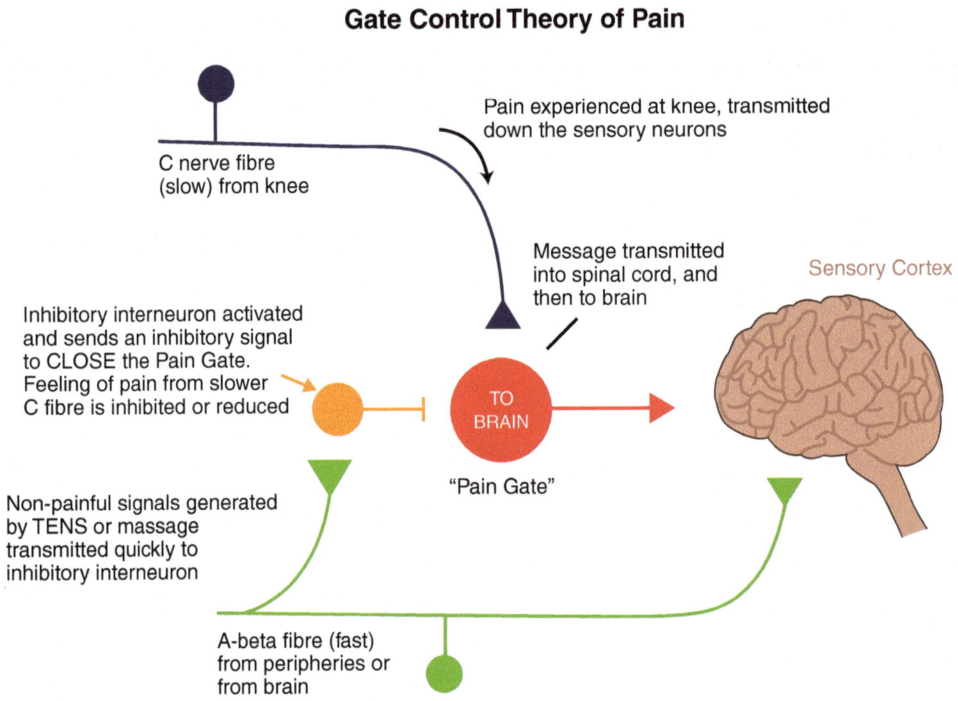

Gate Control Theory of Pain

Figure 3.3.8 Gate control theory of pain

APPLICATION TO PRACTICE

During labour, various non-pharmacological methods may be employed to provide pain relief. The mechanism for how many of these work is thought to be grounded in the gate control theory of pain. Use of massage, hot packs and transcutaneous electrical nerve stimulation (TENS) are all thought to reduce pain perception by 'closing the gate'.

Autonomic nervous system

The key function of the autonomic nervous system is to mediate changes in tissue function which are under involuntary control. Thus, the autonomic system has a key role to play in maintaining homeostasis, achieved by the **sympathetic** and **parasympathetic** divisions of the autonomic nervous system working in a complimentary way to either increase or decrease activity of target cells. The sympathetic division is often associated with the 'fight or flight' response to danger, whereas the parasympathetic division is often referred to as being the 'rest and digest' response. Tissues are often innervated by each division, and this determines the activity. For example, cardiac muscle is innervated by both the sympathetic and parasympathetic divisions. The sympathetic will cause the heart rate to increase (ready to respond to danger), the parasympathetic to decrease (rest and digest). In this way, the two divisions can work together to maintain homeostasis. Table 3.3.3 summarises how the two systems work on some of the key body systems.

Table 3.3.3 Effects of the sympathetic and parasympathetic nervous system

Structure	Sympathetic innervation	Parasympathetic innervation
Eye	Dilates pupil; accommodation for distance vision	Constricts pupil; accommodation for near vision
Salivary glands	Concentrated secretion stimulated	Watery secretion stimulated
Sweat glands	Increased secretion	Not innervated
Cardiovascular system		
Blood vessels		Not innervated, except in penis and clitoris: dilation
To skin	Vasoconstriction	
To skeletal muscles	Vasodilation	
To digestive viscera	Vasoconstriction	
Heart, rate and force of contraction	Increases	Decreases rate
Blood pressure	Increases	Decreases*
Adrenal gland	Medulla secretes adrenaline + noradrenaline	Not innervated
Respiratory system		
Diameter of airways	Increases	Decreases
Respiratory rate	Increases	Decreases
Digestive system		
Sphincter muscles	Contract	Relax
General level of activity	Decreases	Increases
Secretory glands	Inhibited	Stimulated
Urinary system		
Kidneys	Decreases urine production	Not innervated
Bladder	Relaxes muscle of bladder, contracts internal sphincter	Contracts bladder muscle, relaxes internal sphincter
Male reproductive system	Increases glandular secretion; ejaculation	Erection through action on blood vessel

*Indirect effect as consequence of actions on heart rate.

3.3

INTERRUPTER

Using the appropriate table in your workbook (or create your own), fill in the blanks using Table 3.3.3 to help you.

Changes and adaptations during pregnancy

Perhaps the most surprising change to the CNS during pregnancy is that the grey matter of the brain has been shown to shrink! Hoekzema et al. (2017) undertook a study demonstrating for the first time that pregnancy led to a substantial reduction in grey matter volume, particularly in regions of the brain associated with social cognition. These changes could still be detected six years later. The authors postulated that this reduction may be linked to maternal bonding with the newborn and highlighted that the reduction should not automatically be assumed to be a negative finding! That this striking change was only discovered for the first time in 2017 demonstrates how much is still to be explored and understood with respect to the human brain overall, but particularly the changes as a result of pregnancy.

Other key changes to the nervous system during pregnancy largely occur as a result of changes to the endocrine system:

▶ There is limited and conflicting evidence of a reduction in cognitive ability during pregnancy. Lesiewska and Bieliński (2021) highlight this in their review and call for further research in this area.

▶ Changes to sleep patterns during pregnancy are under control of the CNS. Up to 80% of women report disturbed sleep during pregnancy (Ohayon et al., 2017). REM sleep has been shown to increase during pregnancy, with a corresponding decrease in slow-wave sleep. Progesterone promotes daytime sleepiness, but night-time sleep fragmentation. In addition, there is increased night wakening in later trimesters due to factors such as nausea, heartburn, nocturia and back pain.

▶ Alterations to sensations received by the sensory organs, such as changes in taste and smell, and congestion of the nasal mucosa occur. This can cause nasal stuffiness, rhinorrhoea and rhinitis. Causes are poorly understood, but likely to be due to hormonal changes due to pregnancy.

References

Hoekzema E., Barba-Müller E. et al. Pregnancy leads to long-lasting changes in human brain structure. *Nat. Neurosci.* [Internet] 2017, 20:287–96. doi:10.1038/nn.4458.

Lesiewska N., Bieliński, M. Cognitive functions in pregnant women. *Donald Sch. J. Ultrasound Obstet. Gynecol.* [Internet] 2021, 15(2):203–14. www.dsjuog.com/doi/pdf/10.5005/jp-journals-10009-1690.

Ohayon M., Wickwire E. et al. National Sleep Foundation's sleep quality recommendations: First report. *Sleep Health* [Internet] 2017, 3(1):6–19. https://pubmed.ncbi.nlm.nih.gov/28346153/.

Further reading

Kember A.J., Elangainesan P. et al. Common sleep disorders in pregnancy: A review. *Front. Med. (Lausanne)* [Internet] 2023. https://pubmed.ncbi.nlm.nih.gov/37671402/.

Martínez-García M., Paternina-Die M. et al. Do pregnancy-induced brain changes reverse? The brain of a mother six years after parturition. *Brain Sci.* [Internet] 2021, 11(2):168. https://pubmed.ncbi.nlm.nih.gov/33525512/.

Sweeney M.D., Zhao Z. et al. Blood-brain barrier: From physiology to disease and back. *Physiol. Rev.* [Internet] 2019, 99(1):21–78. https://pubmed.ncbi.nlm.nih.gov/30280653/.

Won C.H. Sleeping for two: The great paradox of sleep in pregnancy. *J. Clin. Sleep Med.* [Internet] 2015, 11(6):593–4. https://pubmed.ncbi.nlm.nih.gov/25979097/.

CHAPTER 3.4

The endocrine system

Jane Carpenter

LEARNING OUTCOMES

▶ Describe the structure and function of the endocrine system

▶ Understand the function of hormones, and the key ways in which they act

▶ Understand the structure and function of key glands

▶ Understand the how these glands change and adapt during pregnancy, and apply this to practice

Endocrine system overview

Functions of the endocrine system

The endocrine system is a complex network of glands and organs. It controls and coordinates the body's processes, such as metabolism or reproduction, via the use of

hormones, often referred to as 'chemical messengers' that alter the activities of cells.

The functions of the endocrine system are many, but can perhaps be summarised into four key functional headlines:

1. Coordination of homeostatic balance
2. Regulation of various physiological systems throughout the body
3. Sex differentiation facilitation in the embryonic stage, and secondary sexual characteristic development at puberty
4. Induction or modification of behavioural changes within the individual

In order to carry out these functions, hormones are secreted into the blood, and these then travel to 'target destinations' where they effect the required change. In some ways, this is similar to the action of the nervous system covered in the previous chapter. However, key differences are apparent. In the nervous system, the

DOI: 10.4324/9781003227571-15

effects are localised to where the specific nervous response has been activated via neurons and neurotransmitters. Hormones, however, are released into the blood and so will travel throughout the body, meaning that the change will be effected in *any cell* which has receptors for that hormone. The nervous system sends messages directly, via neurons and neurotransmitters, meaning its action is often quick, effecting rapid responses or changes. As hormones need to be secreted into the blood, travel via the blood to target destinations and then effect the response, the endocrine system works more slowly, but tends to effect longer-term changes.

Therefore, the two systems are complimentary and work in conjunction to ensure effective regulation of body systems.

Hormones

We have thus far defined hormones as 'chemical messengers' altering activities of cells – but in order to understand the functioning of the endocrine system, a deeper understanding of how hormones work as 'chemical messengers' is required. A more detailed explanation of a hormone is perhaps as a substance produced by cells in one part of the body, secreted into the blood in response to a specific stimulus and in amounts that vary with the strength of the stimulus, and which acts in the body some distance from the site of secretion. However, even this is problematic as some secretions which may be considered a hormone do not fit this definition – for example, the chemicals may sometimes be secreted into interstitial fluid rather than blood.

Hormones can be divided into four types based on their chemistry: peptides, catecholamines, steroids and eicosanoids.

Peptides, such as insulin and glucagon, are composed of amino acids. As such,

these are soluble in water, but are only poorly soluble in lipids. Once produced in a cell, they are stored in that cell within a membrane bound vesicle. When secretion is required, this can happen quickly via exocytosis, and as they are water soluble they do not require a 'carrier protein' in order to circulate in the bloodstream. This means they can act relatively quickly compared to some other hormones. However, in order to act on target cells, a receptor on the surface of the cell membrane of the target cell is required.

Catecholamines, such as adrenaline and noradrenaline, are derived from an amino acid called tyrosine. They are slightly lipid soluble, but as with peptide hormones can also be contained in vesicles in the cell and released quickly, and require a membrane receptor on target cells. Thyroxine, although not a catecholamine, is also derived from tyrosine and so is similar in structure. However, the hormone-to-target cell receptor relationship is more complex and therefore, it takes longer for responses to occur.

Steroid hormones, such as oestrogens, testosterone, cortisol and aldosterone, act quite differently to the hormones described thus far. Steroid hormones are derived from the lipid cholesterol and as such are highly lipid soluble. Because of this they pass easily through cell membranes (as these are lipid-based) and thus cannot be stored. Instead, they must be produced as required. Again, as they are lipid soluble, they can pass straight into target cells, without the requirement of a membrane receptor, instead there are intracellular receptors. Once inside the cell, steroid hormones can then act as required, but this makes them comparably slower in onset of actions.

Eicosanoids, such as prostaglandins, are derived from a fatty acid called arachidonic acid. They are lipid soluble and so, as with steroid hormones, must be produced as required, and act intracellularly – usually close to their site of production.

Regulation of hormones

Most hormones are regulated by feedback loops. These loops can either be positive or negative, and short or long. Feedback loops are a key concept in how the endocrine system functions.

Most hormones are regulated by **negative feedback loops**. One classic example of a negative feedback loop is regulation of blood glucose levels. Ensuring blood glucose is kept within safe limits is essential for survival – blood glucose which is too high or too low can be dangerous. This regulation is under the control of the endocrine system, with the action of hormones regulated via a negative feedback loop.

Figure 3.4.1 shows the process of blood sugar regulation. Consider that a person eats a carbohydrate rich meal. This will cause the blood glucose level to rise. At a certain threshold, in order to regulate the blood sugar, this will trigger the beta cells of the pancreas to release insulin into the blood. Insulin in the blood will trigger uptake of glucose from the blood into body cells, and also by the liver for storage as glycogen. The blood glucose level will therefore decrease, and at a set point the stimulus for insulin to be released will cease. Blood sugar levels are stable once more.

Now consider that the person does not eat another meal for many hours. This would then cause the blood glucose level to drop. At a certain point, this dropping blood glucose level will trigger alpha cells of the pancreas to release glucagon into the

3.4

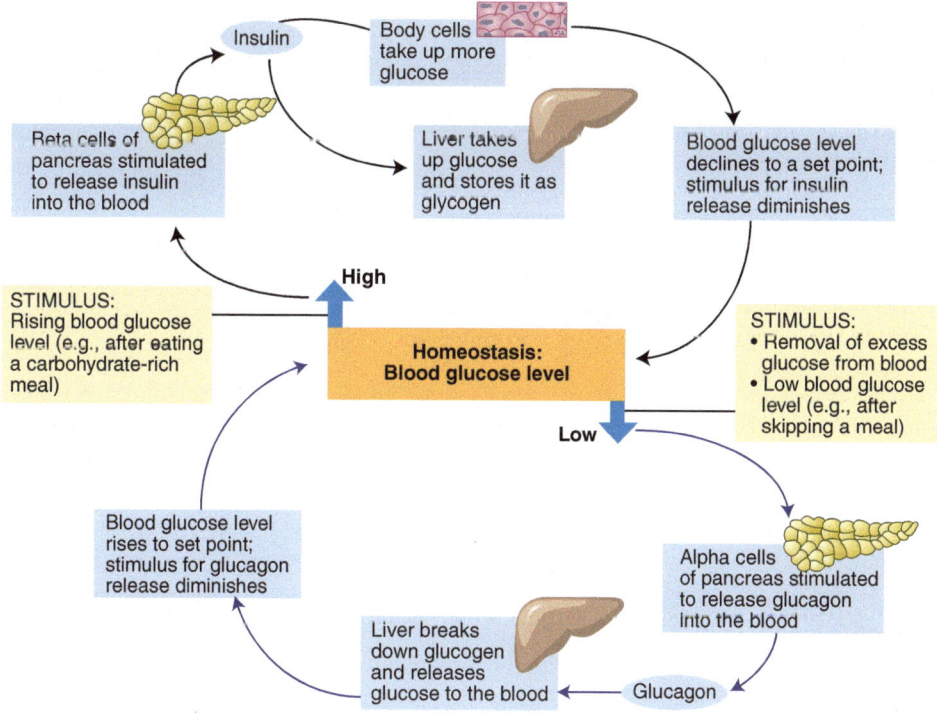

Figure 3.4.1 Hormonal regulation of blood sugar by negative feedback loops

blood. This circulating glucagon will cause the liver to break down its stored glycogen into glucose, and this will be released into the blood. This will increase blood glucose levels, and once these levels rise to a certain threshold, the stimulus for glucagon release will cease. Blood sugar levels are stable once more.

This example demonstrates the classic working of negative feedback loops. This type of feedback loop works to reverse an effect once a threshold is reached – it works negatively.

Positive feedback loops are much less common, as rather than regulating and maintaining stability, they cause ever increasing effects. Two key positive feedback loops in humans are highly relevant to midwifery, being via the hormone oxytocin, causing uterine contractions during labour and birth (see Chapters 4.2 and 4.3), and via the action of prolactin and oxytocin to cause milk production and ejection from the breast.

In response to a baby suckling, prolactin is released from the anterior pituitary gland. Prolactin causes the production of milk. At the same time, suckling stimulates the secretion of oxytocin from the posterior pituitary. This causes contraction of muscle cells in the breast tissue, which contract and squeeze milk down ducts and out of the nipple. This milk feeds the baby, which causes the baby to suckle more. The suckling causes further release of prolactin and oxytocin, which further stimulate the production and ejection of milk, which cause further suckling – and so on. The effect of the positive feedback loop is to ever-increase the effect, rather than to reverse it as in negative feedback. The hormonal control of lactation is further described in Section 6.

INTERRUPTER

Use the relevant section of your workbook to explain in your own words (or with diagrams if you prefer) how feedback loops work. Make sure you distinguish between negative and positive feedback loops.

Location and function of key endocrine glands

Secreting cells are usually collected into discrete areas known as glands. **Exocrine glands** release their secretions onto the surface of the body. **Endocrine glands** release their hormone secretions, in the most part, into the blood. Some glands, such as the pancreas, can have both exocrine and endocrine elements. Figure 3.4.2 shows the location of the major endocrine glands throughout the body, and Table 3.4.1 provides a summary of their hormone secretion, targets and actions.

Key endocrine glands in depth

Hypothalamus and pituitary gland

We have previously noted that homeostasis is the maintenance of a stable internal environment despite changes to the internal or external environment. The endocrine system, along with the nervous system, is key in maintaining homeostasis. Of all the glands, the **hypothalamus** and **pituitary gland** are often considered to be the 'command centre' for the whole of the rest of the endocrine system, as together they control and regulate the action of most of the other endocrine glands. In addition, the hypothalamus has an important role in the nervous system, regulating a number of autonomic mechanisms. This further demonstrates the close link between

3.4

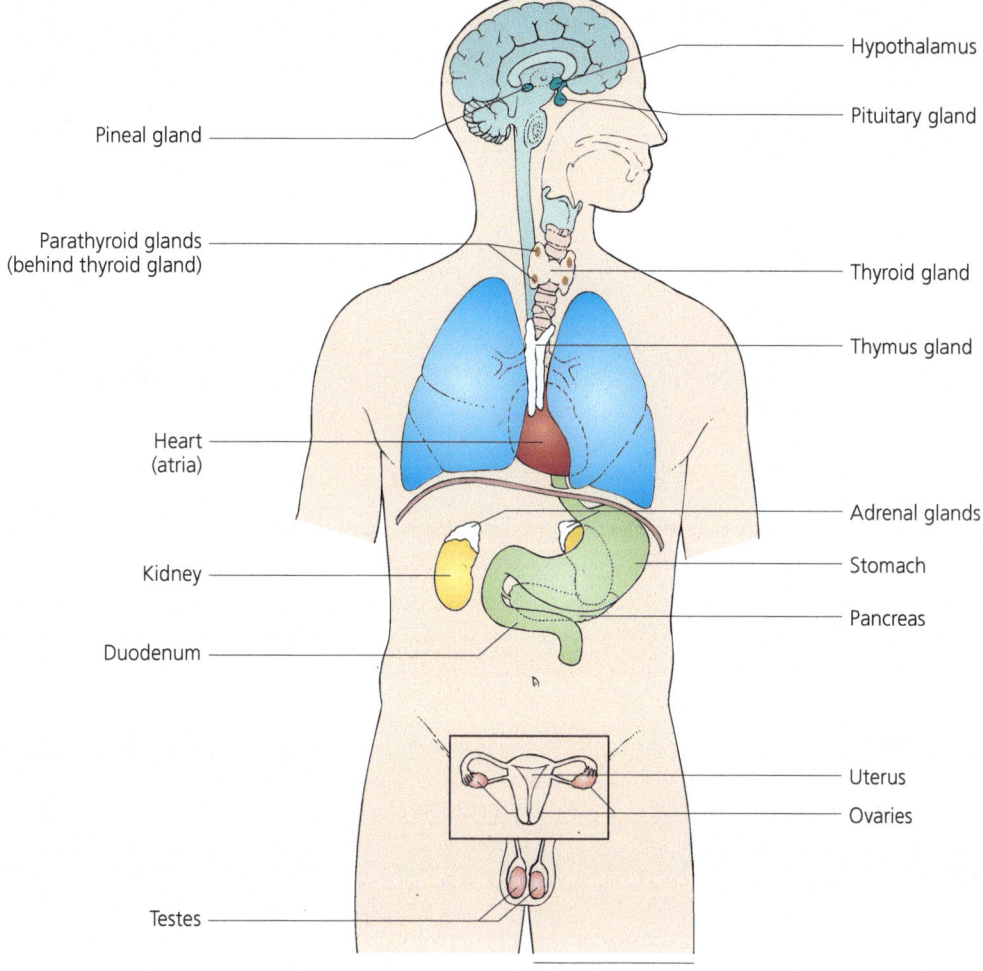

Hypothalamus

Pituitary gland

Pineal gland

Parathyroid glands
(behind thyroid gland)

Thyroid gland

Thymus gland

Heart
(atria)

Adrenal glands

Stomach

Kidney

Pancreas

Duodenum

Uterus

Ovaries

Testes

Figure 3.4.2 Location of major endocrine glands in the human body
Source: Figure 9.3, p.212, Clancy and McVicar (2009)

the endocrine and nervous systems, as highlighted at the start of this chapter.

The hypothalamus and pituitary gland are situated close to each other in the brain, separated by the infundibulum (Figure 3.4.3). The pituitary gland is further split into **anterior** and **posterior** lobes, and these two lobes have different structures and functions, further described below.

The hypothalamus produces a number of key regulatory hormones, and then secretes these into the anterior pituitary via the hypophyseal portal system. Hypothalamic-releasing hormones stimulate the anterior pituitary to release other hormones and include thyrotropin-releasing hormone, gonadotropin-releasing hormone (GnRH), growth hormone-releasing hormone and corticotropin-releasing hormone (CRH). Hypothalamic-inhibiting hormones inhibit the release of manufactured hormones from the anterior pituitary gland and include growth hormone inhibiting hormone and dopamine (or prolactin inhibiting hormone, PIH).

Table 3.4.1 Summary of hormones secreted, and their targets and actions, for the major endocrine glands

Gland	Hormone	Target	Action
Hypothalamus	*Releasing hormones	Anterior pituitary	Release of various hormones (see text)
	*Inhibitory hormones	Anterior pituitary	Inhibit release of various hormones (see text)
Anterior pituitary	Corticotropin (ACTH)	Adrenal cortex	Release of glucocorticoid hormones
	Thyrotropin (TSH)	Thyroid follicles	Release of thyroxine
	Gonadotropins, i.e. luteinizing hormone (LH), follicle-stimulating hormone (FSH)	Gonads	Oestrogens and progestins (female), testosterone (male)
	Growth hormone (GH, somatotropin) Prolactin	Various tissues	Metabolic (see text)
	Melanocyte-stimulating hormone (MSH)	Breast (female) Unclear in male	Lactation (role in male unclear)
	Melanocytes in skin	Promotes melanin synthesis	Unclear Hypothalamic regulatory hormones
Posterior pituitary	Vasopressin (antidiuretic hormone, ADH)	Kidney, arterioles	Water retention Vasoconstriction (blood pressure regulation)
	Oxytocin	Breast and uterus (unclear in male)	Lactation, labour Promotes bonding
Thyroid	Thyroxine (T3, T4)	Various tissues	Metabolic, especially role in basal metabolic rate
	Calcitonin	Bone	Promotes calcium deposition
Parathyroid	Parathyroid hormone (PTH)	Bone, kidney	Promotes calcium resorption from bone Activates vitamin D in kidney (i.e. promotes calcium uptake from bowel)
Adrenal cortex	Glucocorticoids, e.g. cortisol	Various tissues	Metabolic, permissive influence on other hormones
	Mineralocorticoids, e.g. aldosterone	Kidney	Promote sodium reabsorption from renal tubule, promote potassium secretion (i.e. excretion)
	Gonadal steroids	Gonads	Influence on reproductive tract, but not regulatory
Adrenal medulla	Catecholamines (adrenaline, noradrenaline)	Heart and circulation, also various other tissues (see text)	Promote cardiac function Promote vasoconstriction (blood pressure regulation)

(Continued)

Table 3.4.1 (Continued)

Gland	Hormone	Target	Action
Duodenum	Secretin and CCK–PZ	Digestive glands, gall bladder, pancreas, stomach	Promote secretion of pancreatic fluid and enzymes, bile secretion, regulate gastric emptying
Pancreas	Insulin	Liver, skeletal muscle	Promotes glucose utilization
	Glucagon	Liver, skeletal muscle	Promotes glucose mobilization from stores
	Somatostatin	Insulin- and glucagonsecreting cells of pancreas	Modulates release of insulin and glucagon
Gonads: ovaries (female)	Oestrogens (e.g. oestriol), progestins (e.g. progesterone)	Reproductive tract, breast and secondary sexual characteristics	Regulation of menstrual cycle. Behavioural effects
Gonads: testes (male)	Androgens (e.g. testosterone)	Reproductive tract and secondary sexual characteristics	Regulation of spermatogenesis, and accessory glands of reproductive tract Behavioural effects

*Hypothalamic regulatory hormones include specific releasing and inhibitory hormones that act on the secretion of individual hormones from the anterior pituitary gland. CCK–PZ, cholecystokinin–pancreozymin

Source: Table 9.1, p.211, Clancy and McVicar (2009)

The anterior pituitary is made largely of glandular tissue and produces and releases a number of **tropic** hormones. The Greek word *tropos* means 'change' or 'turn' – and indeed these tropic hormones act to stimulate or inhibit endocrine glands elsewhere in the body. These hormones are growth hormone, thyroid-stimulating hormone, adrenocorticotropic hormone, prolactin, melanocyte-stimulating hormone, follicle stimulating hormone and luteinising hormone. Thus, the anterior pituitary manufactures and releases its own hormones, but this process is regulated by hormones secreted from the hypothalamus.

The posterior pituitary is structurally quite different to the anterior pituitary, comprising of nervous tissue, and secretes only two hormones – oxytocin and anti-diuretic hormone. These two hormones are produced in the hypothalamus and released via the posterior pituitary. The posterior pituitary does not produce hormones, but instead stores and secretes hormones produced by the hypothalamus.

The number of hormones produced, stored and released by the hypothalamus and pituitary gland, and then their ongoing action, is summarised in Figure 3.4.4. This complexity reflects the importance of these structures as the 'command centre' from which many endocrine and nervous responses are controlled.

Adrenal glands

The two adrenal glands lie on top of each kidney. Structurally and functionally, the adrenal glands are split into an inner **medulla** and an outer **cortex**. Cells located in the adrenal medulla secrete catecholamine hormones, whereas cells in the adrenal cortex secrete steroid hormones (Figure 3.4.5).

The **adrenal medulla** secretes the catecholamines adrenaline and noradrenaline. The cells which produce

153

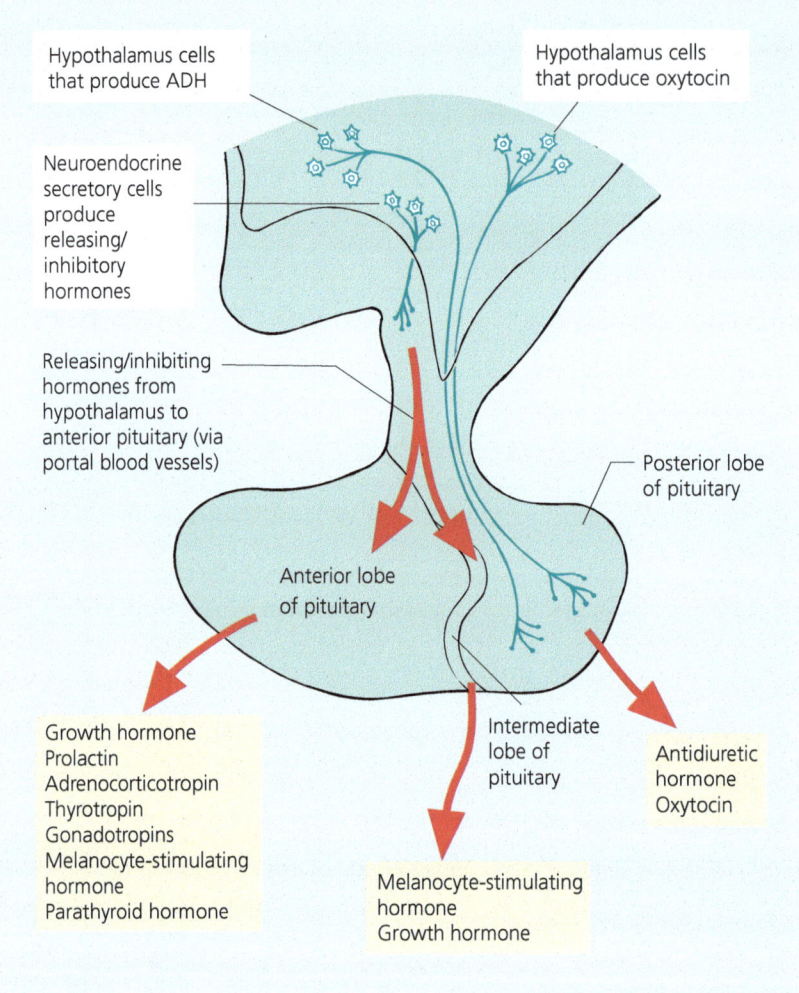

Figure 3.4.3 The hypothalamus and pituitary gland
Source: Figure 9.5, p.214, Clancy and McVicar (2009)

and secrete these hormones originally developed from embryonic neural crest cells, giving the close link between the nervous and endocrine system here. The release of catecholamines is triggered when sympathetic nerves to the adrenal glands are stimulated – the so-called fight or flight response. Therefore, these hormones stimulate the required responses to facilitate escape from danger. Such changes include:

▶ Increase in heart rate and contractility of heart muscle, leading to greater cardiac output.
▶ Vasoconstriction of certain vessels with vasodilation of others – this allows blood flow to be concentrated in places it is needed such as the heart and active tissues.
▶ Reduction in gut motility as digestion is not a priority. Instead, blood flow is diverted to other active tissues.

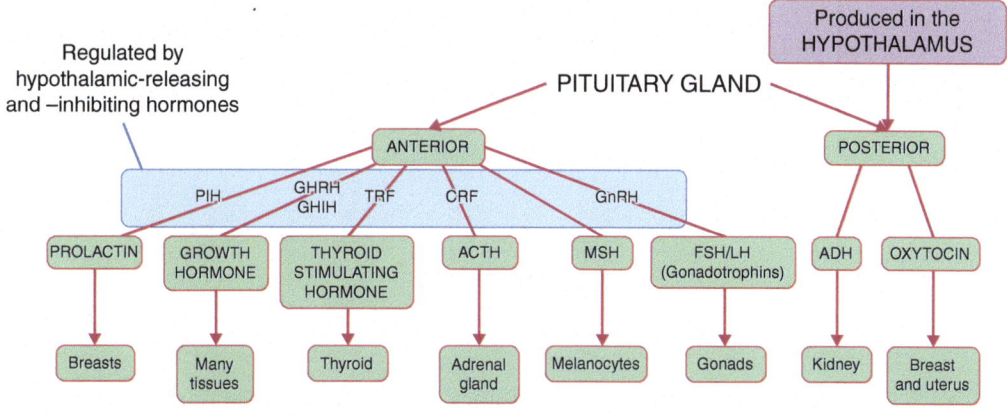

Figure 3.4.4 Hormonal secretions of the pituitary gland

▶ Bronchodilation to facilitate alveolar ventilation in the lungs.

The **adrenal cortex** secretes steroid hormones, usually divided into three groups **(glucocorticoids, mineralocorticoids and gonadocorticoids)**, but collectively referred to as **corticoids**. Glucocorticoids, such as **cortisol** and **corticosterone**, have wide-ranging effects on the body and are considered pivotal in protein, glucose and fat metabolism, as well as reducing inflammation. They are necessary for normal body functions, but stress induces significant secretion of cortisol. As such, cortisol is often referred to as the 'stress hormone'.

Mineralocorticoids, such as **aldosterone**, have a role in maintenance of electrolyte composition in plasma. Aldosterone works mainly in the kidney, but also in sweat, saliva and in the gut, to balance sodium (and therefore water) and potassium. Aldosterone is a key part of the Renin-Angiotensin-Aldosterone System described in more depth in Chapter 3.6.

Finally, gonadocorticoids **(androgens/ oestrogens)** are also secreted by the adrenal cortex, but in very small amounts compared to the amounts produced by the gonads. The amounts produced in the

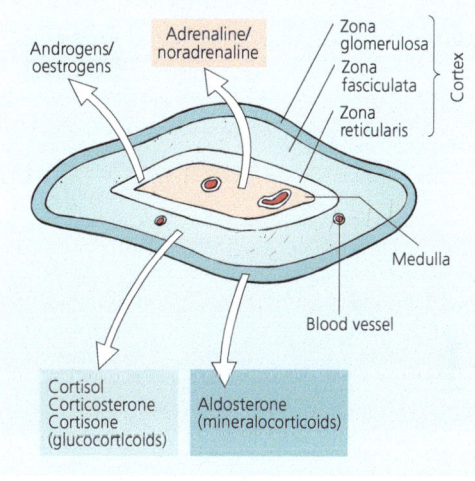

Figure 3.4.5 Diagrammatic cross-section of an adrenal gland
Source: Figure 9.11, p.219, Clancy and McVicar (2009)

cortex are probably of little consequence in adulthood but are more important during fetal development and pre-pubertal childhood.

The hypothalamic-pituitary-adrenal axis (HPA)

The HPA axis has a fundamentally important role is the body's management of stress. Now that we have considered the hypothalamus, pituitary and adrenal glands separately, we can look at how these function together in order to regulate the stress response.

The immediate response to stress is mediated by the autonomic arm of the sympathetic nervous system (see Chapter 3.3). This nervous response is immediate and triggers the release of adrenaline and noradrenaline.

The HPA axis is then activated soon after, as rising levels of noradrenaline are detected by the hypothalamus. This leads the hypothalamus to secrete CRH. This further increases the action of the sympathetic nervous system, but in addition triggers the pituitary to secrete **adrenocorticotropic hormone (ACTH)** into the blood. This hormone is detected by the adrenal cortex and leads to the release of **cortisol**. Cortisol is thought to be important in the management of longer-term stress (rather than the rapid action of the autonomic nervous system) and induces effects such as an increase in blood pressure, cardiac output and blood glucose, but also inhibits non-essential body functions – for example, reproductive activity.

Healthy functioning of the whole HPA axis is important in order for the body to react to short- and longer-term stress. However, over-stimulation of this axis (e.g. in someone faced with persistently high levels of stress on a daily basis) may cause both physical and mental health issues. Elevated cortisol levels may lead to suppression of the immune response and has been linked to type 2 diabetes, obesity, cardiovascular disease and depression.

Thyroid gland

The thyroid gland is situated just below the larynx and on top of the trachea and is often described as being 'butterfly-shaped' (Figure 3.4.6). The thyroid gland produces and releases triiodothyronine (T3)

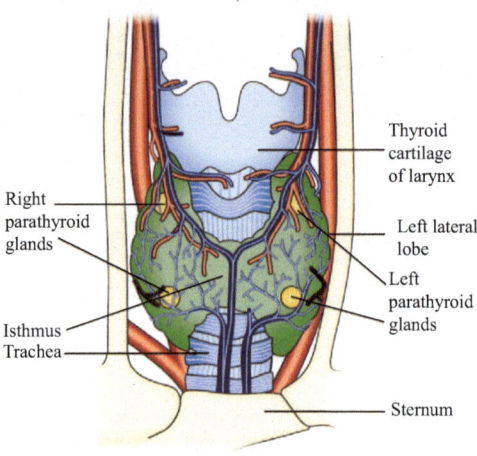

Figure 3.4.6 The thyroid gland

and thyroxine (T4). These two hormones are formed from thyroglobulin, iodine and tyrosine. Iodine cannot be produced by the body, and so must be obtained from dietary sources. Although the thyroid gland produces much more T4 (90%) than T3 (10%), the latter is much more potent. Both T3 and T4 have a number of important functions, including promoting normal bone development in childhood, regulation of bone density in adulthood, and regulation of fat, protein and carbohydrate metabolism. This makes them essential for normal cell development and differentiation. They also have a role in regulating body temperature, as they increase oxygen consumption and energy production in cells. This increases the basal metabolic rate, which generates heat and hence, regulates temperature.

If the thyroid is unable to produce enough T3 and T4, this results in **hypothyroidism**. Poor dietary intake of iodine can ultimately result in hypothyroidism; iodine deficiency during pregnancy can result in developmental delay in the child. Hypothyroidism can also be caused by the autoimmune condition Hashimoto's thyroiditis, in which antibodies are produced that attack the thyroid tissue, leading to enlargement of the thyroid gland (known as goitre). There are various other potential causes of hypothyroidism – including surgical removal of the thyroid gland (often to manage hyperthyroidism). Hypothyroidism causes symptoms such as fatigue, weight gain, feeling cold, dry skin and constipation.

Hyperthyroidism occurs where too much T3 and T4 are secreted by the thyroid gland, thereby leading to increased metabolism and cellular activity. Hyperthyroidism is most often caused by Grave's thyroiditis, an autoimmune condition where antibodies mimic the action of thyroid-stimulating hormone and hence, cause overproduction of T3 and T4. Symptoms include restlessness, weight loss, palpitations, tachycardia and goitre. Hyperthyroidism can sometimes be treated with medication to regulate production of T3 and T4, however, in some cases partial or total removal of the thyroid (thyroidectomy) may be necessary. This will then lead to hypothyroidism.

Pancreas

The banana-shaped pancreas can be found located behind the stomach. Only about 1% of this organ is dedicated to producing hormones, and this 1% is organised into 'clusters' of cells known as pancreatic islets (or islets of Langerhans). Although only 1% of the organ, this still equates to c. two million islets in a healthy pancreas. Within the islets are four different cell types: alpha, beta, delta and pancreatic polypeptide (PP) cells.

Alpha cells produce glucagon and **beta cells** produce insulin. As the role of these hormones is considered above (see *Regulation of hormones*) they are not considered further here. **Delta cells** produce **growth hormone inhibiting hormone** (**GHIH**), although this is also produced elsewhere in the body such as the hypothalamus). The role of GHIH in the pancreas is to inhibit the secretion of insulin and glucagon when blood sugar levels are within their homeostatic range. **PP cells** produce **pancreatic polypeptide**, the primary role of which is to modulate digestion of food.

Ovaries/testes

The endocrine function of the ovaries and testes is considered in Chapter 2.3, and so is not considered again here even though the endocrine function of these structures is of high relevance to midwifery.

Changes and adaptations during pregnancy

Changes in hormone production during pregnancy

Hormones to maintain the pregnancy

One of the key ways in which the endocrine system changes during pregnancy is the production of key hormones that develop and sustain the pregnancy:

Human chorionic gonadotropin hormone (hCG) is only made during pregnancy, almost exclusively by the placenta. hCG levels peak during the first trimester, as it stimulates the corpus luteum to produce progesterone to maintain the pregnancy. hCG has often been linked to nausea and vomiting in pregnancy as both peak at a similar time. No causal pathway has been found, and recent research (Fejzo et al., 2023) has identified that abnormally high levels of the hormone GDF15, and increased sensitivity to it, are the major factors contributing to hyperemesis gravidarum (severe nausea and vomiting in pregnancy).

Human placental lactogen (hPL) provides nutrition to the fetus. It also stimulates milk glands in the breasts for breastfeeding.

Oestrogen, actually a group of hormones, is made by the placenta during pregnancy to help maintain a healthy pregnancy.

Progesterone is a key pregnancy hormone, produced by the ovaries and placenta during pregnancy. It stimulates the thickening of the uterine lining for implantation of a fertilised egg. It comes from the Latin pro-, meaning 'for' and gest-, referring to pregnancy (gestation). Progesterone levels remain high throughout pregnancy due to its role in maintaining the uterus in a quiescent state, stopping the uterus from contracting and entering labour. This effect of 'relaxing' the smooth muscle, although aimed at the uterus, has far reaching consequences across many of the other body systems as you will read in the other chapters of this section of the book.

Changes to the HPA axis

The maternal HPA axis undergoes substantial change across the perinatal period, with changes across all three components of the axis. Key changes are summarised below.

Hypothalamus

Due to high levels of cortisol during pregnancy (see below), hypothalamic CRH secretion is suppressed.

Pituitary

It is thought that the pituitary gland increases in weight by up to 50% during pregnancy – this is largely due to the required increase in prolactin-secreting cells for lactation (see Section 6). Growth hormone producing cells fall in number during pregnancy, returning to normal within a few weeks. During pregnancy, the fetoplacental hormones exhibit substantial changes to hormone production and release from the pituitary, for example, follicle stimulating hormone (FSH) and luteinising hormone (LH) are inhibited.

Adrenal gland

By the end of the third trimester, cortisol levels have increased threefold compared to pre-pregnancy levels (Duthie and Reynolds, 2013). This increase is due to the placenta secreting CRH, which further stimulates ACTH with the consequence of an increase in cortisol levels. This rise in cortisol further stimulates release of placental CRH secretion.

The fetus is usually protected from these higher levels of cortisol by an enzyme which converts it to cortisone. However, a small amount of cortisol may reach the fetus, and this can be increased in the presence of maternal illness or infection.

There is evidence that high maternal cortisol levels are negatively associated with birth weight and gestation at birth (Duthie and Reynolds, 2013), demonstrating that excess levels of cortisol may slow growth of the fetus *in utero* and shorten gestation. There is also growing evidence that high maternal cortisol can alter the neurodevelopmental trajectory of the infant, with a possible epigenetic role here (Kassotaki et al., 2021).

Thyroid gland

Changes to the thyroid gland during pregnancy tend to mimic hyperthyroidism, although overall, thyroid function remains within normal levels. Although the thyroid tends to slightly enlarge during pregnancy, this is usually not detectable via a physical examination.

Thyroid hormones are essential for fetal development, particularly of the brain and nervous system. The embryo is entirely reliant on maternal thyroid hormones via the placenta for development. After this, the fetus will start to develop its own thyroid hormones, although it will still require input from the maternal system until c. 18–20 weeks gestation. After this point, the fetus can develop and use its own.

Pancreas – insulin resistance and gestational diabetes

As explored above, the pancreas secretes key hormones to regulate blood glucose levels. During pregnancy some of the placental hormones released to maintain and develop the pregnancy (oestrogen, cortisol and human placental lactogen) can have a blocking effect on insulin. This **contra-insulin** effect starts to happen at around 20–24 weeks gestation and leads to higher levels of maternal blood glucose after eating a meal (as the insulin is less able to perform its function). Normally, the maternal beta cells will then produce additional insulin to overcome the **insulin resistance** which has developed. However, if the production of insulin is not great enough to overcome the insulin resistance, gestational diabetes will develop.

APPLICATION TO PRACTICE

Gestational diabetes (GDM)

GDM develops where the maternal beta cells in the pancreas are no longer able to produce enough insulin to overcome the insulin resistance caused by certain placental hormones.

Risk factors include

▶ Obesity – usually determined as a body mass index (BMI) over 30 at the start of pregnancy

▶ Family history of diabetes (type 1, 2 or gestational), or GDM in a previous pregnancy
▶ Previous baby of over 4.5 kg
▶ South Asian, Black, African-Caribbean or Middle Eastern origin

Diagnosis

If a woman has any of the risk factors for developing GDM, or if glucosuria is detected, a screening test known as an **oral glucose tolerance test** will often be offered. This involves having a period of fasting, a blood test to check blood glucose, a glucose drink and then another blood test after two hours. This can be used to observe how the body is able to manage the raised glucose. If there is evidence that the body is unable to effectively manage this, this indicates GDM.

Treatment

The multidisciplinary team, often consisting of specialist midwives and obstetricians but also potentially including anaesthetists, public health specialists and others, will determine the treatment in partnership with the woman. However, the focus of treatment is around management of blood glucose levels, and often women are given kits to test their blood glucose levels several times per day. It may be possible to keep blood glucose within optimal levels by making changes to diet and undertaking gentle exercise. If this does not work, however, medications can also be prescribed. These can be in tablet or injection form.

Complications

Polyhydramnios (too much amniotic fluid), premature birth and pre-eclampsia are all risks from having GDM.

Macrosomia can occur if maternal blood glucose levels are not well controlled. If maternal blood glucose levels are higher than normal, the fetal pancreas will produce more insulin to regulate this. The fetus will convert the extra blood glucose to fat. This causes the fetus to be excessively large.

Hypoglycaemia at birth may then follow, as the fetus has had high levels of insulin *in utero* to regulate the higher blood glucose levels. However, after birth, the newborn will still have high levels of insulin, but will no longer receive the high level of blood glucose via the placenta. This can mean that the newborn may develop very low blood sugar after birth. For this reason, in many settings infants born to women with GDM will have their blood sugar levels checked in the early postnatal period. If low blood sugar is detected this can be treated, either via a breastfeed, expressed breastmilk (women with GDM are often encouraged to hand express antenatally for this reason), a glucose gel or, in severe situations, a glucose intravenous drip.

CHAPTER CHALLENGE

Diabetes is increasingly a feature of pregnancy, presenting both gestational and longer-term challenges for women. Have a look at the paper below and consider which women are at increased risk of developing problematic levels of insulin resistance in pregnancy. Consider the ways in which you could help people in your care avoid and manage this.

Kampmann U., Knorr S. et al. Determinants of maternal insulin resistance during pregnancy: An updated review. *Diabetes Res.* [Internet] 2019, 5320156. www.ncbi.nlm.nih.gov/pmc/articles/PMC6885766.

References

Duthie L., Reynolds R. Changes in the maternal hypothalamic-pituitary-adrenal axis in pregnancy and postpartum: Influences on maternal and fetal outcomes. *Neuroendocrinol.* 2013, 98(2):106–15. doi:10.1159/000354702.

Fejzo M., Rocha N., Cimino I. et al. GDF15 linked to maternal risk of nausea and vomiting during pregnancy. *Nature* 2023. doi:10.1038/s41586-023-06921-9.

Kassotaki I., Valsamakis G., Mastorakos G., Grammatopoulos D.K. Placental CRH as a signal of pregnancy adversity and impact on fetal neurodevelopment. *Front. Endocrinol. (Lausanne)* 2021 Aug 2, 12:714214. doi:10.3389/fendo.2021.714214.

The musculoskeletal system

Giada Giusmin

LEARNING OUTCOMES

▶ Describe the structure and function of the musculoskeletal system
▶ Describe some of the physical changes to the musculoskeletal system which occur during pregnancy
▶ Understand the effects of key hormones on the musculoskeletal system, and apply this to practice

Musculoskeletal system overview

The musculoskeletal system is made of bones, muscles and joints, some of which are shown in Figure 3.5.1. Its main function is to provide structural support and allow movement. This chapter provides an overview of the three main components of the musculoskeletal system before discussing changes during

pregnancy and the postnatal period and some common musculoskeletal conditions affecting women.

Skeletal system

The skeletal system, or skeleton, is made up of bones, ligaments and joints, as well as cartilage. Overall, these constitute around 12–15% of the total body weight. As bones are the principal component of the skeletal system, they will be discussed first.

Bones

Bones are far more than inert structural features. Bone functions include:

▶ Shielding of vital organs contained within their boundaries, for example, the brain contained in the cranium, or lungs and heart contained in the thoracic cavity
▶ Hosting haematopoiesis (see Chapter 3.1) in their red bone marrow

DOI: 10.4324/9781003227571-16

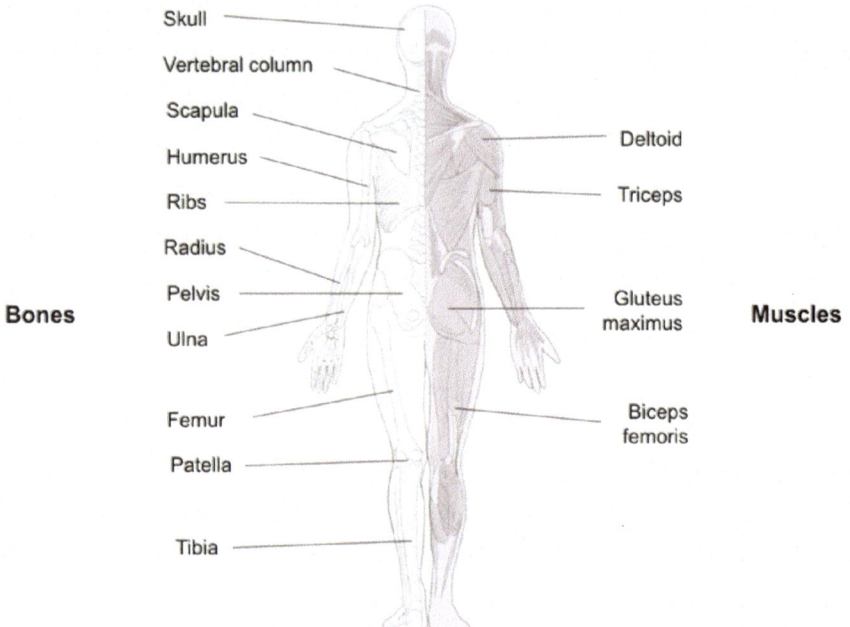

Bones / Muscles

Skull
Vertebral column
Scapula
Humerus
Ribs
Radius
Pelvis
Ulna
Femur
Patella
Tibia

Deltoid
Triceps
Gluteus maximus
Biceps femoris

Figure 3.5.1 Overview of some important bones and muscles

▶ Storing minerals, especially calcium, important for neuromuscular function, and storing fats in the yellow bone marrow

▶ Acting as a framework to which muscles and tendons attach, allowing movement

Microscopic anatomy

Bones are a form of connective tissue made of two-thirds of a mixture of calcium salts, mostly calcium phosphate, and one-third of osteoid, an organic material made predominantly of bone cells and collagen fibres. Calcium salts give bones firmness, whereas collagen gives some slight flexibility.

There are three types of bone cells:

▶ **Osteoblasts**. These build bone by depositing calcium salts and osteoids in bone tissue.

▶ **Osteocytes**. Matured osteoblasts that have become trapped by new ones. Their function is to maintain bone tissue.

▶ **Osteoclasts**. Large cells which break down bone and ensure healthy remodelling of bones. Their activity is balanced with the bone-forming activity of osteoblasts.

Osteoblasts and osteocytes all originate from the osteoprogenitor cell, an active stem cell. Osteoclasts derive from the same lineage as white blood cells.

There are approximately 270 bones in infants, but the number reduces to 206–213 in adults as they fuse together. The fetal skeleton is initially made of **cartilage** before bone replaces the structure. Cartilage, compared to bone, is mainly made of water and has some resilience to return to its original shape. It has no blood vessels or nerves and is nourished by a surrounding layer of connective tissue.

Bone comprises **compact** and **spongy bone**, making up 80% and 20%, respectively, of the total bone mass. Compact bone (see Figure 3.5.2) consists of a number of central

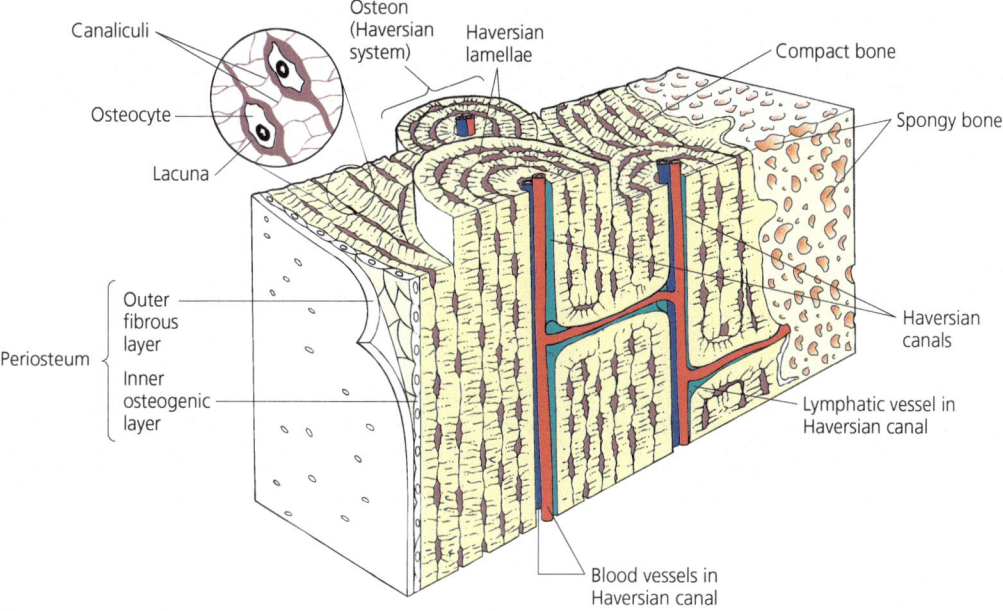

Figure 3.5.2 Magnified view of compact bone
Source: Figure 3.1(b), p.62, Clancy and McVicar (2009)

elongated canals, which contain blood, lymphatic vessels and nerves, surrounded by concentric rings, forming units all parallel to each other. The parallel structure running from one bulky end to another gives it strength. Within the small cavities in compact bone, osteocytes are found. Compact bone generally surrounds and protects spongy bone, which gets its name from its spongy, or honeycomb, structure. It consists of beams and plates surrounded by irregular cavities containing red bone marrow. Due to the different structure, spongy bone is much lighter than compact bone, and does not require vessels within central canals to nourish the osteocytes, as nourishment occurs by simple diffusion.

Macroscopic anatomy

Bones can be categorised by their shape into five groups (see Figure 3.5.3).

▶ **Long bones**, for example, femur, are generally found in limbs and are longer

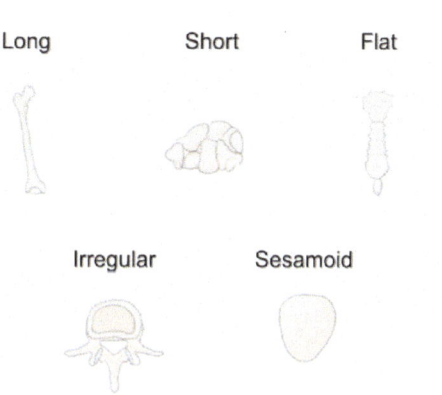

Figure 3.5.3 Five types of bones according to their shape

than they are wide. Long bones have a shaft and two bulky ends. The shaft (called diaphysis) contains mostly compact bone and has a hollow cavity that contains yellow bone marrow. The bulky ends (called epiphyses) are made of spongy bone wrapped by compact bone (see Figure 3.5.4). The shafts of long

163

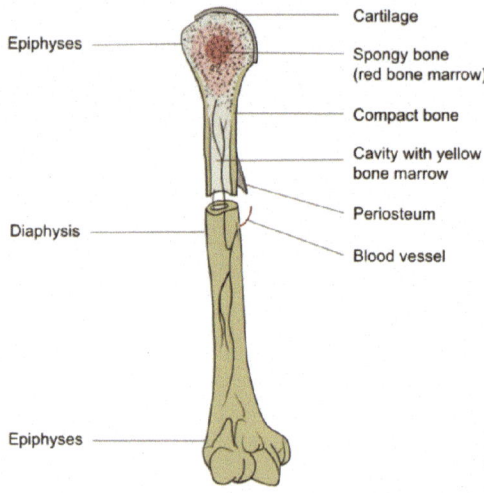

Cartilage

Epiphyses

Spongy bone
(red bone marrow)

Compact bone

Cavity with yellow
bone marrow

Periosteum

Diaphysis

Blood vessel

Epiphyses

Figure 3.5.4 Structure of a long bone

bones are protected by the periosteum, a
vascular membrane which also contains
cells responsible for bone production
and breakdown. The periosteum does
not fully line long bones, as at the level
of joint cavities it allows the tendons to
attach. Cartilage covers the bulky ends
of the bones to ensure a cushioning
function between opposing bones.

Short, flat, irregular and sesamoid bones
consist of red-marrow-containing spongy
bone surrounded by a layer of compact
bone. Similar to long bones, they are
covered by periosteum, with the exception

of the cranial bones' inner layer, which is
covered by dura mater.

▶ **Short bones**, are cuboidal in shape and
found in the hands and feet
▶ **Flat bones** include scapulae (shoulder
blades), skull and ribs
▶ **Irregular bones** include vertebrae,
sacrum and coccyx
▶ **Sesamoid bones** are round bones
usually found in the hands, feet and
knees (e.g. the patella)

Haematopoiesis in adults, the creation
of blood, occurs in the red bone marrow,
mostly in flat bones and the bulky ends of
the thigh and arm bones. During childhood,
red bone marrow is stored in the shafts of
long bones before becoming yellow bone
marrow around the age of 6–7 years.

Muscular system and tendons

Skeletal muscle was introduced in Chapter 1.2.
It is striated and its function is to move the
skeleton under voluntary nervous system
control. It also maintains body posture and
position, stabilises joints and generates heat.

Microscopic anatomy

Muscle fibres that make up skeletal
muscle are surrounded by a network
of connective tissue, blood vessels and
nerves (see Figure 3.5.5). In particular, each

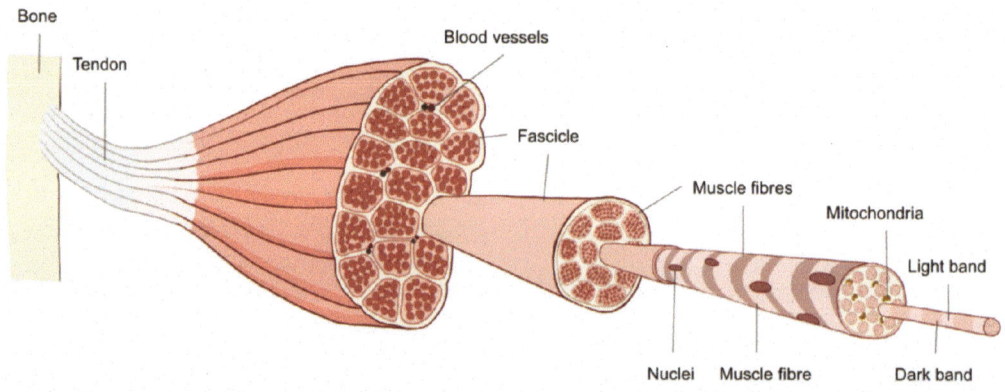

Bone

Tendon

Blood vessels

Fascicle

Muscle fibres

Mitochondria

Light band

Nuclei   Muscle fibre   Dark band

Figure 3.5.5 Organisation of skeletal muscle

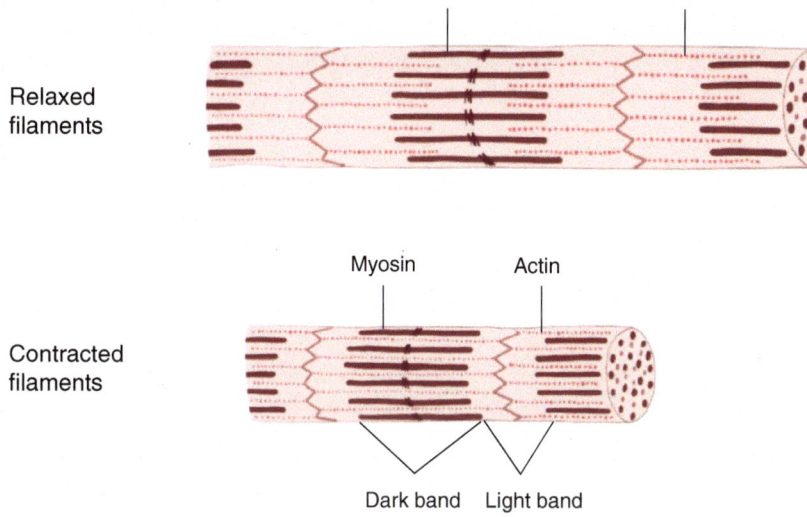

Relaxed filaments

Contracted filaments

Myosin

Actin

Myosin

Actin

Dark band   Light band

Figure 3.5.6 Relaxed and contracted fibres

bundle of muscle fibres, called fascicles, is covered by a connective tissue sheath, and each individual muscle cell is also enclosed within a layer of connective tissue throughout its whole length. This connective tissue layer provides some structure and, at both extremities, it merges with tendons, whose function is to connect muscle to bone. Tendons are stiffer than muscles and transmit the force generated by the contraction of muscles to the skeleton, which enables movement or maintenance of body posture.

On a more structural level, skeletal muscle cells have a cylindrical shape and run parallel to each other. Each individual cell can have a number of nuclei as they can be extremely long, up to 30 cm, although the vast majority are around 2–3 cm. Skeletal muscle fibres look striated because they contain myofilaments, the thick and dark ones are made of a protein called myosin. These also contain enzymes that can split energy-containing adenosine triphosphate (ATP) molecules to release energy and contract muscle. The thin and lighter in colour myofilaments are made of a protein

called actin. The extremities of the myosin filaments overlap with the actin filaments so they can allow contraction to occur (see Figure 3.5.6). A simplified version of this process is described below.

Contraction of the skeletal muscle cells occurs when a neurotransmitter called acetylcholine (ACh), is released (see Figure 3.5.7). The ACh release occurs at the neuromuscular junction, which is where the thin filaments of the nerve fibre (the axon) are approximated to the muscle cell; however, these two do not directly touch each other. Before ACh is released by the axon terminal, calcium is released from the intercellular stores and enters the axon; this allows the release of ACh towards the muscle fibres. Here, ACh causes the release of potassium ions and the entry of sodium ions into the muscle fibre, however, due to the greater intake of potassium ions, this causes depolarisation. The movement of ions causes an electrical current that travels from one end of the muscle fibres to the other, causing the muscle to contract. The muscle then relaxes when the released ACh is broken down by an enzyme. During

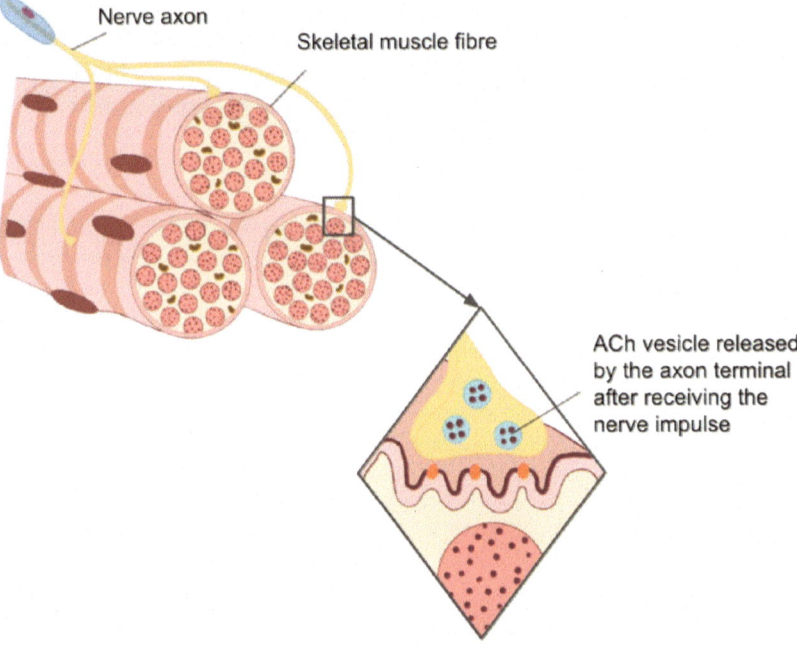

Nerve axon

Skeletal muscle fibre

ACh vesicle released
by the axon terminal
after receiving the
nerve impulse

Figure 3.5.7 Neuromuscular junction

contraction, actin and myosin bind to each other, and slide over each other, as shown in Figure 3.5.6. ATP (see Chapter 3.2) is broken down to give energy to actin and myosin, a process that also requires calcium ions. Calcium ions are released by the cells and trigger the actin and myosin to slide on each other. When the electrical current ends, calcium ions are returned to their stores, this causes actin and myosin to slide back to their original position and allows for the muscle to return to its resting state and initial length.

A more in-depth exploration of specific muscles related to pregnancy and childbirth can be found throughout the textbook, such as in Chapters 4.2 and 4.6.

Joints and ligaments

Joints, also called articulations, are the areas where two or more bones come together, and the bones' edges are bound together by connective tissue. Most joints are flexible and allow the body to

move, such as hip or shoulder joints, however, in some cases, the bones are so strongly held together that movement is impossible, for example, sutures between skull bones. There are three main types of joints: fibrous, cartilaginous and synovial:

▶ **Fibrous joints** are immoveable and do not allow for movement between the presenting bones. Functionally, the bones have fused together.

▶ **Cartilaginous joints** can also not allow for movement, but there are some exceptions, for example, the symphysis pubis that, when subject to pregnancy hormones, can expand. Functionally, these are semi-moveable.

▶ **Synovial joints** are the most moveable, and their main functions are to reduce friction and prevent wear due to bone-to-bone contact, as well as distribute weight. The parts of the bones facing each other are covered in hyaline cartilage to provide a smooth surface

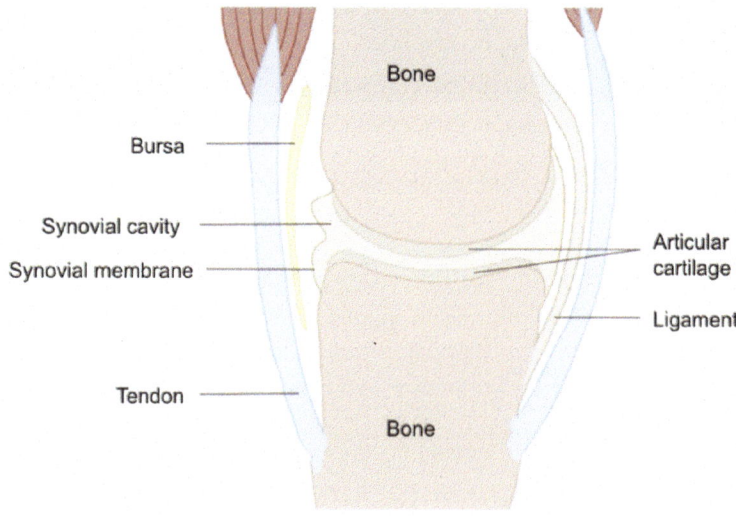

Figure 3.5.8 Synovial joint

and are surrounded by a synovial membrane containing synovial fluid. Its role is to ensure lubrication and the provision of nutrients to the joint cavity. The synovial membrane is wrapped further by the capsular ligament (see Figure 3.5.8). In some joints, there are additional sacs of synovial fluid, called bursae, which act as a cushion to prevent friction between structures such as the bone and the ligaments.

Ligaments are made of strong connective tissue and often connect bones to other bones. Ligaments can be described as 'straps', and their function is to stabilise the bones and the joint to ensure there is no excessive movement that could cause a dislocation. Ligaments can also be found around internal organs, and their function here is to keep them in place. For example, ligaments are responsible for keeping the uterus and other structures in the right position within the pelvis. The broad ligaments, see Figure 3.5.9, are a double-layer of peritoneum that hang like sheets from the fallopian tubes and

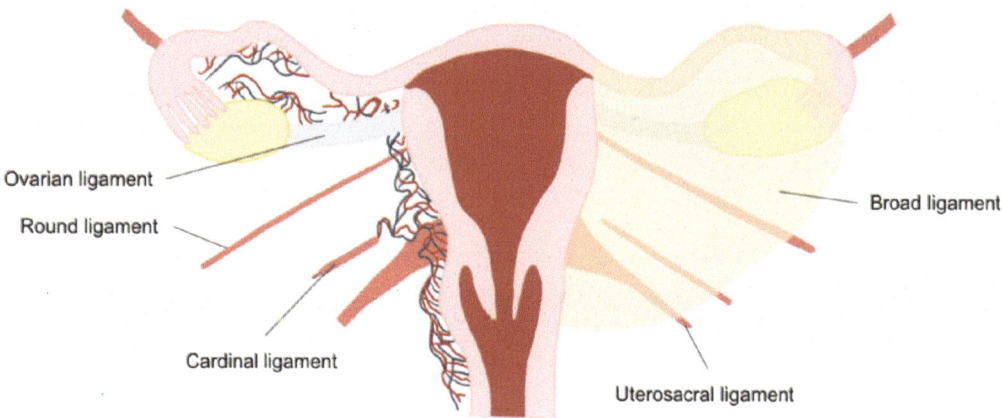

Figure 3.5.9 Ligaments of the uterus

are attached to the pelvis by their sides. Broad ligaments enclose the ovaries, the major blood vessels and nerves to the reproductive organs and other ligaments, as well as the fallopian tubes. For example, round ligaments and uterosacral ligaments are included within the broad ligaments, these both originate from the uterus and respectively reach the labia majora and the sacrum. Other important ligaments include the cardinal ligaments, which connect the cervix/vagina to the sides of the pelvis, and the pubocervical ligaments, which extend from the cardinal ligaments, go around the bladder and attach to the pubic bones. However, it is important to note that only uterosacral ligaments, cardinal ligaments and pubocervical ligaments help keep the uterus in the pelvis, whereas broad ligaments and round ligaments act as secondary support.

Changes and adaptations during pregnancy

Physical changes due to pregnancy

Weight gain in pregnancy, including the weight of the growing uterus, causes a shift in the woman's centre of gravity, which causes the pelvis to tilt forward. The woman's lower back, the lumbar portion of the spine, which is already normally curved anteriorly, due to the effect of the hormones and the shifting centre of gravity, becomes even more curved, also known as **lumbar lordosis**. This could cause lower back pain and strained muscles. In addition to this, women might also extend their necks, hold their shoulders backwards and present a waddling gait when walking. The growing uterus, especially towards the end of the pregnancy, can also compress nerves or blood vessels, resulting in tingling or numbness of the limbs. Leg cramps or restless leg syndrome can also present in pregnancy.

Bone composition is potentially challenged by pregnancy, as calcium, which is needed to make bones strong, is in high demand by the growing fetus. The maternal body adapts to enable more calcium absorption, but circulating calcium levels are generally lower in the mother than in the fetus, suggesting that calcium is crossing the placenta to promote fetal skeletal mineralisation. On the maternal side, there might be a rise in calcium storage to prepare for lactation, as the bone mineral density falls. To protect maternal bone health at this time, oestrogen inhibits osteoclasts (slowing bone reabsorption) and promotes osteoblasts (responsible for new bone). Unless the dietary intake of calcium is inadequate, dietary supplementation does not increase bone density. It has, however, been shown to decrease blood pressure and reduce the rate of pre-eclampsia (Hofmeyr et al., 2019). This is likely because calcium controls the contractility of smooth muscle cells in the blood vessels, which in turn, adjusts peripheral vascular resistance. It is important to note that, despite the fall in calcium levels during lactation, this does not lead to permanent osteoporosis when breastfeeding is prolonged.

Increased levels of progesterone, oestrogen and relaxin in pregnancy have an impact on the cartilage and connective tissue present in **joints**, making these **laxer** with the goal of preparing the woman's body for childbirth. For example, the symphysis pubis and the sacroiliac joints (see Chapter 4.1) become more flexible to allow the pelvis to expand in diameter, and this can cause muscle and ligament strain.

APPLICATION TO PRACTICE

Pelvic girdle pain

Pelvic girdle pain (PGP), also known as symphysis pubis dysfunction (SPD), occurs when the pubic bones, under the effect of relaxin and oestrogen, have increased mobility and separate. Women are likely to report burning or stabbing pain on the symphysis pubis, but the pain can radiate to the inner thigh area (see Figure 3.5.10). Around one-fifth of pregnant women may suffer from PGP, and a high body mass index (BMI,) smoking and multiparity are some of the risk factors that can accelerate its onset. Some women might alter the way they move, by adopting a sideways motion, or require the use of crutches to reduce weight-bearing activities to improve the situation. A prompt referral to the physiotherapy service may be recommended.

Ligament pain

The most common type of ligament pain that can be experienced by pregnant women is round ligament pain. This can present as a sharp or stabbing pain that affects one side or both, around the lower abdomen and groin area, and should resolve spontaneously. This occurs because the round ligament stretches, growing

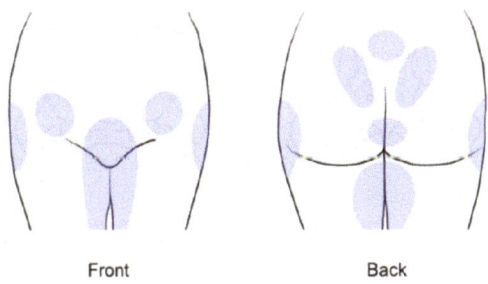

Front   Back

Figure 3.5.10 Pelvic girdle pain areas

3.5

in length and diameter; for this reason, it is considered a physiological pain in pregnancy.

Varicosities

Varicose veins can affect between 20% and 40% of pregnant women, and they develop because of two main pregnancy adaptations. Anatomically, the growing uterus can compress veins from the lower part of the body and reduce the venous return, creating congestion and more pressure on the veins. Hormonally, high levels of progesterone have a relaxing effect on smooth muscle, which causes vasodilation of the blood vessels. Together, anatomical and hormonal changes cause an incomplete valve closure at the level of the veins, leading to backflow of blood and stasis (see Figure 3.5.11). Varicose veins are more likely to be seen on lower limbs but can also occur in the pelvic area as vulvar varicosities and haemorrhoids. When affecting the legs, it is recommended that women wear compression stockings, mobilise regularly and elevate the legs when possible. Haemorrhoids occur because of the same mechanism described above, plus constipation that affects many pregnant women. Haemorrhoids affect around 30% of pregnancies, women may report pain and a burning sensation in the area. Topical medications might be applied in pregnancy, and haemorrhoids are likely to resolve postnatally. Vulvar varicosities are rare but can be extremely painful. Relief to the congested area can be achieved by lifting the lower body and avoiding standing for long periods. Congested vulvar varicosities can bleed significantly during birth if trauma occurs to the tissues.

Carpal tunnel syndrome

This syndrome occurs when the median nerve, which innervates the thumb, index,

169

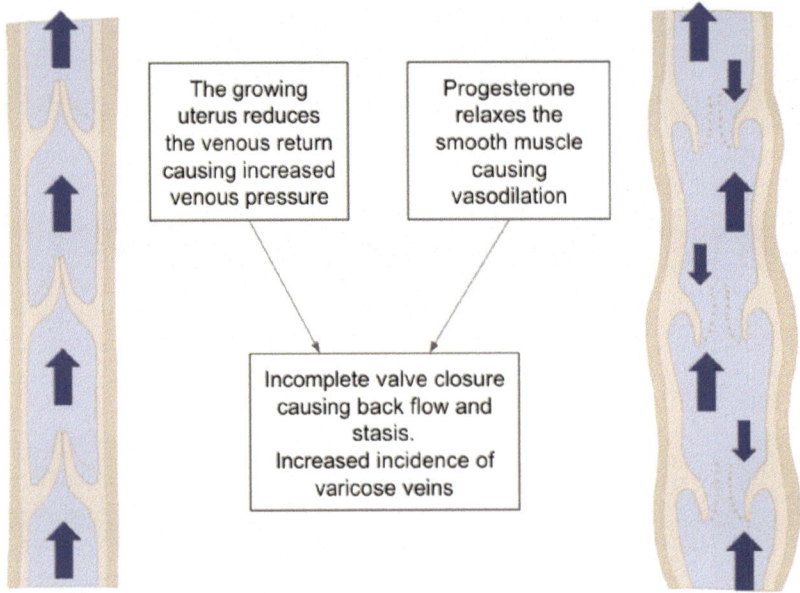

The growing uterus reduces the venous return causing increased venous pressure

Progesterone relaxes the smooth muscle causing vasodilation

Incomplete valve closure causing back flow and stasis.
Increased incidence of varicose veins

Figure 3.5.11 Varicose veins in pregnancy

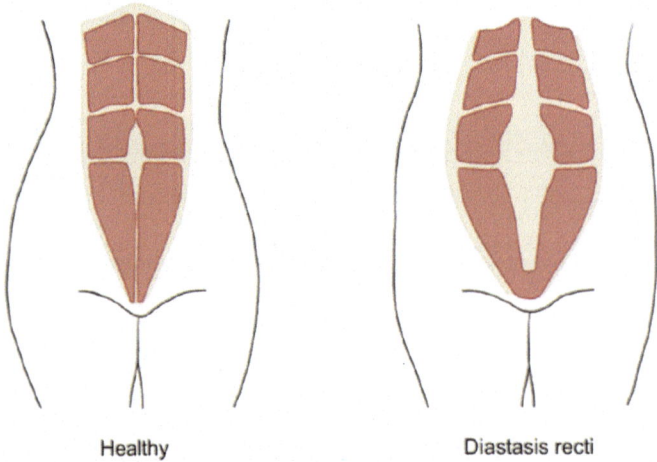

Healthy

Diastasis recti

Figure 3.5.12 Diastasis recti

middle and ring fingers, is compressed in the wrist as it passes through the carpal tunnel. It can affect up to 50% of pregnant women, mostly in the second and third trimesters. As the top of the carpal tunnel is made of connective tissue, it is stiff; therefore, it does not allow much flexibility to stretch. Due to hormonal changes in pregnancy and the build-up of fluid around the body, there is an increase in pressure on the median nerve, causing carpal tunnel syndrome. Women might experience pain, tingling or numbness, affecting mostly the first four digits of the hand. Women may be advised to wear a splint and raise the affected hand at night to reduce the swelling.

Diastasis recti

Diastasis recti, also known as divarication of the recti, is the increased distance between the muscles that run vertically down the middle of the abdomen due to weakness of the abdominal wall. This occurs in pregnancy due to the pressure of the growing uterus causing the linea alba, the connective tissue band that connects the sternum to the pubic bone and the abdominal muscles, to stretch and separate (see Figure 3.5.12).

Reference

Hofmeyr G., Betran A. et al. Prepregnancy and early pregnancy calcium supplementation among women at high risk of pre-eclampsia: a multicentre, double-blind, randomised, placebo-controlled trial. *Lancet* [Internet] 2019, 393:330–9. www.thelancet.com/journals/lancet/article/PIIS0140-6736(18)31818-X/fulltext#%2.

3.5

Further reading

Fiat F., Merghes P. et al. The main changes in pregnancy – Therapeutic approach to musculoskeletal pain. *Medicina (Kaunas)* [Internet] 2022, 58(8):1115. www.ncbi.nlm.nih.gov/pmc/articles/PMC9414568/.

The renal system

Jane Carpenter and Louise Hunter

LEARNING OUTCOMES

▶ Describe the structure and function of the renal system
▶ Understand the key processes in the kidney which lead to the formation of urine
▶ Understand how urine moves from the kidneys to the bladder, and then out of the body
▶ Explain the key changes to the renal system in pregnancy, and apply these to practice

Renal system overview

Structure and function of the renal system

The renal system is composed of the kidneys, ureters, urinary bladder and urethra (see Figure 3.6.1). The kidneys are a pair of bean-shaped, purplish-brown organs situated just below the ribs towards the middle of the back. In an adult, they are roughly fist sized. The right kidney is located

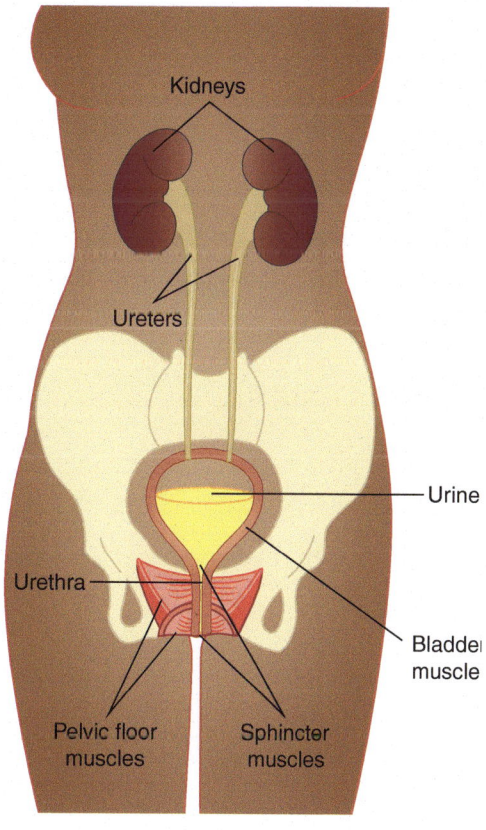

Figure 3.6.1 The renal system

DOI: 10.4324/9781003227571-17

a little lower than the left as it is displaced by the liver. Each kidney is attached to a tube, or ureter, which leads down to the top of the bladder. The bladder is situated at the brim of the pelvis, in front of the uterus and vagina. A further tube, the urethra, extends from the base of the bladder to the urethral opening located in an area between the labia minora, known as the vestibule.

A key function of the renal system is to maintain homeostasis of body fluids, ensuring optimal volume and composition. This is achieved by filtering out excess and unwanted substances, maintaining acid-base balance, and either conserving or eliminating excess fluid and solutes from the body as urine, via the bladder. Waste solutes can include byproducts of metabolism, inactivated or 'used' hormones, and dietary substances that are either of no biochemical value or cannot be stored (such as water-soluble vitamins and minerals).

The renal system has a number of other essential functions, most of which are undertaken by the kidney.

The kidneys

The kidneys have a number of important functions in addition to producing urine:

▶ Regulation of fluid and electrolyte balance
▶ Excretion of waste and toxic chemicals
▶ Regulation of blood pressure
▶ Control of formation of red blood cells
▶ Conversion of vitamin D to its active form

We will explore many of these functions throughout this chapter, although the focus will be on the homeostatic functions of regulation of fluid and electrolyte balance and excretion of waste.

Kidney structure

In order to understand how the kidney functions, it is important to explore its internal structure. This can be seen in Figure 3.6.2.

▶ The outer surface of each kidney is formed of a connective tissue capsule.
▶ Beneath this is the **cortex**, which supports an extensive vascular system and contains over a million **nephrons**.
▶ Under the cortex is the **medulla**. There are around eight **renal pyramids**, or lobes in the medulla.
▶ At the centre of each kidney, attached to the ureter, is the **renal pelvis**.

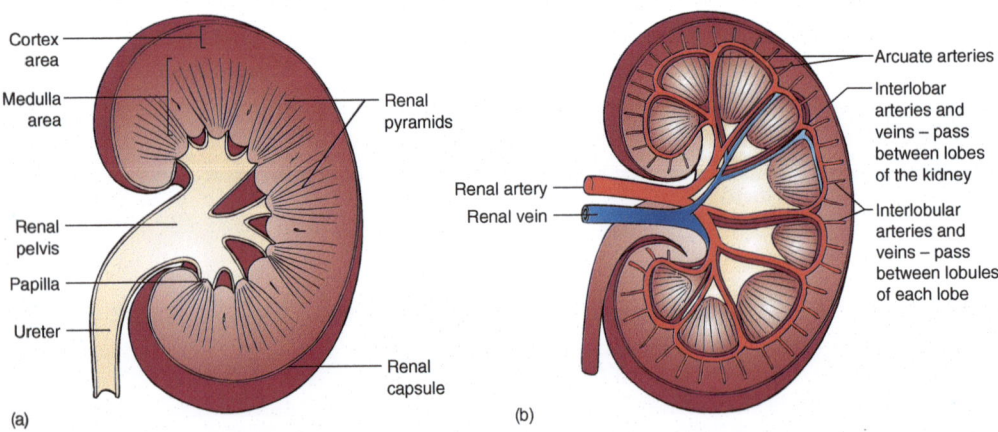

Figure 3.6.2 a) Anatomy of the kidney; b) Vasculature of the kidney
Source: Figure 15.3(a) and (b), p.424, Clancy and McVicar (2009)

Blood supply to the kidney is via the **renal artery**, which branches off from the abdominal aorta. Blood leaves the kidney via the **renal vein**, which drains directly into the vena cava.

Kidney function: Fluid homeostasis and excretion of waste

In this functional role, the kidneys are essentially filtration beds, and this filtration occurs via the nephron. Via this complex process, the kidneys can regulate volume, pH and electrolyte balance as well as excrete waste products. For ease of learning, this has been broken down into a number of steps, essentially following the structure of the nephron. In reality, this is one continuous process, constantly changing and adapting to the needs of the body:

Step 1: The glomerulus

Step 2: The proximal convoluted tubule

Step 3: The loop of the nephron (Loop of Henle)

Step 4: The distal convoluted tubule

Step 5: The collecting ducts

Step 6: Peritubular capillaries and vasa recta

The structures of the nephron and its associated blood supply are shown in Figure 3.6.3, which should be referred back to throughout the following sections.

3.6

Step 1: The glomerulus

Around 1.2 L of blood (about 20% of cardiac output) enters the kidneys every minute via the **renal artery**, which stems directly from the aorta (See Figure 3.6.2b). The renal artery branches into a number of vessels that carry blood between the renal pyramids to the cortex of the kidney, where it is diverted into smaller and smaller vessels, or arterioles. These culminate in an **afferent arteriole**, which leads into a nephron. The blood travelling within the afferent arteriole enters the **glomerulus**, a ball of blood

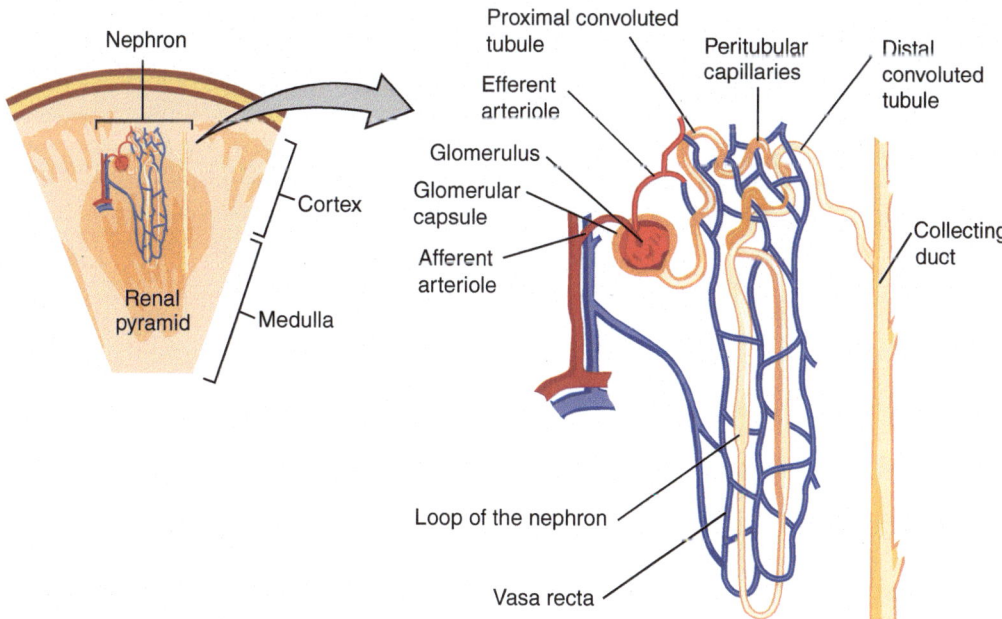

Figure 3.6.3 Process of filtration and urine formation in the kidney

capillaries that provides a large surface area for filtration.

The glomerulus is highly adapted to its function; the capillaries in each glomerulus are **fenestrated** – they have tiny holes in them. These holes are large enough to allow the passage of small molecules such as glucose, electrolytes, waste products and water, but stop larger proteins such as immune cells and blood cells from entering. The larger molecules and blood cells remain inside the capillary and travel out of the glomerulus via the **efferent arteriole**. The smaller molecules which pass through the fenestrations are known as '**the filtrate**', and we will continue on our journey through the nephron with the filtrate, returning to consider what happens to the remaining blood in our efferent arteriole later.

Each glomerulus is situated within the cup or goblet-shaped structure of the **glomerular (Bowman's) capsule**. The glomerular capsule also has pores between its cells, meaning that the two layers of cells (of the glomerulus and glomerular capsule) with a permeable basement membrane between them, enable the passage of the filtrate from the glomerulus into the glomerular capsule of the nephron. This filtration occurs surprisingly quickly and in a surprisingly large volume – for a young adult, the **glomerular filtration rate** (GFR) is around 125 ml/min.

Step 2: The proximal convoluted tubule

From the glomerular capsule, the filtrate funnels into a tube known as the **proximal convoluted tubule** (proximal = 'nearer', convoluted = 'intricately folded'). As we have already determined, it is quite some volume of filtrate which has moved from the bloodstream into the nephron and is now moving into the proximal convoluted tubule. The convolutions increase the surface area of this

section of the nephron, and microvilli on the inner surface further increase the surface area. This supports the key function of the proximal convoluted tubule – which is **tubular reabsorption**. Thus, via active transport, much of the filtrate is reabsorbed via the interstitium into the peritubular capillaries. Indeed, approximately 65% of water, sodium, potassium and chloride, 100% of glucose, 100% amino acids and 85–90% of bicarbonate is reabsorbed during this step.

Step 3: The loop of the nephron

The next step on the journey is the **loop of the nephron** (loop of Henle). A long, thin descending loop makes its way from the cortex into the medulla, before a narrow hairpin bend in the tube and a thicker ascending loop returns to the cortex. The remaining filtrate (although most has already been reabsorbed in the previous step) makes its way around this loop. Here, an interesting concept comes into play – that of '**countercurrent multiplication**'.

As the filtrate moves through the descending loop into the medulla, the surrounding interstitial fluid is highly concentrated – more concentrated than any other tissue in the body. Therefore, remaining water in the filtrate passes out into the surrounding fluid via osmosis. The remaining filtrate in the loop is now highly concentrated.

As the filtrate then moves through the ascending limb, solutes, in particular sodium ions, are pumped out of the loop by active transport (causing the highly concentrated interstitial fluid which caused the osmotic effect in the descending limb). However, the ascending loop is not permeable to water and so osmosis does not continue here. As the solutes are pumped out, the remaining fluid in the ascending loop becomes less concentrated again. By the time it reaches the end of the loop of the nephron, the filtrate is dilute and about 85% of the filtrate overall has been reabsorbed.

Step 4: The distal convoluted tubule

Now back in the cortex, the filtrate moves into the **distal convoluted tubule** (distal = 'furthest'). Here, the movement of solutes into the interstitial fluid via active transport continues. At this point, the permeability of the tubule to water can be modified, and this modification is under the influence of antidiuretic hormone (ADH). If dehydrated, ADH will increase the permeability of the tubule and thus, water will be reabsorbed into surrounding interstitial fluid via osmosis, leaving a more concentrated fluid in the tubule. Without the action of ADH, the permeability of the tubule remains low, and so any remaining water in the tubule stays there.

Step 5: The collecting ducts

From the distal convoluted tubule, the filtrate moves through a collecting tubule into the collecting duct. Several tubules will connect to a single collecting duct. This collecting duct descends back into the medulla. This duct has variable permeability to water, and it is here that the final concentration of the fluid, now urine, is determined. If ADH was acting on the distal convoluted tubule and collecting tubule, this permeability to water continues in the collecting duct, leading to a small volume of very concentrated urine – particularly as the medulla has the very high solute concentration in the surrounding interstitial fluid. If permeability of the distal tubule was low, then this continues in the collecting duct and water cannot pass out of the duct, leading to a higher volume of dilute urine.

The urine passes out of the duct into the renal pelvis, and then drains into the ureter.

Step 6: Peritubular capillaries and vasa recta

Now we return to our efferent arteriole. Back at Step 1 we followed our filtrate as it moved into the glomerular capsule of the nephron – but what happens to the larger molecules and blood cells which remained in the efferent arteriole? Figure 3.6.3 shows the efferent arteriole moving into the **peritubular capillaries** and **vasa recta**. It can be seen how this network of vessels moves in, around and between the nephrons. Peritubular capillaries surround parts of the proximal and distal tubules in the cortex, while the vasa recta go into the medulla to approach the loop of the nephron. This allows ongoing tubular reabsorption and **tubular secretion**. As solutes and water either move or are pumped out of the nephron, they can be reabsorbed by the peritubular capillaries and vasa recta. Equally, these vessels can continue to secrete into the interstitial fluid and nephron; this can include waste products such as creatinine, many drugs, toxins and poisons, and much of the urea that was reabsorbed into the blood in the proximal tubule. These vessels then unite into a venule and return to the renal vein.

Kidney function: Regulation of blood pressure

Another key function of the kidney is its role in the regulation of blood pressure, which happens via the Renin-Angiotensin-Aldosterone System (RAAS).

If blood pressure falls below a certain threshold, which the kidneys will detect as a decrease in blood flow to them, they will release the enzyme **renin** into the bloodstream. Renin acts on **angiotensinogen**, a large protein that circulates in the bloodstream which produces **angiotensin I**. Angiotensin I is relatively inactive, but **angiotensin-converting**

enzyme (ACE) converts angiotensin I to the hormone **angiotensin II**.

Angiotensin II causes the muscular walls of arterioles to constrict, and this increases blood pressure. In addition, angiotensin II triggers the release of the hormone **aldosterone** from the adrenal glands and ADH from the pituitary gland, as well as triggering thirst, encouraging drinking to add fluid volume.

Aldosterone causes the kidneys to retain sodium and excrete potassium. The increased sodium causes water to be retained, thus increasing blood volume and blood pressure. ADH, as discussed previously, also causes water to be retained at the point of the distal convoluted tubule and collecting ducts, which also then increases blood volume and blood pressure.

INTERRUPTER

Using the appropriate section of the workbook (or your own paper) draw your own flow diagram of the RAAS to show how this mechanism works to maintain blood pressure.

APPLICATION TO PRACTICE

ACE-inhibitor hypertension medication

Hypertension (high blood pressure) is highly relevant in midwifery practice, due to the potential for development of pre-eclampsia and then eclampsia during the perinatal period. Midwives become very familiar with the recognition and management of raised blood pressure during pregnancy – and the range of medications available to manage hypertension.

ACE-inhibitors are one such type of medication – and their name gives a strong clue to their method of action! Indeed, these medications do inhibit the action of ACE, which then inhibits the conversion of angiotensin I to angiotensin II. This then stops the later stages of the RAAS and hence, lowers blood pressure.

Other functions of the kidney

Juxtaglomerular cells (juxta = next to) in the kidney produce erythropoietin, a hormone which causes the bone marrow to increase production of red blood cells. Therefore, the kidney has an important role in controlling the formation of red blood cells, meaning the kidney regulates both the volume of the blood and the number of red blood cells. This is important, as maintaining the optimal ratio of these two enables maximal oxygen delivery.

The kidney also converts vitamin D to its active form. Vitamin D is either synthesised in the skin or ingested in the diet and is then transported to the liver where it is metabolised into a metabolite of vitamin D for storage. The kidney converts this metabolite to the active form, where it plays a role in the reabsorption of calcium.

APPLICATION TO PRACTICE

Urine

Human urine is around 95% water, 2% urea (a byproduct of amino acid metabolism), 0.1% creatinine and 0.03% uric acid. It also contains very small amounts of chloride, sodium, potassium, sulphate, ammonium, phosphate and other ions and molecules.

As the end product of a complex filtration process, a person's urine can tell us something about their state of health:

▶ If very little urine (less than 30 ml an hour) is being produced, then either the person is dehydrated (deep yellow and concentrated urine) or in renal failure.

▶ Urine can be deep yellow (due to the presence of urochromes produced by the breakdown of old blood cells) to almost colourless if someone is very well hydrated. It is usually clear but can sometimes be a little cloudy due to the presence of mucins secreted by the urinary tract lining. It can be affected by pigments in food – eating beetroot or blackberries, for example, can result in reddish coloured urine.

▶ Unusually coloured urine can indicate a health problem: some urinary tract infections can turn urine milky white. Conditions such as kidney stones, and some cancers, can cause blood to be present in urine, turning it red. Dark or orange urine can indicate liver failure.

▶ Urine has a characteristic odour and will start to smell of ammonia if it is very concentrated or is left standing for a while. Ammonia-smelling urine can also be a sign of a urinary tract infection. If urine smells sugary or fruity, this could indicate diabetes or hyperglycaemia, both of which will result in the body excreting excess glucose. If someone eats asparagus, sulphur byproducts are produced in the digestion process which can give their urine a distinctive smell. Coffee, alcohol and medicines can also give urine a different smell.

▶ Protein should not be able to pass through the glomeruli into the filtrate. Its presence in urine usually results from kidney damage or high blood pressure, which forces larger molecules into the glomerular capsule (which can then cause kidney damage). Proteinuria can be a sign of kidney damage or infection, fever, strenuous exercise, high blood pressure and pre-eclampsia.

3.6

After the kidneys

In Step 5, above, the urine had passed from the renal pelvis into the ureter. We now continue the journey of urine through the rest of the renal system.

Ureters

The ureters are narrow tubes composed mainly of smooth muscle, which carry urine from the kidneys to the bladder. The smooth muscle cells continually tighten and relax in a peristaltic motion, forcing the urine downwards. Small amounts of urine are emptied into the bladder from the ureters approximately every 10–15 seconds.

Micturition

Micturition is the process of excretion of urine from the **bladder** via the **urethra**. There are two discrete phases to micturition, the **continence phase** where urine collects and is stored in the bladder and the **voiding phase**, where urine is released through the urethra.

Continence phase

The bladder is a hollow organ composed of a wall of specialised smooth muscle called **detrusor muscle** (Figure 3.6.4). The fibres of the detrusor muscle run in multiple directions, allowing the bladder to retain structural integrity when stretched and enabling it to reduce in both length and diameter to ensure efficient and effective emptying when in the voiding phase. The muscle has an inner lining of epithelial cells which are folded into rugae when the

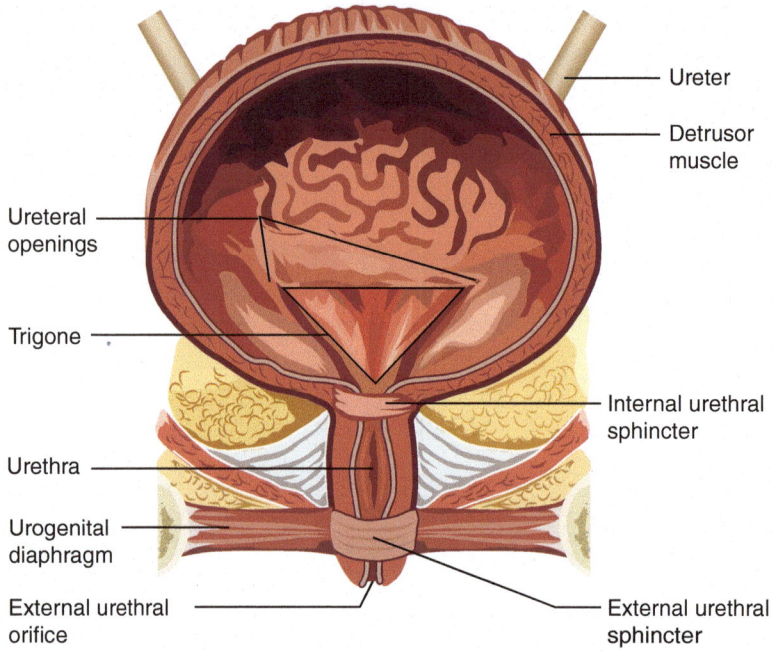

Figure 3.6.4 The bladder

bladder is empty and flatten but do not tear when it is full. The area between the ureter entry points and the urethral exit, known as the **trigone**, lacks rugae. Its smooth, funnel-shaped surface facilitates bladder emptying. An adult female bladder can hold around 500 ml of urine, although the sensation of needing to urinate will be triggered at around 250 ml of urine.

The storage of urine during the continence phase requires relaxation of the detrusor muscle and contraction of both the internal and external urethral sphincters. This is controlled by the sympathetic nervous system in the case of the detrusor and internal urethral sphincter, and the somatic nervous system for the external urethral sphincter. As filling continues, pressure in the bladder rises, eventually signalling a sensation of needing to pass urine. Pain receptors will be activated if this is ignored, and the bladder will continue to fill.

Voiding phase

Movement of the urine out of the bladder is controlled by two sphincters, the **internal urethral sphincter** at the neck of the bladder, under the control of the autonomic nervous system, and the **external urethral sphincter** formed by the pelvic floor which is under voluntary control. When voluntary muscles release the external sphincter and allow urination to commence, the detrusor muscle contracts and the internal sphincter dilates. Urine will then pass out of the bladder and down the urethra to the urethral opening located in an area between the labia minora. The urethra is lined with stratified columnar epithelium and is protected from the corrosive urine by mucus secreting glands.

In females, the urethra is 3–5 cm long, whereas in males it is much longer (15–20 cm). This makes women more vulnerable to urinary tract infections such as cystitis, as the distance is much shorter for bacteria to travel from the anus and enter the bladder via the urethra.

Changes and adaptations during pregnancy

During pregnancy, the kidneys adapt to cope with increased blood flow, and to ensure that the right mix of substrates is available to the growing fetus. Perhaps the most noticeable difference is the increase of sodium (essential for fetal development) in the circulation, which goes hand in hand with fluid retention. Women with pre-existing kidney disease are more likely to struggle with the normal physiological changes of pregnancy, and can develop high blood pressure early on:

- Rising **oestrogen** levels in pregnancy trigger **increased amounts of the hormone angiotensin II** to be produced. Angiotensin II increases thirst and a desire for salt and stimulates the release of other hormones involved in fluid retention such as aldosterone, which causes the retention of sodium and loss of potassium from the kidneys. Angiotensin II also causes vasoconstriction, increasing blood pressure. This may go some way to compensate for the relaxing effect of progesterone on vessel walls.
- **ADH** tends to be released at lower plasma osmolarity in pregnancy. This change is thought to be triggered by hCG and further contributes to enhanced fluid retention. Retained fluid will cause sodium to be pulled into the circulation due to osmolarity.
- Increased fluid retention is probably responsible for the increased blood volume needed in pregnancy. As a result of the additional volume, **blood flow through the kidneys increases** by up to 50%. To cope with this, the kidneys,

which are usually around 10 cm long, enlarge by around 1 cm in length and 30% in volume.

- Increased blood volume produces a **rise in GFR** and a fall in the blood concentration of substances such as creatinine and urea, which are excreted in proportion to the filtration rate. It is thought that the improved removal of these substances facilitates their removal from the fetus across the placenta.
- Paradoxically, serum creatinine and urea levels in urine also fall – if prepregnant levels are maintained this can indicate renal impairment or pre-eclampsia.
- Increased GFR and fluid and sodium retention can also result in drugs being excreted differently from the body, so long term medications may need to be modified.
- Circulating **glucose can increase** later in pregnancy when women can become insulin resistant. Like sodium, glucose is crucial for fetal growth and development. More circulating glucose and increased GFR lead to increased levels of glucose in filtrate. However, there is a reduction of the number of transport sites in the proximal tubule, meaning that it may not be able to reabsorb all of the glucose in the filtrate, leading to glucose being present in the urine (glycosuria). Glycosuria can also be indicative of high levels of plasma glucose, a symptom of diabetes.
- High levels of glucose in urine make it a breeding ground for bacteria, increasing the likelihood of a urinary tract infection (UTI).
- Rising **progesterone** levels in pregnancy affect smooth muscle tone, including in the ureters and bladder. Peristaltic contractions in the ureters are likely to be less efficient. The ureters also elongate and can curve and twist and

are further displaced as the uterus grows and pushes on the bladder. This can alter the angle at which the ureters enter the bladder and allow urine to track back up towards the kidneys. Decreased muscle tone in the bladder almost doubles its capacity and can result in incomplete emptying. These ureter and bladder changes increase the likelihood of urine staying in the body for longer, which increases the chance of a UTI.

▶ In early pregnancy (when the uterus is still in the pelvic cavity) and towards the end of pregnancy, the enlarged uterus can press down on the bladder, reducing its capacity and causing urinary frequency.

Further reading

Sparks M.A., Crowley S.D. et al. Classical renin-angiotensin system in kidney physiology. *Compr. Physiol.* 2014, 4(3):1201–28. https://pubmed.ncbi.nlm. nih.gov/24944035/.

The gastrointestinal system

Claire Smith

LEARNING OUTCOMES

- ▶ Describe the structure and function of the gastrointestinal system
- ▶ Understand the difference between peristalsis and segmentation
- ▶ Understand key changes to the gastrointestinal system during pregnancy, and apply this to practice
- ▶ Describe the importance of nutrition during pregnancy
- ▶ Understand key macronutrients and micronutrients, and how requirements change in pregnancy

Gastrointestinal system overview

Structure

Often known as 'the gut' or alimentary canal, the gastrointestinal tract (GIT) is a

tube of approximately 9 metres in length. It begins at the mouth, passes through the chest, abdomen and pelvis, and ends at the anus. Its principal function is the processing of ingested food.

The GIT consists of the mouth, pharynx, oesophagus, stomach, small intestine, large intestine, rectum and anus. Additionally, there are several **accessory organs** which are essential to its functioning including the salivary glands, liver, gallbladder and pancreas (see Figure 3.7.1).

Blood supply

The GIT has a rich blood supply from branches of the abdominal aorta, the coeliac artery, the superior mesenteric artery and the inferior mesenteric artery (see Figure 3.7.2). The portal vein is the main vessel draining blood from the GIT, transporting venous blood to the liver.

DOI: 10.4324/9781003227571-18

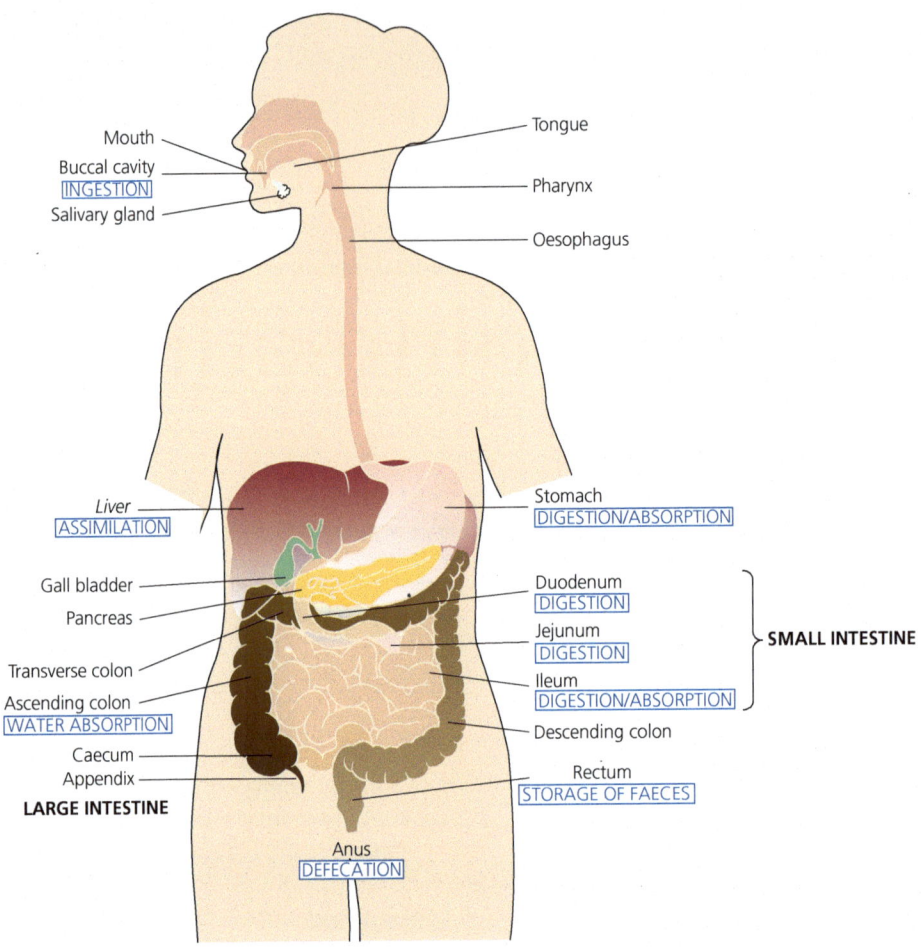

Mouth
Buccal cavity
INGESTION
Salivary gland

Tongue

Pharynx

Oesophagus

Liver
ASSIMILATION

Gall bladder
Pancreas

Transverse colon

Ascending colon
WATER ABSORPTION

Caecum
Appendix
LARGE INTESTINE

Stomach
DIGESTION/ABSORPTION

Duodenum
DIGESTION

Jejunum
DIGESTION

Ileum
DIGESTION/ABSORPTION

SMALL INTESTINE

Descending colon

Rectum
STORAGE OF FAECES

Anus
DEFECATION

Figure 3.7.1 The gastrointestinal tract

Nervous system supply

Extrinsic or autonomic system: this is external to the bowel. It contains parasympathetic nerves that stimulate movement and activity, and sympathetic nerves that inhibit movement and activity.

Intrinsic or enteric system: this internal system, embedded in the gut walls, is often known as the 'brain of the stomach'. It is composed of two plexi (branching networks of nerves) – the Meissner and the Auerbach – which regulate

segment-to-segment movement along the GIT. They produce peristaltic waves, and coordinate gut secretions and blood flow.

Physiology

Each element of the GIT plays a specialised role in the ingestion, digestion and/or absorption or excretion of food.

The mouth

The mouth, or buccal/oral cavity, is where food is ingested (Figure 3.7.3). It is comprised of:

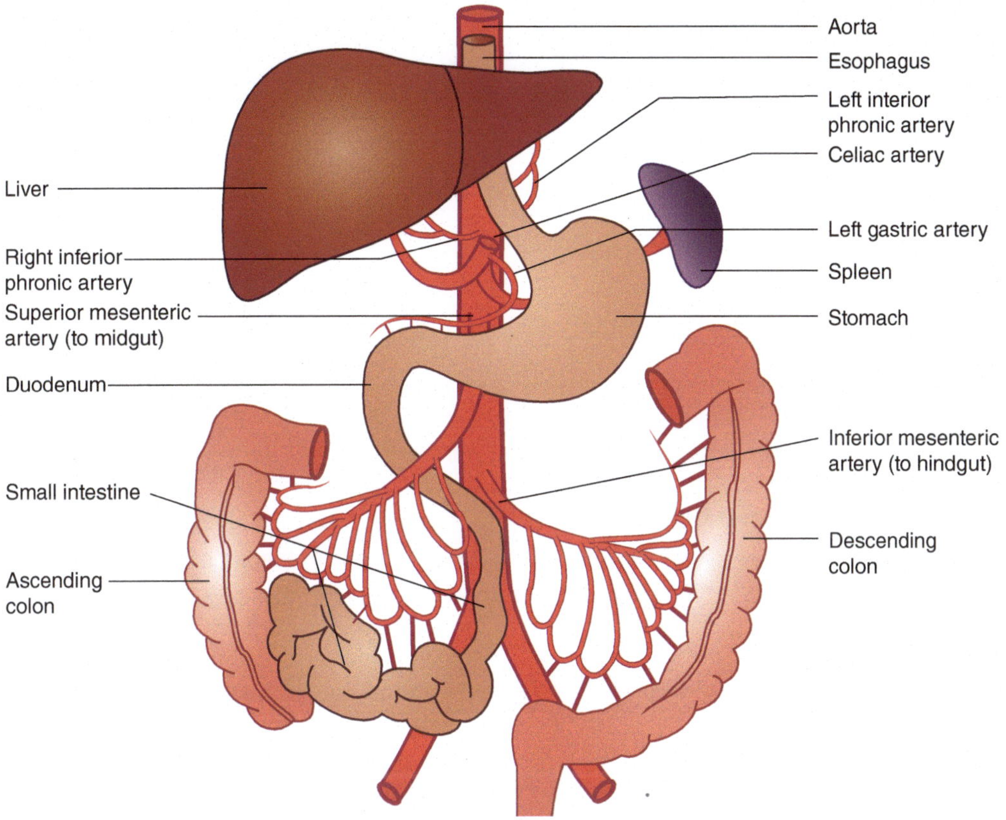

3.7

Aorta

Esophagus

Left interior phronic artery

Celiac artery

Liver

Left gastric artery

Right inferior phronic artery

Spleen

Superior mesenteric artery (to midgut)

Stomach

Duodenum

Inferior mesenteric artery (to hindgut)

Small intestine

Descending colon

Ascending colon

Figure 3.7.2 Blood supply to the GIT

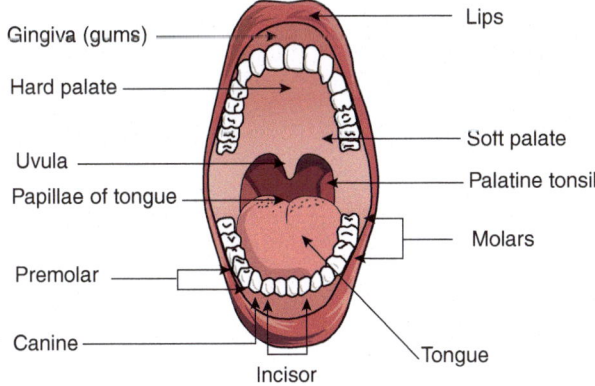

Gingiva (gums)

Lips

Hard palate

Uvula

Soft palate

Papillae of tongue

Palatine tonsil

Premolar

Molars

Canine

Tongue

Incisor

Figure 3.7.3 The mouth (oral cavity)

- **Lips and cheeks** – these help keep food in the mouth. Sensory receptors in the lips judge the temperature and texture of food.
- **Teeth** – Incisors and canines pierce and cut, and molars grind ingested food to break it down and form it into a bolus for swallowing. This process, known as mastication or chewing, is aided by the jaw muscles and the tongue.
- The muscular **tongue** moves food around the mouth. The tongue takes up most of the internal space in the oral cavity. It is coated with thousands of papillae which provide friction and contain taste buds important in detecting sweet, salty, savoury (umami) and sour tastes.
- **Hard and soft palates** – these form the roof of the mouth. The hard palate at the front is a bony structure, while the soft palate is skeletal muscle and connective tissue. The soft palate terminates at the back of the mouth in a projection called the uvula.
- The powerful muscles in the **jaw** bring the teeth into opposition and with the aid of the muscular tongue, push the bolus of food back towards the pharynx (throat).

Oral saliva assists with chewing and swallowing by moistening and lubricating food, softening rougher food in the process to prevent damage to the gut's mucus membrane. Saliva also facilitates taste by dissolving certain molecules and contains **amylase** which begins the chemical digestion of starches, breaking down polysaccharides into disaccharides. Saliva is made up of water, mucus and enzymes. There are three principal pairs of **salivary glands** in the mouth: parotid, sublingual and submandibular (see Figure 3.7.4). They release saliva into the mouth via

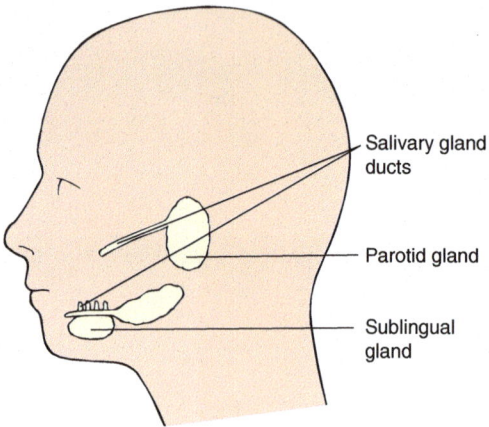

Figure 3.7.4 Salivary glands

Labels: Salivary gland ducts; Parotid gland; Sublingual gland

ducts. Salivation, the act of producing saliva, is often a response to hunger, or the sight or smell of food. Lysosyme and immunoglobulins present in saliva combat invading microbes. Saliva adds increased clotting factors to the bolus and improves the functioning of inflammatory cells which aid healing.

The pharynx

The pharynx or throat is a muscular tube-shaped passageway, which connects the mouth to the oesophagus. The walls of the pharynx are composed of circular and longitudinal muscles: the circular muscles assist in moving the food towards the stomach, whereas the longitudinal muscle fibres aid swallowing. Food passes through the pharynx into the oesophagus during **swallowing**. Swallowing (deglutition) has three phases: oral, pharyngeal and oesophageal (Figure 3.7.5):

- In the **oral** phase, the tongue voluntarily moves the moistened food to the back of the mouth.
- Sensory receptors then trigger an involuntary swallowing reflex, where the

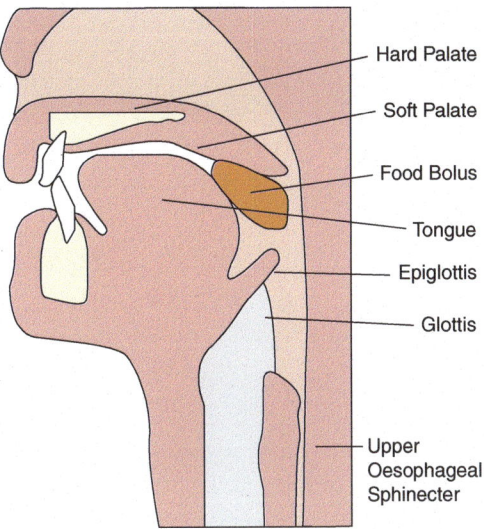

Hard Palate

Soft Palate

Food Bolus

Tongue

Epiglottis

Glottis

Upper Oesophageal Sphincter

Figure 3.7.5 Anatomical features involved in swallowing

soft palate and uvula move up to direct food away from the nasal cavity and into the **pharynx**, and the epiglottis moves down to prevent the bolus from entering the glottis and larynx (the passageway directing air to the lungs and producing sound).

▶ Peristaltic muscle movements then propel the food into the **oesophagus**.

The oesophagus

The oesophagus is a tube lined with smooth muscle, which contracts behind the food bolus, sending it downwards and into the stomach. Glands within its mucosa secrete mucus which moistens and lubricates the lining, easing the passage of food.

The oesophagus features two muscular sphincters, one at the top and one at the bottom. The upper sphincter is under voluntary control and assists with swallowing, the lower oesophageal sphincter (or cardiac sphincter) responds to peristalsis and allows food content into the stomach at the gastro-oesophageal junction. Both sphincters are closed when not involved with digestion, however weakness or disorders of the lower oesophagus can result in gastric reflux (heartburn).

The stomach

The stomach is a 'J' shaped bag situated in the upper left quadrant of the abdomen and is divided into three sections: the fundus, the body and the pylorus (Figure 3.7.6). Its walls are made up of three layers of differently oriented smooth muscle fibres. The stomach expands and acts as a repository where food is further digested.

The stomach lining (mucosa) is formed of epithelial cells and cavities leading to gastric glands. Some of glands secrete the ingredients of **gastric juice** into the stomach, while others secrete the hormone **gastrin**, which helps regulate gastric activity, directly into the bloodstream. Gastric juices start to build up in the stomach as soon as an individual starts to think about or smell food. More are released when food enters and expands the stomach walls. Forceful **peristaltic contractions** in the muscular walls then churn the food (as the differently oriented muscle fibres act like a washing machine drum), mixing it with the gastric juices to form a milky mixture known as **chyme**. About 2 litres of gastric juices are released daily. It is typically very acidic, with a pH of around 1.8, but is quickly diluted by ingested food. Acids and enzymes in the gastric juices continue to break down ingested food: hydrochloric acid in particular denatures protein, which is then further broken down by the enzyme pepsin.

Two common lipid-soluble substances – alcohol and aspirin – pass easily through the stomach mucosa into the blood.

3.7

187

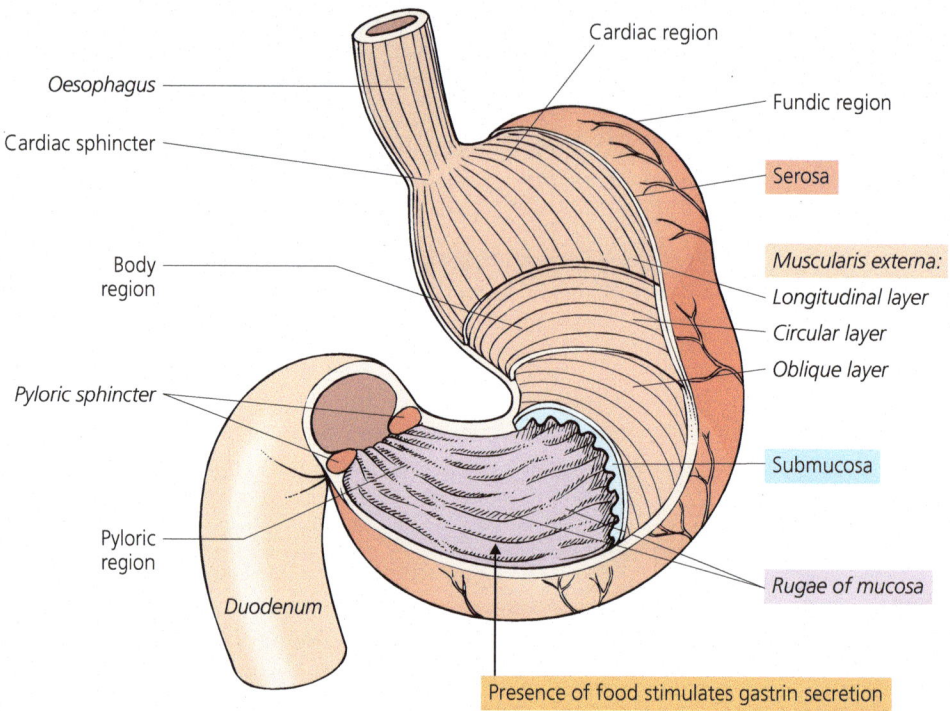

Cardiac region

Oesophagus

Fundic region

Cardiac sphincter

Serosa

Body region

Muscularis externa:
Longitudinal layer
Circular layer
Oblique layer

Pyloric sphincter

Submucosa

Pyloric region

Duodenum

Rugae of mucosa

Presence of food stimulates gastrin secretion

Figure 3.7.6 The stomach

Peristaltic contractions are stronger in the lower parts of the stomach. As pressure within the stomach builds, a small amount of chyme is released into the duodenum with each peristaltic wave. As the duodenum fills, however, it puts pressure on the **pyloric sphincter**, causing it to close.

The small intestine

The 6–7 metres of the small intestine are where digestion is completed, nutrients are absorbed into the body and waste is passed into the large intestine, regulated by the **ileocecal valve**.

It can be divided into three parts:

▶ **The duodenum** begins at the pyloric sphincter. Although it is only approximately 25 cm long, more digestion occurs here than anywhere else in the digestive tract. Ducts from the pancreas and gallbladder open into the duodenum, carrying enzyme-rich **pancreatic juice** and **bile** which mixes with the chyme, chemically breaking down carbohydrate, protein and fat into small, absorbable molecules.

▶ **The jejunum** is approximately 2 metres long. Its surface area is massively increased by deep, circular folds which cause the chyme to spiral, slowing it down and allowing time for full nutrient absorption.

▶ **The ileum**, the longest portion of the small intestine, is approximately 3 metres in length. The jejunum and ileum contain specialised features for digestion and absorption:

   ▶ Tiny **villi** line the jejunum and ileum, in the centre of which is a dense capillary bed and wide lymphatic capillary. This allows for absorption of nutrients.

▶ **Microvilli** are long, slightly woolly-looking, densely packed extensions of the absorptive cells of the mucosa, featuring brush border enzymes, which complete the digestion of carbohydrates and proteins.

▶ A further system of lymphatic vessels (**lacteals**) drain absorbed lipids from the small intestine.

Large intestine

The large intestine, approximately 1.5 metres long, is wider than the small intestine, with a diameter of around 6.5 cm. There are no villi on its mucosa, and the large intestine does not produce any digestive enzymes. Instead, it contains a relatively large population of **bacteria** which feed on the chyme and break it down further, producing energy (used by the bacteria itself and surrounding cells) and vitamins B and K. The large intestine features four main components:

▶ The **caecum** is around 15 cm long and is the widest part of the large intestine. It functions as a reservoir, receiving waste from the small intestine and triggering peristaltic muscle movements when it is full.

▶ The **colon** has ascending, transverse and descending sections which frame the small intestine. Water and electrolytes are absorbed in the ascending and transverse sections, so that faeces are generally pretty solid when they reach the descending colon. Located under the spleen, the descending colon sits on the left of the abdomen and descends

for approximately 12 cm. The colon features three bands of longitudinal muscle fibres along its length (the **teniae coli**) which form a series of pouches when they contract. The pressure of the contraction assists in the absorption of water and salts from the chyme, gradually converting it into pockets of faecal matter (a process called **segmentation**). In tandem with this, slow but strong **peristaltic contractions** shift the developing faeces along the length of the colon to the rectum (a process called **mass movement**).

▶ The **rectum** is approximately 16–22 cm long, ending at the anal canal. It has a thick layer of smooth muscle and follows the curvature of the sacrum, to which it is firmly attached by connective tissue. The rectum ends around 5 cm below the tip of the coccyx, at the anal canal. It temporarily stores faeces, and, when full, triggers the urge to defecate and eliminate waste through the anus.

▶ The **anal canal** is 2–3 cm long and features an internal sphincter formed of smooth muscle which is under involuntary control, and an external, skeletal muscle sphincter under voluntary control.

The products of an ingested meal can spend 2–6 hours in the small intestine and 12–36 hours in the large intestine, meaning that it can take between 2–5 days for food to move through the GIT.

Accessory organs

The liver

The liver receives nutrient-rich blood from the digestive system via the hepatic portal vein. It is situated in the upper right side of the abdominal cavity and is a multifunctional organ, effectively creating a stable environment for the body by metabolising important nutrients, detoxifying unwanted chemicals and producing **bile**. Bile is a yellowish-green fluid containing **salts** which, when mixed with chyme in the duodenum, neutralises stomach acid and acts as an emulsifying agent for fat, breaking it into tiny particles; and **cholesterol** and **pigments** from the breakdown of haemoglobin, which are then excreted from the body in faeces. Bile salts also aid absorption of some cholesterol and the fat-soluble vitamins A, D, E and K by making them water soluble.

The gallbladder

A golf ball sized structure attached to the surface of the liver; the gallbladder is the main storage unit for bile.

The pancreas

The pancreas is a gland situated within the curve of the duodenum. It is approximately 12–15 cm long and contains both exocrine and endocrine glands. The exocrine glands assist in digestion via acini cells which secrete the digestive enzymes **lipase** (assists bile to break down fats), **amylase** (which breaks down carbohydrates) and **protease** (which breaks down proteins). The endocrine glands feature cells known as the **Islets of Langerhans** which secrete **glucagon**, **insulin** and **somatostatin** into the blood. These hormones are crucial in the regulation of blood sugar levels (see Chapter 3.4).

Changes and adaptations to the GIT during pregnancy

Hormonal changes and the physical pressure exerted by the growing fetus result in significant alterations in the anatomy and functioning of the GIT during pregnancy, many of which are experienced as uncomfortable, inconvenient or even painful by women. The principal changes and their impact are summarised in Table 3.7.1.

APPLICATION TO PRACTICE

Oral cavity changes in pregnancy mean that optimising oral health at this time is paramount. Periodontal disease not only increases the likelihood of teeth needing to be extracted but is also linked with poor pregnancy outcomes including pre-eclampsia, preterm birth and low birth weight. Furthermore, children of mothers with untreated cavities or tooth loss are over three times more likely to have cavities in childhood.

Smoking further aggravates gestational dental issues, including delaying the healing of any gum wounds. Alcohol use is associated with tooth decay.

Advice for pregnant women includes:

► Regular dental check ups
► Using a soft-bristled tooth brush
► Floss and brush teeth at least twice a day
► Gargle with mouthwashes or warm salty water to reduce acidity in the oral cavity (this is particularly important after vomiting)
► Wait for at least an hour after vomiting before brushing your teeth (as stomach acid in the mouth increases the likelihood of brushing scratching tooth enamel)
► Eat a healthy diet
► Avoid sugary foods, particularly between meals, and brush teeth after consuming them

Table 3.7.1 GIT system alterations in pregnancy

Event	Consequence	Impact on GIT
Human chorionic gonadotropin (hCG) is produced by the placenta	Sustains early pregnancy, for example by stimulating production of oestrogen and progesterone. Decreases osmotic threshold for thirst.	hCG levels have been linked to increased sensitivity to smell, food cravings and aversions, and nausea and vomiting in pregnancy. Nausea and vomiting are more prevalent in multiple pregnancies where there are high levels of hCG. No causal pathway has been found, however, and recent research has identified abnormally high levels of the hormone GDF15, and increased sensitivity to it, as the major factors contributing to hyperemesis gravidarum (see Chapter 3.4). hCG and nausea have also been linked to the production of excess saliva in pregnancy (a condition known as **pytalism** when it becomes extreme), as this usually occurs in the first trimester. Increased fluid intake (progesterone, angiotensin and relaxin also play a part in this).
Increased levels of progesterone	Causes smooth muscle to relax. Stimulates appetite. Causes increase of bifidobacteria in the gut microbiome.	Reduced peristalsis, leading to poor gut motility. This sluggish behaviour, together with increased water absorption in the colon, often results in constipation. Heartburn is a common complaint in pregnancy and the risk of hiatus hernia is increased due to relaxation of the cardiac sphincter. This may also contribute to nausea and vomiting, and to an increased acidity of oral saliva, which increases the likelihood of dental caries. Gastric emptying is delayed, meaning chyme stays in the stomach for longer, increasing the potential for heartburn. The relaxation of smooth muscle fibres results in an increased surface area in the small intestine, including longer villi, which, together with increased transit time, enhances absorption of nutrients and water. Tone in the gallbladder is also affected, resulting in incomplete emptying, which increases the risk of gallstones. Changes in the gut microbiome promote increased energy storage and a rise in proinflammatory mechanisms which protect against invading pathogens, counteracting the effects of immune system suppression.
Increased levels of oestrogen	Increases vasodilation and blood perfusion of organs. Leads to increased levels of angiotensin and aldosterone. Softens consistency of connective tissue. May have a role in insulin resistance. Suppresses appetite.	Gums become swollen and bleed easily, predisposing pregnant people to gingivitis and periodontal disease. Increased angiotensin and aldosterone lead to water and sodium retention; sodium is a key building block for fetal growth. Increased blood flow, coupled with pressure from the growing uterus and straining due to constipation, can trigger or worsen haemorrhoids.
Increased levels of relaxin	Acts with hCG to reduce threshold for thirst.	Increased fluid intake.

3.7

(Continued)

Table 3.7.1 (Continued)

Event	Consequence	Impact on GIT
Insulin resistance increases as pregnancy progresses	A greater share of glucose is diverted to the fetus, for whom it is a vital energy source.	Most women's bodies will produce sufficient insulin in the pancreas to compensate, but women with type I diabetes are likely to require around 70% more insulin during pregnancy, and women with type 2 diabetes may require even more. Women who are predisposed to type 2 diabetes may develop gestational diabetes (about 50% of women contracting gestational diabetes go on to develop type 2 diabetes in later life).
Leptin resistance develops	Prevents leptin from suppressing appetite.	Food intake and fat deposition increase.
Uterus enlarges	Liver is displaced. Stomach is displaced upwards and compressed. Colon is compressed.	Angle at which the oesophagus enters the stomach is altered, potentially limiting the effectiveness of the pyloric sphincter. Alkaline duodenal content may flow back into the stomach, reducing its acidity. The stomach has a reduced capacity. Transit through the digestive system is further slowed, increasing feelings of bloating and constipation.

Nutrition

A well-balanced diet is essential for optimal fetal growth and development, as well as supporting maternal health during pregnancy and the postnatal period. Maternal malnourishment has been shown to have a direct link to intrauterine growth restriction, leading to small, underweight babies. Key macro- and micronutrients are outlined below.

Macronutrients

Protein requirements increase in pregnancy, as protein is key for tissue growth and repair. A restricted protein intake has been associated with intrauterine growth restriction and metabolic disorders in later life. Beans, pulses, meat, fish and dairy products are all rich sources of protein.

Carbohydrates are the main food support for fetal and placental development. They provide fuel for maternal and fetal brain function, and are required for the development and growth of fetal tissue. They are also an important source of folate (see below), and contribute to glucose and insulin metabolism. There are two important types of carbohydrates: polysaccharides (complex carbohydrates) and monosaccharides (simple carbohydrates). Monosaccharides, such as those found in fizzy drinks and sweets, are absorbed and processed quickly, having a greater impact on insulin levels. They are therefore best avoided during pregnancy. Polysaccharide-dense foods include vegetables, some fruits, dairy and wholegrain products.

Fats: Although too much fat consumption is adverse to both maternal and fetal health, fats and fatty acids play an important role in the development of the fetal brain, eyes and nervous system. Furthermore, fats assist in the absorption of vitamins A, D, E and K, and boost the immune system. A healthy pregnancy diet should include omega-3 fatty acids (essential for brain and eye development), and monounsaturated and polyunsaturated fats such as those found in oils, some nuts and seeds, and oily fish. A diet high in saturated fats such as red meat, whole dairy milk and butter, has been linked to heart disease and diabetes.

Fibre: Although not strictly a nutrient, fibre consumption helps to offset some of the pregnancy-related issues in the GIT. It reduces the likelihood of constipation and haemorrhoids by adding bulk to stools and absorbing water; facilitates stomach emptying and slows down the postprandial insulin response by delaying the absorption of carbohydrates. Fibre is also a source of B vitamins and helps control weight gain by inducing feelings of satiety. Low maternal fibre intake in pregnancy has been associated with children developing allergies (Hajhoseini, 2013). Too much fibre, on the other hand, can cause diarrhoea.

Micronutrients

Vitamin D is important for fetal bone development and helps to regulate calcium and phosphate within the body. Dietary vitamin D is found in oily fish, fat spreads, eggs and fortified food. Absorption of sunlight through the skin assists in the production of vitamin D. As the sun in more northerly climates such as the UK is rarely strong enough to produce vitamin D in the winter months, pregnant and breastfeeding women are advised to take a daily supplement of vitamin D between September and March. Pregnant women with darker skin tones, or who have a raised body mass, are not exposed to sunlight or live in areas where there is reduced sunlight, may also benefit from ongoing vitamin D supplementation.

Folates and folic acid (vitamin B9) assist with fetal cell development (including red blood cells) and have been shown to reduce the incidence of neural tube defects such as spina bifida. It is therefore recommended that women take folic acid supplements preconception and in the first trimester. Folates (the natural form of folic acid) are found in green leafy vegetables, nuts, beans, citrus fruits and wholemeal bread.

Other **B vitamins**, particularly B1, 2, 6 and 12, are also key in pregnancy. They provide energy, maintain the nervous system and contribute to vision, red blood cell and placental development. They are found in yeast extract, bananas, some meats and cereals.

Vitamin C boosts the immune response, and aids tissue repair and wound healing. It also boosts the absorption of iron from plant sources. Citrus fruits, broccoli and tomatoes are rich sources of vitamin C.

Vitamin A: Although harmful and even teratogenic at high doses, especially in early pregnancy, vitamin A is nevertheless essential for bone development, the functioning of reproductive organs, and healthy skin, as well as strengthening the immune system. Vitamin A deficiency blindness is still the biggest cause of preventable blindness globally. It is found in leafy green, orange and yellow vegetables and dairy produce.

Table 3.7.2 Food and drink to avoid during pregnancy

Food and drink	Concern	Adverse effect
Raw/partially cooked hen, duck, goose, quail eggs	Salmonella	Extreme sickness and diarrhoea
Liver, supplements containing vitamin A	High levels of vitamin A	Birth defects, especially of the nervous and cardiovascular systems Spontaneous abortion
Undercooked steak/raw meat Game Cured meats	Toxoplasmosis Lead shot	Stillbirth Blindness
Unpasteurised milk, mould ripened cheese such as brie, stilton. Caution with soft-serve ice cream	Listeriosis	Miscarriage Stillbirth
No more than x 2 portions of oily fish per week	Mercury	Adversely affects fetal brain, nervous system, hearing and vision
Raw shellfish	Harmful bacteria/viruses/toxins e.g. listeriosis	Miscarriage Stillbirth
Restrict intake of tea, coffee, energy drinks and other foods containing caffeine (such as chocolate) to no more than 3 servings (200 mg) per day	Pregnancy complications	Miscarriage, low birth weight, stillbirth
Alcohol	Harmful to fetus	Miscarriage, premature birth low birth weight, focal alcohol spectrum disorder (FASD)

Iron is essential for the production of haemoglobin, which carries essential oxygen and nutrients to the fetus. Iron is absorbed more readily in pregnancy, but demand from the growing fetus can deplete iron levels. Maternal iron deficiency is linked to preterm birth and low birth weight, and decreases women's tolerance to blood loss after birth. Women with iron deficiency may experience cravings for non-food items (a condition known as **pica**) such as dirt, stones, clay, chalk, charcoal, ice or paper. Red meat, nuts, pulses, dried fruit, green leafy vegetables and wholemeal bread are all sources of iron.

APPLICATION TO PRACTICE

Oral iron supplementation is common in pregnancy, as many women struggle to maintain their haemoglobin levels through diet alone. Iron absorption from oral supplements is maximised when they are taken:

▶ First thing in the morning, when hepcidin levels are lower. Hepcidin is a hormone that regulates iron absorption. Counterintuitively, it does this by preventing the body from absorbing iron
▶ On an empty stomach
▶ With water or a vitamin C drink

Other medication should not be taken at the same time, and caffeinated and dairy drinks should be avoided as tannins and polyphenols found in tea and coffee, and calcium in all forms have been found to reduce iron absorption by up to 65%.

Calcium is important for bone and tooth development. Calcium requirements increase in the third trimester, when the fetal skeleton becomes substantially larger. Maternal capacity for calcium absorption and storage increases throughout pregnancy. A diet low in calcium may result in the fetus taking calcium from the mother's bones leading to later life osteoporosis. The recommended daily calcium intake for women is 1000 milligrams which equals three servings of milk or other dairy produce. Non-dairy sources of calcium include canned oily fish such as sardines or pilchards, kale, watercress, almonds, Brazil nuts, sesame seeds and fortified cereals and dairy alternatives.

Microbial communities

3.7

The **gut microbiome** – the extensive and diverse community of microbes that inhabits the gut – impacts metabolism, immune function and mental well-being. As outlined above, progesterone initiates gut microbiome changes in pregnancy that boost its immune capabilities. An unfavourable maternal gut microbiome composition has been linked to pre-eclampsia and macrosomic infants. Probiotic and fermented foods such as kimchi, miso and yogurt, and a Mediterranean, plant-based diet are believed to optimise microbiome health and diversity (Miller at al., 2021). On the other hand, a western diet, typically high in fat and low in fibre, can reduce the diversity of

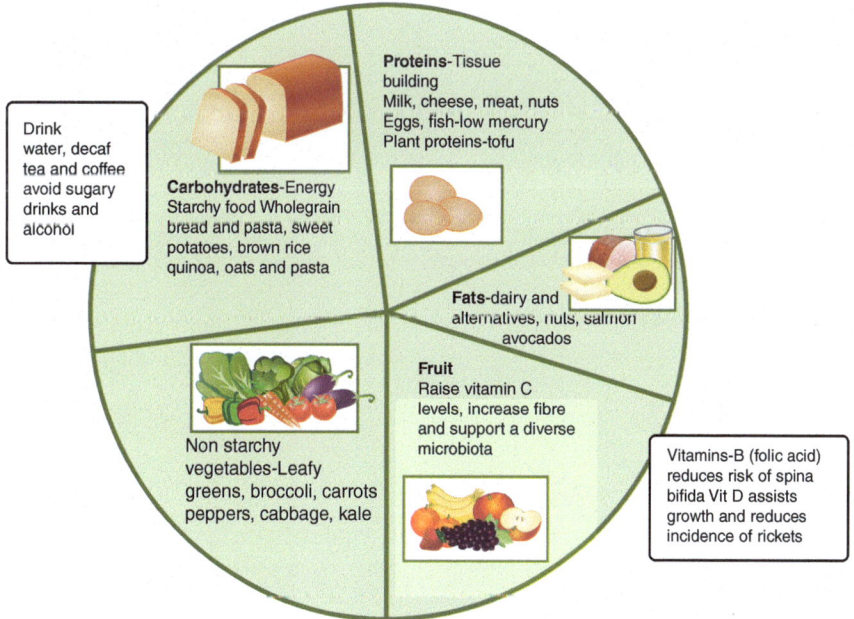

Figure 3.7.7 Healthy eating in pregnancy visual aid

the gut microbiome, leading to an increased risk of obesity and lower immunity (Cruickshank et al., 2019). Antibiotic therapy has also been associated with a lowered microbiome diversity. Foods to avoid in pregnancy are listed in Table 3.7.2.

APPLICATION TO PRACTICE

Talking to women about what they eat can be challenging – our diets are constrained by financial, as well as cultural, religious and personal factors. Think about how you might have open, non-judgemental and enabling conversations around food, using the information in this chapter. A visual aid, such as the pie chart in Figure 3.7.7, might help, as might starting with small changes to an existing diet.

References

Cruickshank S. Immunology, the Microbiome and Future Perspectives [e-video]. Henry Stewart Talks, 2019. https://hstalks-com.oxfordbrookes. idm.oclc.org/t/3927/immunology-the-microbiome-and-future-perspectives/ ?biosci.

Hajhoseini L. The importance of optimal fibre consumption during pregnancy. *Int. J. Women's Health Reproduction Sci.* [Internet] 2013, 1(3). www.ijwhr. net/pdf/pdf_IJWHR_13.pdf.

Miller C., Benny P. et al. Adherence to Mediterranean diet impacts gastrointestinal microbial diversity throughout pregnancy. *BMC Pregnancy Childbirth* [Internet] 2021, 21(558). https://bmcpregnancychildbirth.biomed central.com/articles/10.1186/s12 884-021-04033-8.

Further reading

Gorczyca K., Obuchowska A. et al. Changes in the gut microbiome and pathologies in pregnancy. *Int. J. Environ. Res. Public Health* [Internet] 2022, 19(16):9961. www.ncbi.nlm.nih.gov/pmc/articles/ PMC9408136/.

CHAPTER 3.8

The immune system

Giada Giusmin

LEARNING OUTCOMES

▶ Describe the structure and function of the lymphatic system
▶ Describe the structure and function of innate and adaptive immunity
▶ Understand the causes and symptoms of hypersensitivity and anaphylaxis
▶ Describe the key methods of vaccination
▶ Understand the broad mechanisms which ensure maternal acceptance of the fetus, and passive immunity to the fetus and neonate
▶ Understand the cause of rhesus incompatibility, and describe the use of anti-D prophylaxis

Immune system overview

In this chapter, we will first explore the structure and function of the lymphatic system, then discuss three lines of defence that our bodies put in place when attacked by foreign substances. After discussing the role of antibodies, we will briefly cover different types of immunity, including vaccinations. To conclude this chapter, we will focus on the changes that happen to the immune system in pregnancy. A number of war-related metaphors will be used to simplify some of the concepts discussed in this chapter, however, no disrespect is meant towards people affected by war.

Structure and function of the lymphatic system

The lymphatic system is made up of two main structures, the **lymphatic vessels** and the **lymphoid tissue and organs**.

The lymphatic vessels

The key function of the lymphatic vessels is to return the fluid that has exited the cardiovascular system back to it. In Chapter 3.1, we discussed how tissue cells receive gases and nutrients from the capillaries via the interstitial fluid, now some

DOI: 10.4324/9781003227571-19

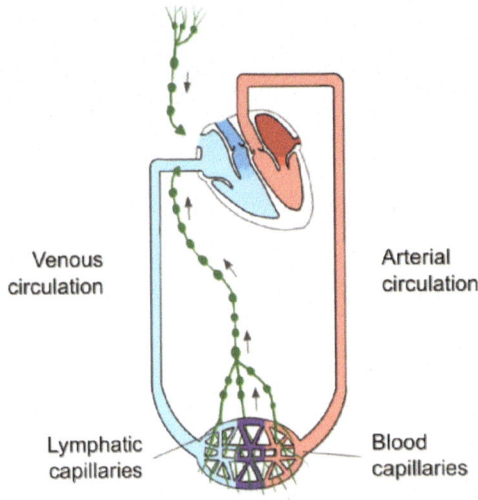

Venous circulation

Arterial circulation

Lymphatic capillaries

Blood capillaries

Figure 3.8.1 Lymphatic system overview

of this fluid left behind in the tissue spaces needs to be returned back to the blood to ensure the cardiovascular system maintains a stable volume to function correctly. Therefore, the role of the lymphatic vessels is to form a plumbing system that collects the surplus of interstitial fluid, called lymph, and returns it into blood circulation.

The lymphatic vessels are structured in a one-way system, as shown in Figure 3.8.1, which transports the lymph from the body back to the heart, and not the other way around. Lymph capillaries are closely intertwined among blood capillaries and tissue cells, which allows them to soak up the leaked fluid. In addition to their strategic position, lymph capillaries are also permeable due to their thin walls, with endothelial cells that slightly overlap, allowing the fluid to enter but not escape back, see Figure 3.8.2. As well as lymph, the lymphatic vessels also collect large particles like bacteria, viruses and cell debris, playing a vital role in immunity.

If this complex drainage system does not work properly, there is the risk of excessive lymph accumulating in the tissues, which becomes visible from the exterior as

swelling, also known as oedema. This excessive amount of oedema can hinder the ability of blood capillaries and tissue cells to exchange nutrients and gases.

As shown in Figure 3.8.1, lymph is transported to the heart in larger and larger lymphatic vessels using a similar mechanism to venous return, as the lymphatic system is also pumpless and relies mostly on skeletal muscle movement, as well as pressure changes in the chest during breathing movements, to push the lymph to the heart. The lymphatic vessels return lymph to the venous system via the right lymphatic duct, which drains the upper right side of the body, and the thoracic duct, which drains lymph from the rest of the body, as shown in Figure 3.8.3.

The lymphoid organs

Lymph nodes are probably the most known lymphoid organ. Their function is to filter lymph going towards the heart and to protect the body by removing pathogens, which are organisms that are harmful to the host such as bacteria and viruses. This happens thanks to white cells roaming the lymph nodes, namely macrophages and lymphocytes (more details on this later in the chapter). Most lymph nodes are approximately 1 cm in size and located, in large clusters, in the groin and underarm areas. During an infection, the lymph nodes can swell temporarily, making them palpable through the skin.

The other lymphoid organs include:

▶ The **spleen** is located in the abdomen and clears the blood of bacteria, viruses and other debris rather than filtering lymph. The spleen also has other functions, including the breakdown of red blood cells and the proliferation of some white blood cells.

▶ The **tonsils**, located in the throat, have the function of filtering pathogens

3.8

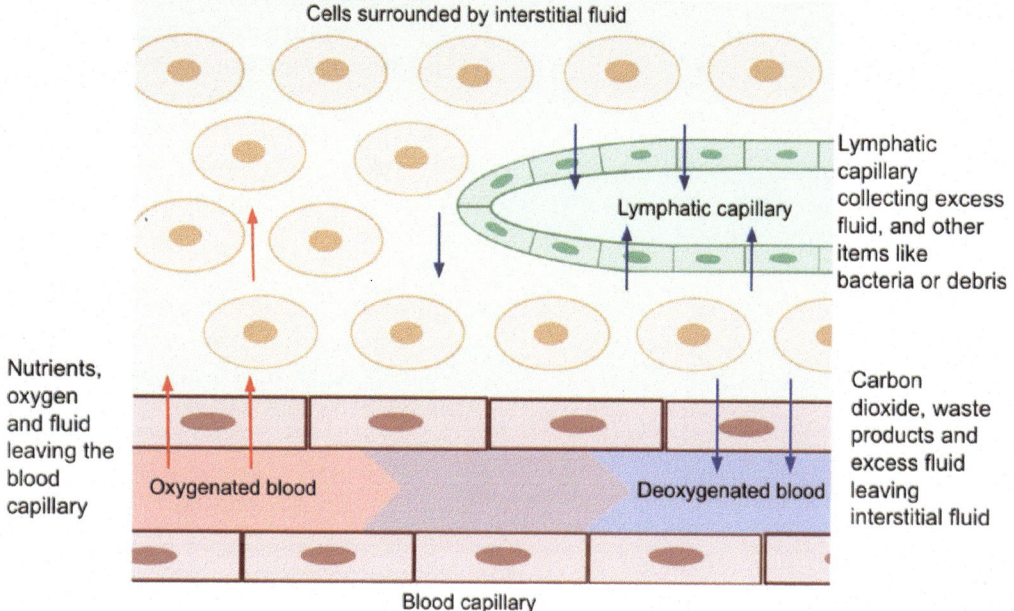

Figure 3.8.2 Lymphatic capillary

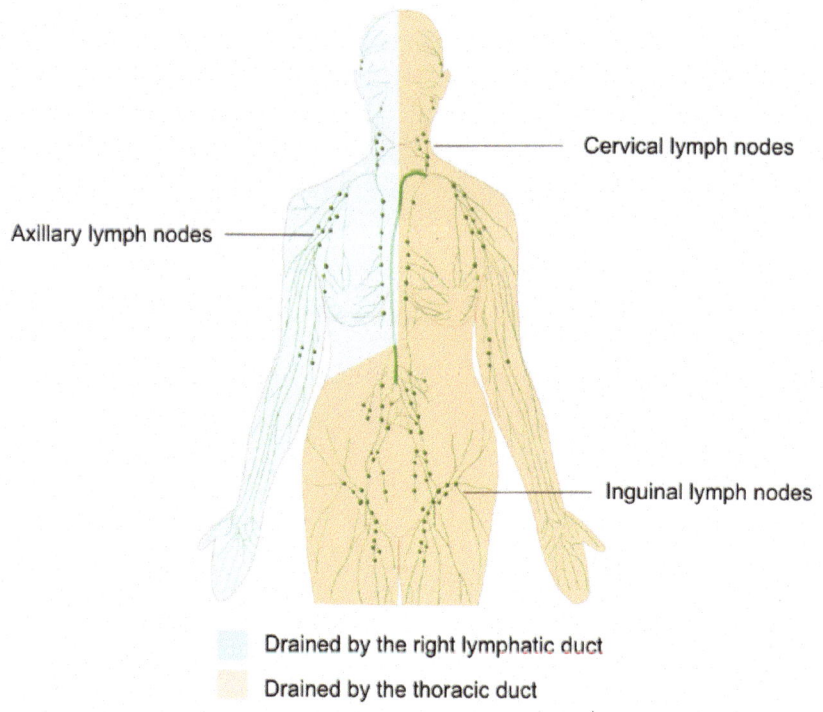

Figure 3.8.3 Areas drained by different ducts and some lymph nodes

entering them. When the tonsils are congested because of their trapping function, they become inflamed (tonsillitis).

▶ The **appendix**, located in the lower abdomen, contains lymphoid tissue.
▶ The **thymus** is a gland in between the upper lungs which functions fully only until puberty. It then slowly decreases in size and is replaced by fat.

There is also other lymphoid tissue around the body, for example, in the intestine (Peyer's patches).

Defence mechanisms

The immune system functions to protect the body from harmful invaders, and employs two mechanisms to do so, the **innate** and **adaptive** defence mechanisms (Figure 3.8.4).

Innate (non-specific) defence mechanism

The innate defence mechanism, as the name might suggest, is made up of defence systems all individuals are born with, such as intact skin, white cells and automatic responses, like macrophages and the inflammatory response, respectively. It can be further divided into the **first line**

and **second line** of defence. The main focus of the innate defences is to prevent the entrance and the proliferation of microorganisms. The innate defences are always ready to defend the body against invaders, they do not need to be 'sensitised' by exposure before they can operate. Overall, innate defences' characteristics can be summarised as follows:

▶ They include surface membrane barriers, but also cells and chemicals
▶ They act within minutes of the invader entering the body and can cause pyrexia (fever), they are 'feverishly fast'
▶ The cells belonging to this type of defence are **non-specific** – they have no memory, and they do not distinguish between invaders

APPLICATION TO PRACTICE

What is the difference between a bacterium and a virus?

A bacterium is a living organism, usually made of one cell, and has a cell membrane and DNA. Antibiotics are used against bacteria because they block biochemical processes that occur inside the bacteria and keep them alive.

Innate (non-specific) defence mechanisms		Adaptive (specific) defence mechanisms
First line of defence	Second line of defence	Third line of defence
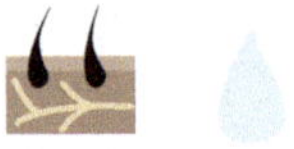 Includes: • Skin • Mucosa • Secretions produced by the skin and mucosa	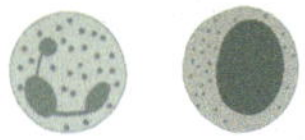 Includes: • Phagocytic cells (like neutrophils) • Natural killer (NK) cells • The inflammatory response • Pyrexia	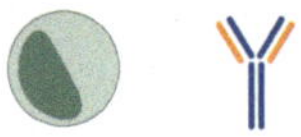 This consists of: • Lymphocytes • Macrophages and other antigen-presenting cells (APCs) • Antibodies

Figure 3.8.4 Overview of innate and adaptive defence mechanisms

A virus does not have biological processes, therefore, is considered a non-living organism. This is why antibiotics do not work in the case of viral infections. Viruses are much smaller than bacteria and need a host to replicate. Viruses can be found dormant even outside living cells, like on soil.

First line of defence

The first line of defence is made of intact skin and intact mucous membranes, the latter covering all the surfaces of body cavities that open to the exterior. The skin is a mechanical barrier that stops harmful organisms from entering the body. The skin also has secretions that prevent bacterial proliferation. Nasal hair, stomach juices or the acid mantle of the vagina, also prevent pathogen entry, whether by trapping them (nasal hair), destroying them (gastric juices) or inhibiting their growth (acid mantle of the vagina). Tears and saliva also belong

in the mucous membrane category, and they contain an enzyme that kills microorganisms.

Second line of defence

The second line of defence includes cells, chemicals and other non-specific responses. In Chapter 3.1, we introduced white blood cells (neutrophils, eosinophils, basophils, monocytes and lymphocytes), and explained their progenitors and their functions. In this section, we will focus on their role in the immune response and introduce other key components of the immune system, like natural killer (NK) cells. Figure 3.8.5 broadly describes the cells' origin and what type of defences they belong to.

Natural killer (NK) cells

NK cells originate from the lymphoid progenitor, but they belong both to innate and adaptive defences. NK cells circulate in blood and lymph, and their function is to

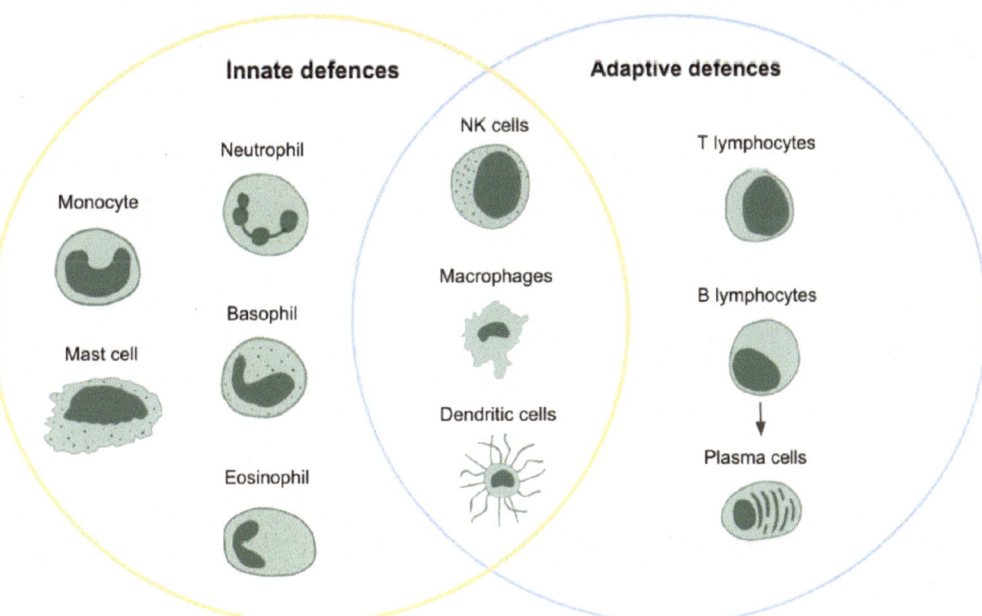

Figure 3.8.5 Overview of white cells and type of defences these belong to

eliminate cancer cells and cells infected by viruses before the adaptive defences are deployed. NK cells eliminate the target cells by infecting them with enzymes that cause the target cell to disintegrate.

Inflammatory response

The inflammatory response is an innate response that occurs anytime the body tissue is injured, for example, during infection or physical trauma. The four most common visible signs of an inflamed area are:

▶ A change in colour – depending on skin tone this could be red, purple or brown colour
▶ Heat
▶ Pain
▶ Swelling

Figure 3.8.6 shows the full inflammatory process and illustrates how the four signs of inflammation occur.

The inflammatory process starts when damaged cells release inflammatory chemicals, such as kinins and histamine. These inflammatory chemicals lead to three different events, which in reality overlap and occur at the same time, and are summarised below for clarity:

▶ The blood vessels near the injured area dilate in order to have a greater blood flow to the area. This is responsible for the **heat** and **skin colour changes**. It also allows oxygen and nutrients to arrive in the area and for the metabolic activity of the cells to increase.
▶ The capillaries become more permeable, which allows for fluid to exit the vascular compartment and enter the interstitial space, accounting for **swelling**. When the pressure of the growing swelling builds up, it triggers pain receptors in the area, accounting for **pain**. In addition to this, if the pain and swelling are localised to particular areas like joints, these can cause a temporary reduction of movement. Moreover, the increased permeability of capillaries also allows

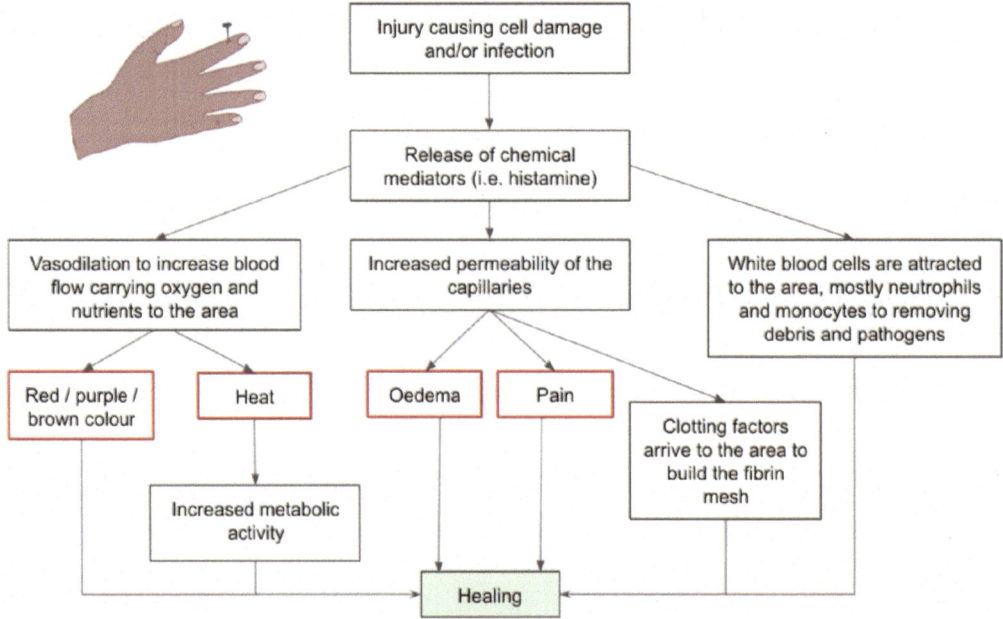

Figure 3.8.6 The inflammatory response

clotting proteins to arrive at the area and to start building a fibrin mesh, which has the dual function of preventing further expansion of the invaders and setting up the structure necessary for repair.

▶ White blood cells are attracted to the area, especially neutrophils and monocytes, for their phagocytic activity. This enables the removal of remaining dead cells and pathogens from the inflamed area. As introduced in Chapter 3.1, leukocytes move out of the blood vessels through a process called diapedesis (see Figure 3.8.7). In the case of inflammation, neutrophils follow chemicals released by the injured site, until they reach the specific area. Where the chemical signal is at its strongest, they flatten and squeeze to pass through the capillary walls. Arriving at the injured area, they readily commence their phagocytic activity.

Pus can form in the inflamed area and cause an abscess (a collection of pus).

Pus is made of a mix of dead cells and phagocytes, inflammatory exudate, living or dead microorganisms.

Pyrexia

Fever or pyrexia is a temporary increase in body temperature that occurs in response to invading pathogens. In particular, fever is caused by chemicals secreted by our white blood cells after encountering harmful microorganisms. These chemicals affect the ability of the hypothalamus to regulate body temperature and cause it to rise. Pyrexia, if mild or moderate, can be beneficial to the body as, during a fever, the liver and spleen accumulate zinc and iron, reducing their availability for bacteria, which need copious amounts to proliferate. However, a high temperature can be life threatening as excessively severe pyrexia damages protein structure, causing cell injury and death. It is important to note that fetal temperature is approximately 0.5°C higher than maternal body temperature, making the fetus more

3.8

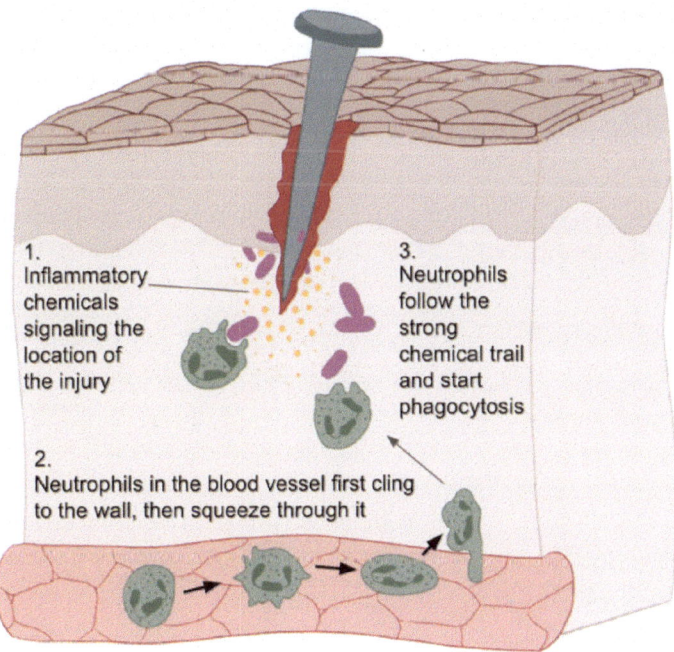

1. Inflammatory chemicals signaling the location of the injury

3. Neutrophils follow the strong chemical trail and start phagocytosis

2. Neutrophils in the blood vessel first cling to the wall, then squeeze through it

Figure 3.8.7 Diapedesis of neutrophils

susceptible to protein structure damage during maternal fever.

Before moving on to adaptive body defences, it is important to clarify that the second line of defences includes other elements, for example, antimicrobial proteins, which have not been covered in this chapter as it is beyond the scope of this textbook to provide extremely detailed information, unlikely to have a practical application in midwifery.

Adaptive (specific) defence mechanism – third line of defence

The adaptive mechanism is also known as **specific**, as it only attacks specific pathogens that have managed to bypass the innate defences. Moreover, the response developed by the adaptive defences is **systemic** rather than being localised to the site of the injury. Lastly, adaptive defences have a '**memory**', which allows them to remember invaders encountered previously and mount a greater and quicker attack when encountered again.

The third line of defence can be subdivided into two types of immunity, **humoral immunity** (also known as antibody-mediated) and **cellular immunity** (also known as cell-mediated). However, it is important to clarify that this distinction is not categorical, as these types of immunity overlap with each other.

Before continuing with humoral and cellular immunity, it is vital to understand more about some critical elements necessary in an immune response: antigens, lymphocytes and antigen-presenting cells.

Antigens

An antigen can be defined as any substance that causes the immune system to react against it, causing an immune response (see Figure 3.8.8). Usually, foreign antigens are much larger than the antigens

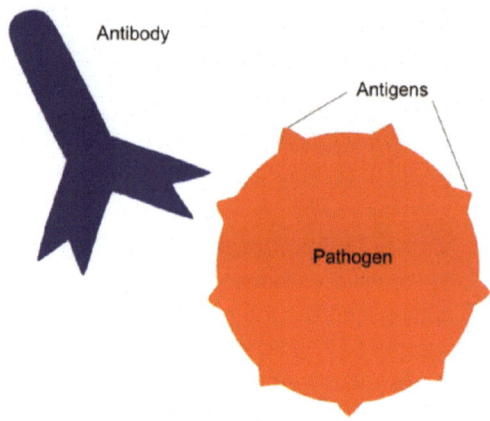

Figure 3.8.8 Relationship between pathogens, antigens and antibodies

present on our own cells; therefore, are recognised as '**non-self**'. Conversely, our immune system is able to recognise our own antigens as '**self**' and not cause an immune response. However, as discussed in Chapter 3.1, self-antigens can cause an immune response if these are encountered by other people, for example, when receiving a blood transfusion of the incorrect blood type.

Lymphocytes

Apart from NK cells, lymphocytes, as discussed in Chapter 3.1, can develop into two main types, B lymphocytes (or B cells) and T lymphocytes (T cells). B cells belong to antibody-mediated immunity as they produce antibodies, whereas T cells belong to cell-mediated immunity because they directly defend the body against invading pathogens.

Lymphocytes originate mostly from the red bone marrow and they leave it as immature, undifferentiated lymphocytes. They then migrate to mature in the thymus if they are destined to be T cells, and in the bone marrow if they are destined to be B cells (**T** cells in the **T**hymus, and **B** cells in the **B**one marrow). In these two locations, T cells and B cells become **immunocompetent**, which means they can react to different antigens. Each lymphocyte will ultimately only actually recognise one particular antigen, and they learn not to react to any self-antigens and erroneously attack their own cells. Therefore, B and T cells become immunocompetent prior to meeting the antigens they might encounter and attack in the future – this means that our immune response is partially predetermined genetically. After B and T cells become immunocompetent, they move to the spleen, lymph nodes and other lymphoid organs to come into contact with antigens, where they will bind with them and finalise their differentiation into mature B and T cells. As mature B and T cells, and in particular for T cells, they roam around the body to increase their chances of encountering antigens.

Antigen-presenting cells

Antigen-presenting cells (APCs) are a group of cells that process and present to antigens the cells with which they will actually interact. The three main cell types that act as APCs are B lymphocytes, macrophages (found in lymphoid organs and connective tissue) and dendritic cells (found in connective tissue and skin). In particular, dendritic cells are extremely good at becoming APCs thanks to their extensions that allow them to capture antigens, digest them by phagocytosis and then present them. Dendritic cells and macrophages unite the innate and adaptive immune mechanisms. More details on the mutual activation of lymphocytes and APCs are discussed in the cell-mediated immunity section below.

Antibody-mediated (humoral) immunity

As previously mentioned, B cells become mature when they become immunocompetent and are then exposed to antigens. When B cells bind to the antigen, this **activates** them, and they undergo **clonal selection** (Figure 3.8.9).

During clonal selection, activated B cells multiply very quickly, creating an 'army' of clones. **Plasma cells** release soluble proteins called **antibodies**. This occurs during the first encounter with an antigen, known as the **primary humoral response**. After an initial lag, the production increases exponentially, with antibody numbers peaking at 10 days post antigen encounter. The majority of B cell clones then become plasma cells and a smaller number who do not become **memory cells**. Memory cells are in charge of the immunological memory as they can respond to the same antigen when encountered again. This process is part of the **secondary humoral response**, which is produced much more rapidly and intensely than the primary one.

Antibodies

As mentioned earlier, antibodies (also called **immunoglobulins** or **Igs**) are secreted by B cells that have been activated or by plasma cells after these have encountered an antigen, and antibodies can only bind to that particular antigen. Antibodies have a similar structure and can be grouped into five different Ig classes (IgM, IgA, IgD, IgG and IgE). The basic structure of antibodies is composed of four chains linked together by bonds, making them resemble the letter Y (see Figure 3.8.10). Two of the chains are identical and are called **heavy chains**, whereas the other two chains are also identical but are half of the size of the heavy chains, these are called **light chains**.

In addition, antibodies have a constant region and a variable region, the latter positioned towards the end of the two upper arms of the letter Y. Different variable regions allow antibodies to respond to the antigens that fit specifically into that shape;

3.8

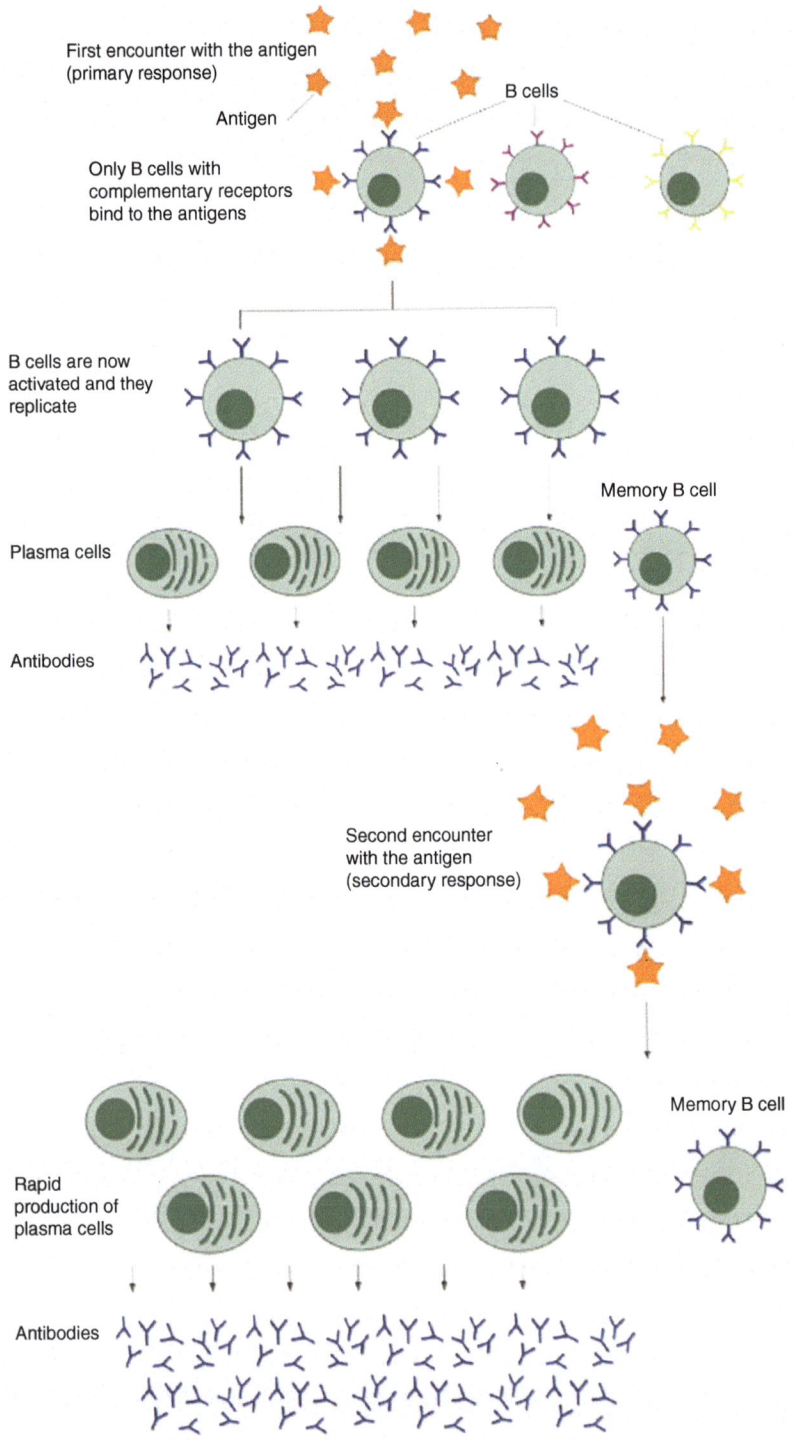

Figure 3.8.9 Antibody production during primary and secondary response

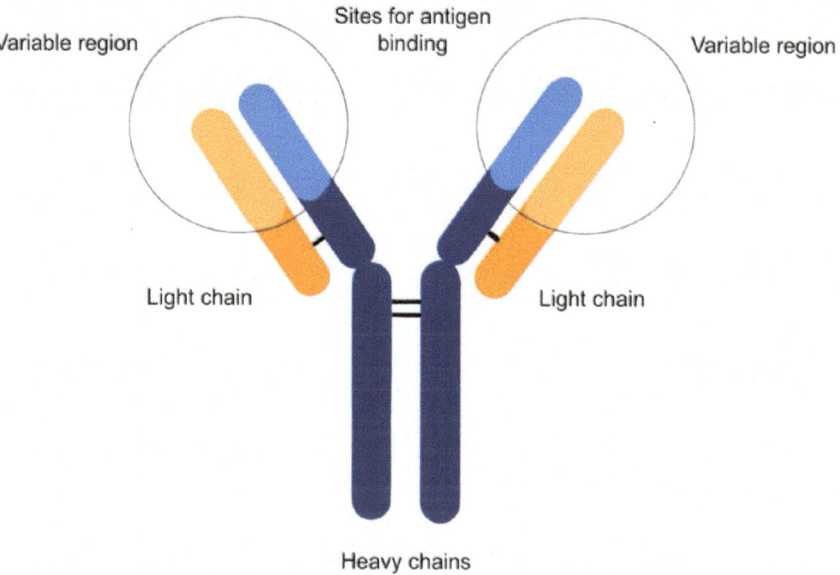

Figure 3.8.10 Simplified structure of an antibody

this area is called the **antigen-binding site**, and each antibody has two sites.

Out of the five Ig classes (IgM, IgG, IgA, IgE and IgD), three are particularly relevant to midwifery:

▶ **IgM** are the first antibodies released by the plasma cells during the first infection (primary response)

▶ **IgG** make up approximately 80% of all antibodies and are present during primary and secondary responses. IgG can cross the placenta and provide immunity to the fetus

▶ **IgA** are important as they get passed through breastmilk and other bodily fluids

There are a number of different ways in which antibodies can inactivate antigens, one of these is **neutralisation**, where the antibodies block harmful effects to body cells by binding to specific sites of bacterial toxins or viruses. Another way is **agglutination**, where antibodies clump antigens together – this is what occurs in the case of incorrect blood transfusions.

Cell-mediated (cellular) immunity

T cells are different from B cells as they are unable to bind directly with antigens, instead the antigens need to be presented by an APC as described above. The APC engulfs the antigen, processes it and then displays the antigen on its exterior surface. Here, the T cell, specifically a **helper T cell**, which is the correct one for that antigen, binds to the antigen and the APC receptor. This enables the T cell to activate (Figure 3.8.11). You could imagine the T cells being customers at a bar, they cannot get up and get their own drinks behind the bar area (binding to antigens), and they need to wait for a waiter to bring them a drink on a tray (the APC presenting the antigen).

Cytokines, which are chemicals released mostly by macrophages being APCs, are released during the activation to enhance this. Cytokines are also released by activated helper T cells, which help other cells proliferate. Helper T cells have a leading role in adaptive immunity, as after activation they recruit other cells in the

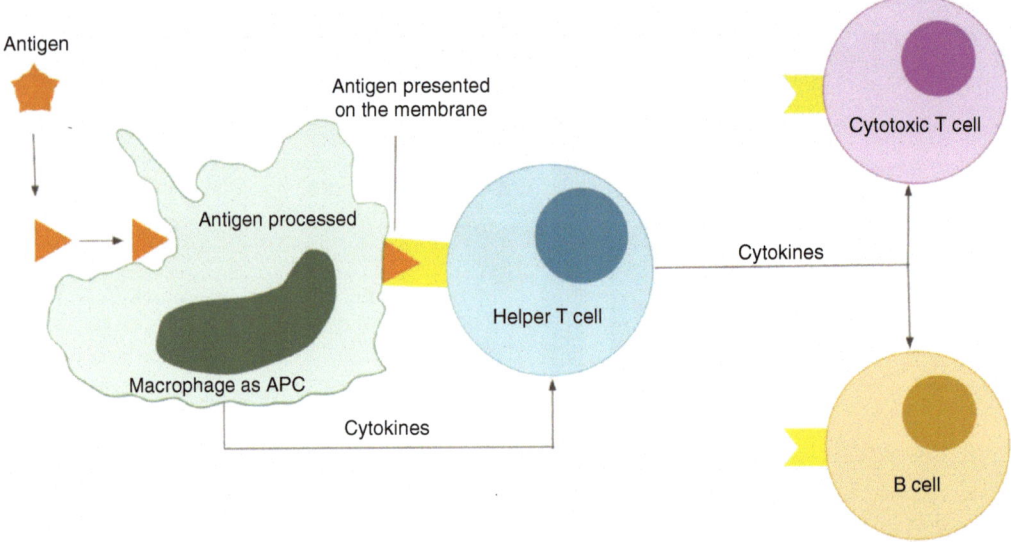

Figure 3.8.11 Cell-mediated immunity

body to fight the invading organisms, and they also help B cells produce more clones. Helper T cells release cytokines that also help **cytotoxic T cells** proliferate. Cytotoxic T cells are specialised in eliminating cancer and virus-infected cells. Lastly, there are **regulatory T cells**, whose job is to regulate the response of B and T cells by slowing down the immune response after an antigen has been dealt with.

Hypersensitivity and anaphylaxis

Hypersensitivities, more commonly known as allergies, are excessive and damaging immune reactions that the body has towards a particular food or substance that would normally be harmless to other individuals. There are three main types of allergic reactions:

▶ **Immediate hypersensitivity**: This type of hypersensitivity occurs after the individual has been sensitised to a particular allergen already, so a subsequent encounter with the allergen triggers a reaction. One of the five types of antibodies, IgE, binds to mast cells and releases histamine, which in turn causes dilatation of blood vessels. This causes some of the typical symptoms of allergy, like watery eyes, skin rash and runny nose. Immediate hypersensitivities usually improve with the use of antihistamine medications.

▶ **Anaphylactic shock** is a rare acute and systemic allergic reaction. It occurs when the allergen moves directly into the bloodstream and circulates through the body. It is the same mechanism that causes immediate hypersensitivity, but on a much larger scale, and it can result in death, especially because of the vasodilation occurring at the respiratory level, causing cardiovascular collapse. Examples include people allergic to specific foods, like peanuts, or medications, like penicillin. Epinephrine, usually known as adrenaline in the UK, is the drug of choice to reverse this process, often referred to as an 'Epi-pen'. People with known severe allergic reactions usually carry the medication with them at all times.

▶ **Delayed hypersensitivities** appear much later than immediate ones, as they are not mediated by histamine but by activated T cells. For this reason, antihistamine medications will not be useful, and corticosteroids are used instead. An example of delayed hypersensitivity is contact dermatitis, which occurs following contact with some particular substances and chemicals.

Acquired immunity and vaccinations

As previously mentioned, after the first exposure to an antigen (primary response) there is an initial lag between the exposure and the rise in antibody level, due to the time needed to mobilise cell-mediated and antibody-mediated immunity. During this time, the majority of antibodies are IgM, but also IgG. In case of subsequent exposure to the same antigen, the immune response is much faster as it builds on existing memory B cells, and much greater. In the secondary

response, the majority of antibodies are IgG (Figure 3.8.12).

Immunity is obtained in two ways, naturally or artificially, and both of these ways can also be active or passive (Figure 3.8.13).

Active immunity

Active immunity occurs when our immune system (B cells) produces antibodies against antigens it has encountered. Active immunity can be acquired in two ways, naturally or artificially. Active immunity is acquired naturally following infection from bacteria and viruses, during which we can present a variety of different symptoms, depending on the disease. Active immunity is acquired artificially through the use of vaccines, whose job is to prime our immune system during a primary response and enable it to set up a vigorous secondary response.

Passive immunity

Passive immunity occurs when it is not our immune system that produces antibodies against a specific antigen, but the antigens are obtained from the serum of an immune

3.8

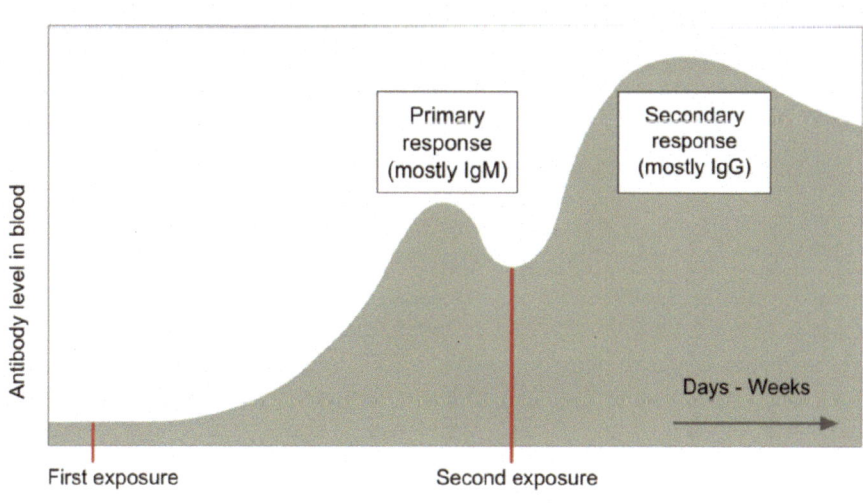

Figure 3.8.12 Antibody level according to the type of exposure

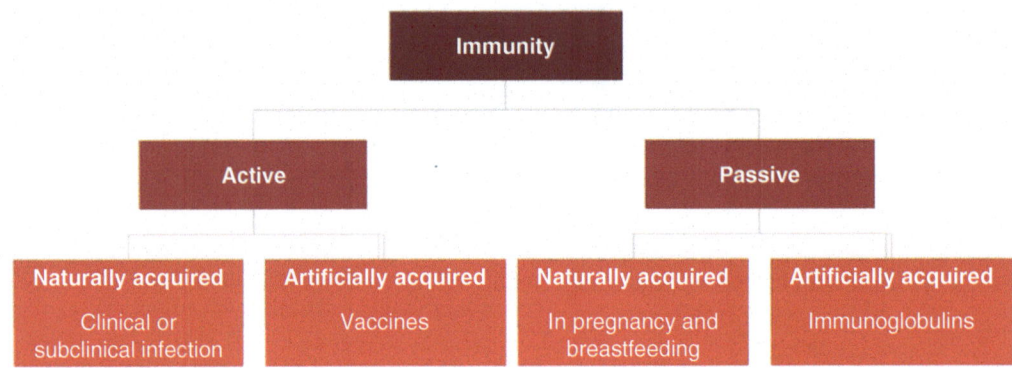

Figure 3.8.13 Four types of immunity

or animal donor. Because the body obtains antibodies without the processes to create them, immunological memory does not occur and the protection is temporary. Passive immunity is acquired naturally during pregnancy, with maternal antibodies crossing the placenta to the fetus, and during breastfeeding. So, for a few weeks and months, the newborn is protected against the same antigens the mother has developed antibodies against.

Passive immunity can be acquired artificially when individuals are given donated antibodies, gamma globulins. These are used in those situations where waiting for active immunity could cost the person their life, for example, after a snakebite, gamma globulins are given to provide immediate protection while the immune system has time to mobilise the immune response.

Types of vaccines

As discussed above, active acquired immunity is obtained following the administration of vaccines. More modern vaccines, such as those employed during the Covid-19 pandemic, use a genetic approach or viral vectors. Traditional vaccines can be either **inactivated** or **live attenuated**. The purpose of vaccines is to encourage the immune response without being exposed to the disease.

Inactivated vaccines have copies of the bacteria or virus that have been killed before being injected into the body. These types of vaccines are not as strong as live attenuated vaccines, therefore they need topping up over time with booster shots. Some examples of inactivated vaccines are pertussis, tetanus, polio, diphtheria and seasonal influenza.

Live attenuated vaccines contain a weakened version of the bacteria or viruses, more commonly used for viruses. Live attenuated vaccines can cause some symptoms of the disease but are not severe enough to cause the full illness or transmit the disease to other people. Live attenuated vaccines offer stronger protection, providing lifelong immunity with one or two doses. Examples of live attenuated vaccines are measles, mumps and rubella (MMR), chicken pox and yellow fever vaccines.

Vaccines offer great protection against some deadly diseases but are not 100% effective. For example, some people fail to build the first immune response to the vaccination, or some people's response could be inadequate due to older age or being poorly nourished. In addition to these, some people are infected by different strains of the disease they have been vaccinated against, even though the disease's presentation is the same, like for seasonal influenza.

Changes and adaptations during pregnancy

Acceptance of the fetus

The fetus has a unique combination of antigens, half obtained from the father, which are recognised as *non-self* by the maternal immune system, and half obtained from the mother. The fetus, therefore, is at an immunological level distinct from both its parents. The fetoplacental unit is classified as an allograft, which is defined as foreign tissue from the same species, but the process is actually more complex. Initially, it was thought that at the level of the implantation site, the immune response was suppressed. However, it is now known that the human decidua contains a high number of leukocytes, like NK cells, macrophages and T cells. Moreover, it appears that the presence of immune cells at the implantation site is not caused by a reaction from the maternal immune system recognising the fetoplacental unit as foreign, but it is in place to protect and facilitate the pregnancy. This makes the immune response at the implantation site active and very carefully controlled, rather than suppressed. As pregnancy is crucial for the conservation of the species, it would be contradictory for the immune system to be suppressed during pregnancy, as it is essential for the mother to be protected against infections and ensure the fetus is protected too.

Additionally, the fetal immune system is antigenically mature and shows immunocompetence from an early stage, and it can modulate how the maternal immune system responds to the environment. Therefore, pregnancy is defined as a state of **immunomodulation**, not immunosuppression. Recent research has shown how it is not just the maternal immune system that is a major player in the implantation and continuation of the pregnancy, but that fetoplacental immune responses are combined with maternal ones.

Pregnancy can be a pro-inflammatory and anti-inflammatory condition, depending on the stage. Early pregnancy requires a strong inflammatory response as the blastocyst implants in the uterus, and an inflammatory environment is necessary to ensure good repair of the endometrium and disposal of debris. For this reason, early pregnancy is classified as a pro-inflammatory phase. The following phase, where the fetus is developing and growing, is an anti-inflammatory phase. The final stage of pregnancy, childbirth, sees another pro-inflammatory phase where the myometrium contracts and the fetus, placenta and membranes are expelled.

There is an association between viral infections, even though these can be asymptomatic for the mother, and preterm birth because these infections have caused acute or chronic placental infections (chorioamnionitis). However, most infections affecting the mother do not affect the baby, which suggests that the placenta plays a vital role as an immune-regulatory interface in order to protect the fetus. Moreover, some studies have shown how viral infections to the placenta could, in fact, activate maternal and fetal immune systems, this shows how the fetus and the placenta are active immunological organs and not passive as was postulated in the past. However, it is important to consider that vertical transmission (from mother to baby), although rare, can be extremely dangerous. For example, cytomegalovirus (CMV), if contracted for the first time by the pregnant mother, could cause fetal congenital abnormalities and developmental delays. Therefore, viral infections that can cross the placenta and reach the fetus can have dangerous consequences. Even viral infections that do not cross the placenta could affect the fetus indirectly, depending on the maternal response to the infection.

Passive immunity to the fetus and neonate

As previously discussed, the fetus receives IgG during pregnancy from the mother as these cross the placenta. The passage of IgG starts at around 20 weeks and increases in the late third trimester. This way, the fetus will be protected via passive immunity from the infections likely to be encountered after birth. The passive protection that the mother gives the fetus is temporary until the newborn starts making its own antibodies. The newborn receives IgA and IgM through colostrum and breastmilk, as these do not cross the placenta. Passive immunity can be hindered by preterm birth, as this causes the fetus to have lower exposure to maternal IgG crossing the placenta. Moreover, the immune system of a preterm newborn is also less developed. Similarly, placental dysfunction with intrauterine growth restriction (IUGR) could also limit the transfer of IgG to the fetus, providing limited protection.

Complications can arise if harmful IgG cross the placenta, as is the case for antibodies the mother has developed against autoimmune conditions (when the immune system mistakenly attacks itself). In these cases, autoimmune antibodies can cross the placenta and attack the fetus, affecting fetal development and growth.

APPLICATION TO PRACTICE
Group B Streptococcus (GBS)

GBS is a bacterium that colonises approximately 20–40% of people, and it is generally harmless. Concerns can arise in pregnancy and childbirth if there is vertical transmission from the mother to the fetus/newborn. In particular, preterm babies are at higher risk of infection because of the limited protection obtained via passive immunity. For this reason, intrapartum antibiotic prophylaxis might be recommended. Term newborns have better rates of protection, and this can be lengthened with breastfeeding.

Rhesus factor and incompatibility

The formerly known **rhesus system**, now called **Rh**, is another antigen system of vital importance during blood transfusions. It was originally named after the rhesus monkey used to discover the antibody, however, in more recent years, that original antibody was found to be different from the one now identified as the Rh factor. Technically, there are 49 Rh antigens known, but the most important in midwifery and obstetrics is the **D antigen**. This is because the D antigen in particular, and the Rh antigens in general, are highly **immunogenic** and can cause transfusion reactions and haemolytic disease of the newborn (HDN).

Approximately 85% of the Caucasian population has the RhD antigen compared to over 92% of Black and Asian populations. When an individual has the RhD antigen on the red blood cell (RBC) surface, they are referred to as **Rh positive**. Rh positive individuals cannot make **anti-RhD antibodies**. Conversely, individuals who do not have the RhD antigen on the RBC surface are considered **RhD negative**. This means that these individuals are capable of generating anti-RhD antibodies if they encounter the RhD antigen on the RBCs present in a blood transfusion or fetal RBCs.

Compared to the ABO blood group system, which is pre-formed, Rh are not, which means RhD antibodies are created if the immune system encounters the Rh antigen as foreign. In clinical practice, this is relevant when a Rh negative mother encounters the Rh antigen on the fetal RBCs and produces antibodies. This happens when the mother is RhD negative, the father RhD positive and the fetus is also RhD positive. The maternal immune system is likely to come into contact with fetal RhD-positive antigens during the third stage of labour when, during placental separation, a millilitre of fetal blood crosses into the maternal circulation. However, there are other potential events when this contamination can happen, such as during abdominal trauma, miscarriage or

termination, antepartum bleeding or during procedures like amniocentesis.

Whenever the maternal immune system is sensitised, or **isoimmunised**, against RhD antigens, this is irreversible and lifelong. If maternal antibodies against the Rh antigen encounter fetal Rh positive RBCs during a subsequent pregnancy, it leads to the fetal blood cells disintegrating. As the adaptive immune response has a lag time, Rh incompatibility is mostly problematic for subsequent pregnancies. Figure 3.8.14 provides an example of the process.

For the fetus, this can cause symptoms ranging from mild anaemia to hydrops fetalis (severe swelling around tissue and organs) or even fetal death. In the newborn, Rh incompatibility can cause HDN, where anaemia caused by RBC breakdown, increases the risk of heart failure, jaundice and kernicterus (see Chapter 5.2 for further information on jaundice in the newborn).

Since the 1960s, severe Rh incompatibility and its consequences have drastically reduced in many counties, as a prophylactic

3.8

First pregnancy

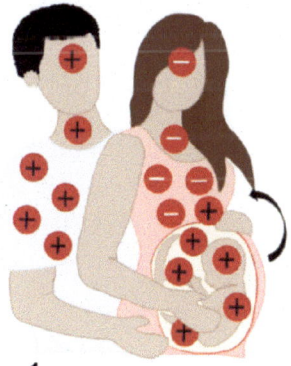

1.
RhD-positive father and RhD-negative mother. The mother carries her first RhD-positive fetus. During childbirth, RhD-positive antigens from the fetus enter into the maternal circulation.

Between pregnancies

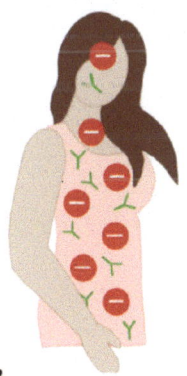

2.
Following fetal RhD-positive antigens being recognized by maternal immune system, the mother will produce antibodies against RhD-positive antigens (Anti-RhD antibodies).

Subsequent pregnancy

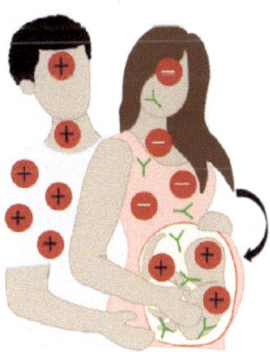

3.
In a subsequent pregnancy with an RhD-positive fetus, maternal antibodies will cross the placenta and attack fetal red blood cells.

Figure 3.8.14 RhD incompatibility

treatment was introduced. The anti-D injection is made of immunoglobulins (antibodies) to anti-D, coming from donated plasma. The job of **anti-D immunoglobulins** is to bind to the fetal RhD antigens when these enter maternal circulation before maternal lymphocytes have the chance to recognise the RhD antigens as foreign. Therefore, currently in England, the anti-D injection is offered routinely to RhD-negative women twice, at around 28–30 weeks and after delivery of the placenta. If the woman has other potentially sensitising events, like abdominal trauma, then this injection can be repeated as required throughout the pregnancy. However, it is important to pair the anti-D injection with a maternal blood test, called the Kleinhauer test, which establishes the presence of fetal RBCs in the maternal circulation. For many years, all women who were RhD negative were routinely offered the anti-D injection. In more recent years, blood tests that can identify the RhD factor of the unborn baby have been developed. This has allowed mothers who were carrying a RhD-negative fetus to avoid unnecessary anti-D administration and potential risks deriving from the use of blood products.

Further reading

Mor G., Cardenas I. The immune system in pregnancy: A unique complexity. *Am. J. Reprod. Immunol.* [Internet] 2010, 63(6):425–33. www.ncbi.nlm.nih.gov/pmc/articles/PMC3025805/.

UK Health Security Agency. The Green Book [Internet]. 2020. www.gov.uk/government/collections/immunisation-against-infectious-disease-the-green-book.

Yong E. Immunology is where intuition goes to die. *The Atlantic* [Internet]. 2020. www.theatlantic.com/health/archive/2020/08/covid-19-immunity-is-the-pandemics-central-mystery/614956/.

Labour and Birth

Giada Giusmin, Louise Hunter,
Katherine Palles-Dimmock, Kirsten Baker,
Jane Carpenter and Claire Smith

Having explored how new life is created from sperm and egg, and develops in utero, nourished and protected by the placenta; we then explored how the systems of the body need to change and adapt to enable growth and development of the fetus. Now, we come to perhaps one of the most awe-inspiring moments of the journey, when the woman births her baby. We explore the dynamic processes of labour and birth, how the anatomy of woman and fetus work together via a range of physiological processes, culminating in the passage of the fetus through the pelvis and down the birth canal to be born. Although awe-inspiring, this is also a time when the midwife is on full alert for deviations from that normal physiology – and we consider this throughout this section.

DOI: 10.4324/9781003227571-20

The maternal pelvis

Katherine Palles-Dimmock and Louise Hunter

LEARNING OUTCOMES

▶ Describe the structure and function of the maternal pelvis, bearing in mind individual variation of pelvic shapes

▶ Explore the role of the maternal pelvis during birth

The female pelvis both supports the upper body and serves as a gateway during physiological birth. During pregnancy it adapts for this second purpose by developing the ability to move and expand as its joints and ligaments soften and stretch under the influence of hormones. Knowledge of pelvic anatomy enables midwives to work with women in labour to adopt positions that maximise the space within the pelvis and facilitate fetal descent. The fetus needs to align itself, as it travels, with the widest diameters of the pelvis, which will vary with different people. Furthermore, as the fetus negotiates a path through the pelvis during labour, knowledge of pelvic anatomy enables assessment of progress by determining the relationship of the fetus to the landmarks of the pelvis.

Structure and function of the pelvis

Function of the pelvis

The pelvis is a strong, basin-shaped ring of bones which contains and protects the pelvic and abdominopelvic organs. It supports the upper body and transmits weight from the axial skeleton to the lower appendicular skeleton. The muscles and ligaments of the legs, back and abdomen are attached to the pelvis, providing strength and power to keep the body upright, enable bending and twisting movements at the waist, and the ability to walk and run. The female human pelvis has evolved to be narrow enough for efficient upright locomotion while still being wide enough to facilitate childbirth.

DOI: 10.4324/9781003227571-21

Structure of the pelvis

In relation to pregnancy and childbirth, the pelvis is often divided into a **true** and **false pelvis**. The false pelvis is located above the pelvic brim and provides support for the lower abdominal organs. The true pelvis is the bony canal through which the fetus must pass during birth. It has a **brim**, a **cavity** (the space between the inlet and outlet) and an **outlet** (Figures 4.1.1, 4.1.2 and 4.1.3). The pelvis consists of **four pelvic bones**: two hip or **innominate bones**, one **sacrum** and one **coccyx** (Figure 4.1.4).

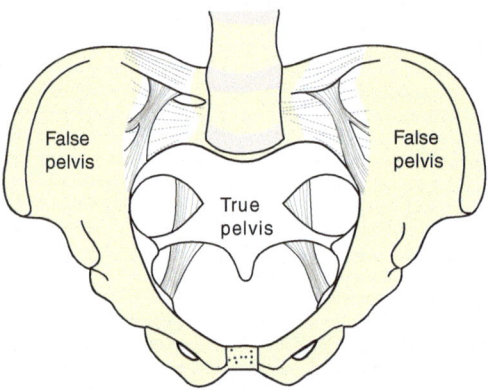

Figure 4.1.1 The true and false pelvis
Source: Figure 4.1, p.91, Clancy and McVicar (2009)

The innominate bones

The two innominate bones join together anteriorly at the **symphysis pubis** (see Figures 4.1.4 and 4.1.5). Each contains a round cup-shaped socket, the **acetabulum**, where the head of the femur articulates to form the hip joint. The innominate bones each consist of three fused bones: the **illum**, **ischium** and **pubis** (Figure 4.1.5). At birth, these three components are separated by hyaline cartilage, and by the end of puberty they will have fused together, but it is not until about 25 years old that the three regions will have fully ossified.

The **ilium** is the upper part of the innominate bone. The concave anterior surface is the iliac fossa and the upper border is the iliac crest. The **ischium** is the thick lower part of the innominate bone. The **ischial tuberosity** is the prominence on which the body rests when sitting. Behind and above each ischial tuberosity is an upward projection called the **ischial spine**, which serves as an attachment point for the sacrospinous ligament. Even though they cannot usually be felt, in labour the ischial spines are used as landmarks to describe the descent of the fetal head through the pelvis (see *Application to practice* box below). The shaft of the ischium meets the inferior ramus of the

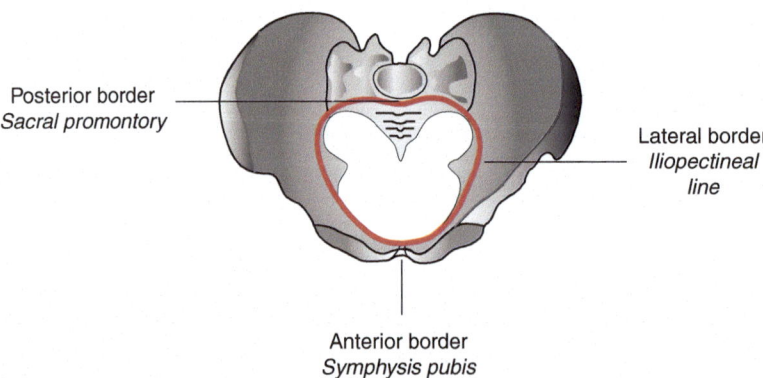

Posterior border
Sacral promontory

Lateral border
Iliopectineal line

Anterior border
Symphysis pubis

Figure 4.1.2 Pelvic inlet/brim
Source: Figure 4.4, p.81, Clancy and McVicar (2009)

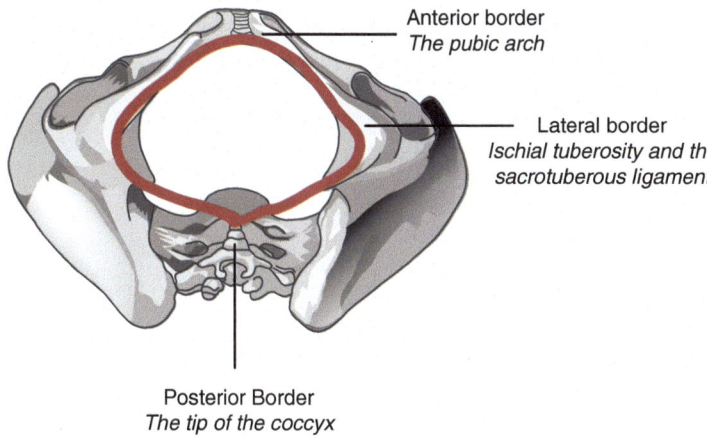

Figure 4.1.3 Pelvic outlet
Source: Figure 12.4, p.195, Kenny and Myers (2017)

4.1

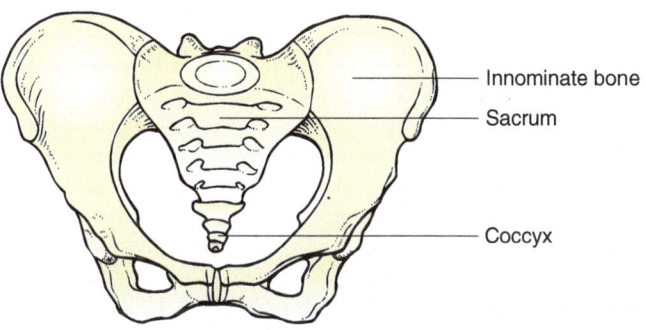

Figure 4.1.4 The pelvic bones
Source: Figure 3.18, p.81, Clancy and McVicars (2009)

pubis to form the **pubic arch**. The angle of the pubic arch varies between individuals and affects the dimensions of the pelvic outlet. The pubis forms the anterior aspect of the innominate bone.

APPLICATION TO PRACTICE

One of the aims of a vaginal examination in labour is to determine how far the fetus has descended through the maternal pelvis. The location of the fetus in the pelvis is referred to as its **'station'** (Figure 4.1.6).

The fetal station is described in relation to the ischial spines, which are visualised rather than physically felt during a vaginal examination. The station is reported in centimetres above (indicated by a minus prefix) or below (indicated by a positive prefix) the spines.

The sacrum

The **sacrum** is made up of five fused sacral vertebrae forming a shield shaped bony mass at the rear of the pelvis. The sacrum strengthens and stabilises the pelvis. The posterior surface is roughened to receive

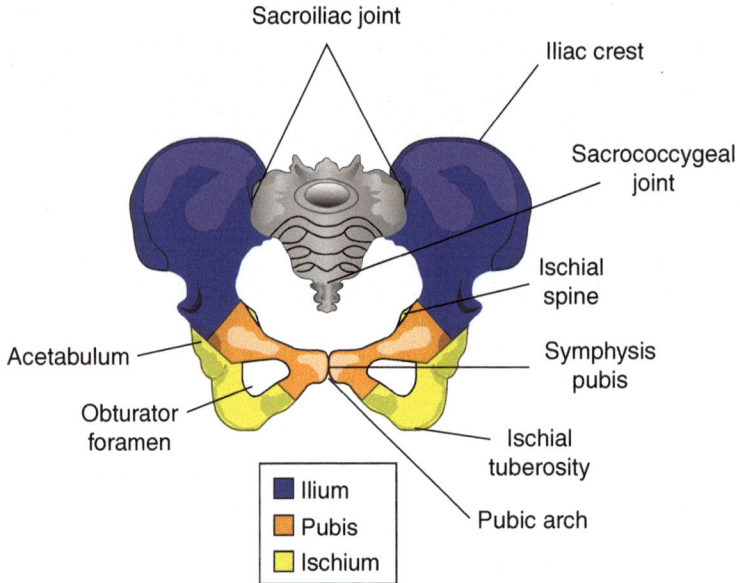

Figure 4.1.5 The components of the innominate bones and the pelvic joints

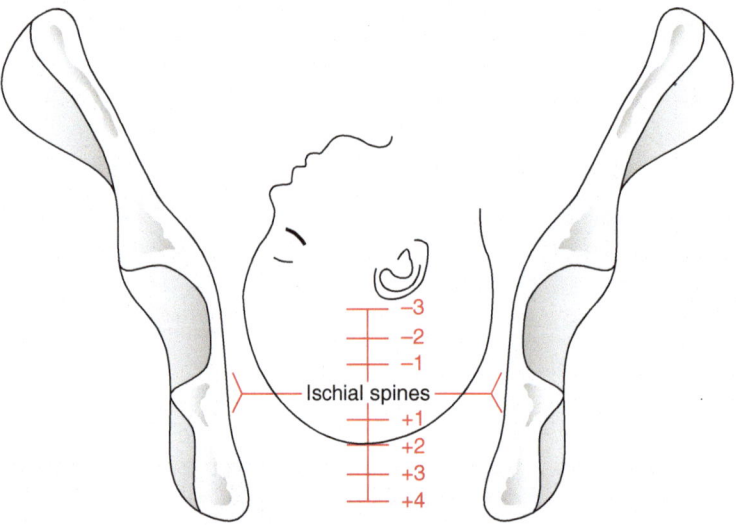

Figure 4.1.6 The station of the fetus

muscle attachments, but the anterior surface is smooth and usually concave. This curvature is referred to as the **sacral hollow**. The sacral nerves pass through the four sets of sacral foramina (openings). The first sacral vertebra projects forward and is called the **sacral promontory** (see Figure 4.1.2).

The coccyx

The **coccyx** is a small triangular shaped bone composed of four fused coccygeal vertebrae. The apex of the coccyx is rounded and the tendon of the external anal sphincter attaches here.

Pelvic joints and ligaments

There are four pelvic joints: two **sacroiliac joints**, one **sacrococcygeal joint** and one **symphysis pubis** (see Figure 4.1.5). These are held together by ligaments (see Figure 4.1.7). The two weight-bearing synovial sacroiliac joints join the sacrum with the ilium, thereby connecting the spine to the pelvis. The **sacroiliac ligaments** span this joint, and usually ensure these joints have only very limited backward and forward movement. In pregnancy, however, the range of movement increases slightly due to the increase in the hormone relaxin. This allows the sacrum to move backwards slightly during labour, to provide more space for the advancing fetus.

The first coccygeal vertebra articulates with the lower end of the sacrum at the **sacrococcygeal joint**, strengthened by **sacrococcygeal ligaments**. The coccyx can also move backwards at this joint to accommodate the birthing baby. Finally, the two pubic bones articulate medially to form the joint called the **symphysis pubis**. This is an oval disc of fibrocartilage reinforced by **inter-pubic ligaments** crossing from one pubic bone to the other. Outside of pregnancy, this joint remains strong and immovable, but again in pregnancy relaxin may enable slight movement of the joint.

This action of relaxin can cause some women to experience pain in the sacroiliac joint or pain and/or misalignment at the symphysis pubis – a condition known as **pelvic girdle pain** (see Chapter 3.5).

Other key ligaments to note are the **sacrotuberous** and **sacrospinous** ligaments which pass between the sacrum and ischium providing additional strength to the pelvis.

4.1

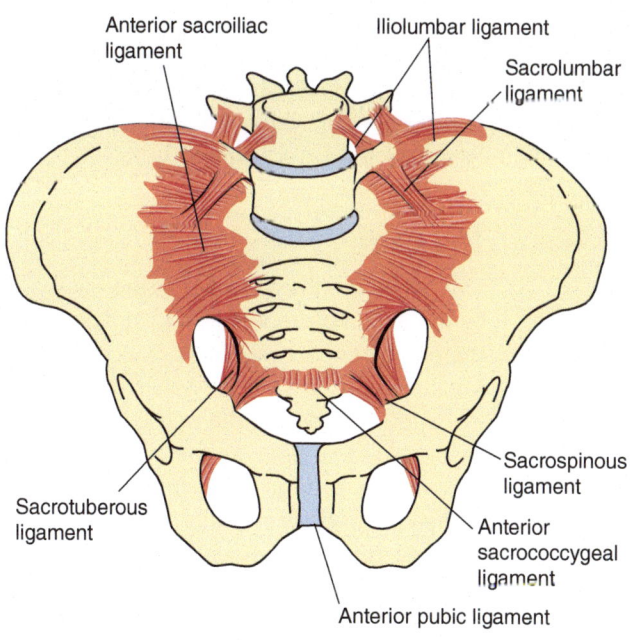

Anterior sacroiliac ligament

Iliolumbar ligament

Sacrolumbar ligament

Sacrotuberous ligament

Sacrospinous ligament

Anterior sacrococcygeal ligament

Anterior pubic ligament

Figure 4.1.7 Pelvic ligaments

APPLICATION TO PRACTICE

If you are able, handle and take a good look at a model pelvis, identifying all the landmarks discussed in this chapter. Think about positions that a woman might adopt to ensure that their pelvis can move and expand to facilitate fetal descent. Which positions might inhibit pelvic movement and why?

Did you know?

It is argued that in people who squat regularly, the sacrum can pivot back further, as the sacrotuberous ligaments will have been stretched (Gorman et al., 2015).

Women in labour will often spontaneously move and sway, which will alter the orientation of the pelvis with respect to the fetus and help it to descend.

The increased mobility of the pelvis in childbirth allows it to be manipulated externally – gentle inward pressure on the hips, for example, can narrow and/ or expand certain dimensions of the pelvis.

Life events such as falls can cause the coccyx to become fused to the sacrum, in which case it may snap as the fetus pushes against it.

Pelvis variations

The pelvis, like the skull, varies structurally with biological sex (Figure 4.1.8). The female pelvis is adapted for childbearing, being generally larger and wider than a male pelvis. The female sacrum tends to be shorter, more curved and have a less pronounced sacral promontory than its male counterpart. Male iliac crests are generally higher, causing the pelvis to look taller and narrower. The female pelvis also generally has less prominent ischial spines allowing for a greater bispinous diameter and a greater angled subpubic arch. Wider hips in females cause an increased angle between the femur and the lower leg called the valgus angle, which can increase the risk of torsional knee injuries.

Additionally, however, not all female pelvises are the same shape. Historically, four different classifications of pelvis have been widely recognised, but these are now widely disputed and discredited (Betti, 2021; Kuliukas and Kuliukas, 2015). A huge variety of pelvic shape exists within (not simply between) female populations (Figure 4.1.9). Pelvic shape can also be influenced by injury or disease, for example rickets. Furthermore, the outward appearance of pelvic shape may not be indicative of internal space and shape. Rather than attempting to categorise and label pelvic shapes, Kuliukas and Kuliukas (2015) argue that it is more helpful to have an awareness that a fetus will negotiate different pelvic shapes in different ways.

The pelvic landmarks that are of particular interest during birth are explored below. Note that it may be useful to refer to Chapters 4.3 and 4.4 alongside this section, in order to understand the terminology related to the fetus here.

The pelvic brim

The pelvic brim is bounded at the back by the sacral promontory, and in front by the pubic bones (see Figure 4.1.2). The fetus passes through the pelvic brim as it 'engages' and enters the pelvic cavity. In order to do this (it is a tight fit!), a cephalic fetus needs to align the widest part of its head (generally the anteroposterior diameter) with the widest part of the pelvic brim, which may be the transverse, oblique or anteroposterior diameter, depending on the woman's shape (Figure 4.1.9).

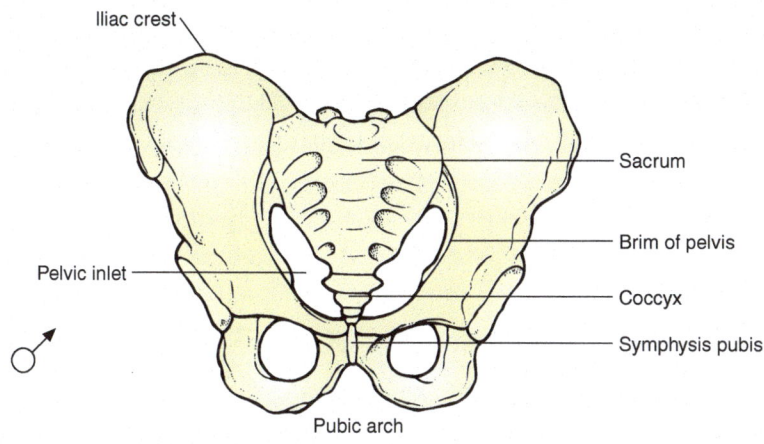

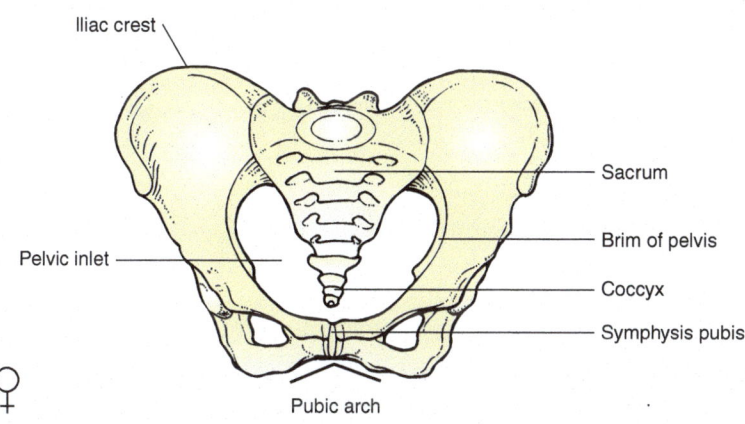

Figure 4.1.8 Female and male pelvises
Source: Figure 3.18b,c, p.81, Clancy and McVicars (2009)

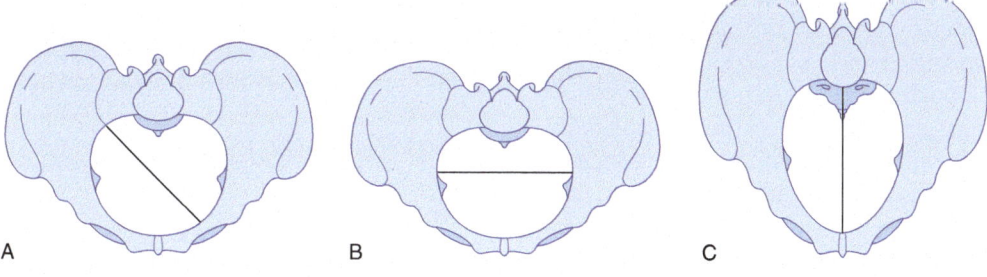

A   B   C

Figure 4.1.9 Some examples of different pelvic shapes. NB The black line denotes the widest diameter
Source: Figure 12.5 (a), p.196, Kenny and Myers (2017)

Where the pelvic brim is an indented circle (Figure 4.1.9A), the fetus may engage in either the transverse or the oblique diameter. In shallower transverse oval shaped brims, the widest diameter of the pelvic brim is the transverse diameter (Figure 4.1.9B). In figure 4.1.9C this pelvic shape is associated with women with

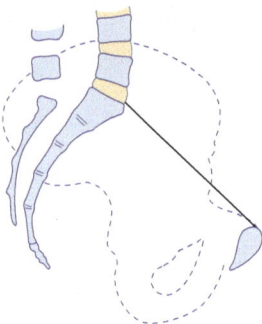

Figure 4.1.10 Pelvic orientation
Source: Figure 12.6(b), p.196, Kenny and Myers (2017)

narrow hips. The widest diameter is the anteroposterior diameter.

The orientation of the pelvic brim is also a consideration. The pelvis is generally tilted at an angle of around 55–60° from horizontal when a woman is standing (Figure 4.1.10). This angle is affected by a woman's posture and muscle tone, and can be exaggerated if she arches her back (not uncommon as the gravid uterus pulls the abdomen forward – see Chapter 3.5). Positions which encourage women to straighten or round their backs can help fetuses to engage.

The pelvic cavity

The anterior wall of the pelvic cavity is formed by the pubic bones and symphysis pubis, giving rise to a depth of around 4 cm. The posterior wall is formed by the sacrum which is around 12 cm in length. The fetus pivots around the symphysis pubis as it descends along the sacrum. If a fetus has entered the pelvis in anything other than a direct occipito-anterior position (where the head will be facing the mother's sacrum), then it will probably need to rotate in the pelvic cavity in order to align itself with the widest diameter of the pelvic outlet (usually the anteroposterior). A fetus entering the pelvis in a direct occipito-posterior position (facing the mother's pubis) may birth in this position, however, particularly if the

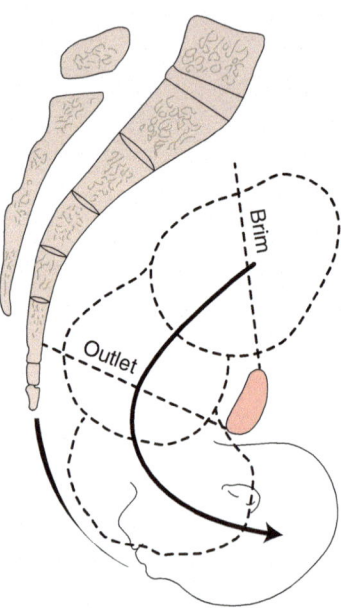

Figure 4.1.11 Descent and rotation in the pelvic cavity

mother's sacrum is also quite straight. The curve of the sacrum along which the baby descends and rotates is hypothetically extended to become the Curve of Carus (Figure 4.1.11). See Chapter 4.3 for a more detailed explanation of the passage of the fetus through the pelvis.

The shape and space available in the pelvic cavity are determined by the shape and orientation of the sacrum, the shape of the sides of the pelvis and the prominence of the ischial spines. It can also be influenced by maternal position and movement, and the degree of laxity in the pelvic joints and ligaments.

The internal surface of the sacrum is usually curved (potentially creating more space) or may be almost straight. A curved sacrum generally inclines backwards, creating a sacral angle of more than 90 degrees, while the **angle of inclination** on a straighter sacrum may be narrower (Figure 4.1.12). While a narrower sacral angle means potentially less space in the pelvic cavity, it can facilitate

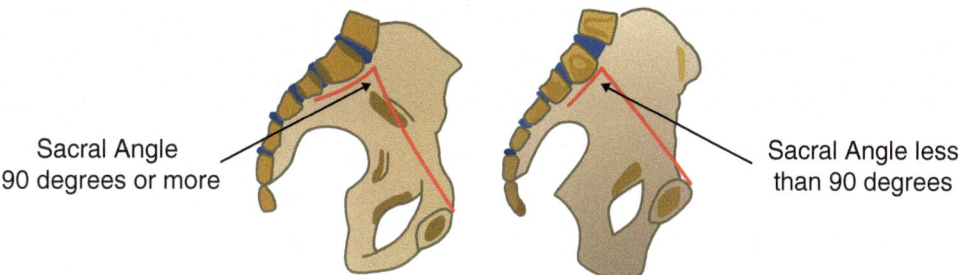

Sacral Angle
90 degrees or more

Sacral Angle less
than 90 degrees

Figure 4.1.12 The sacral angle

Pelvic wall

Straight   Convergent   Divergent

Ischial spines

Not prominent   Prominent   Not prominent

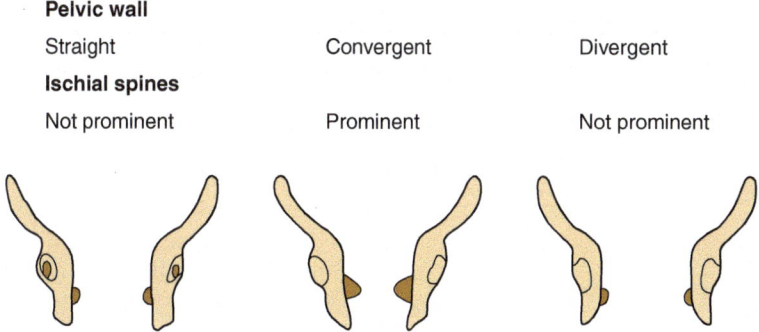

Figure 4.1.13 The internal walls of the pelvis

engagement of the fetal head (as the alignment between the abdominal cavity and the pelvic brim is likely to be greater).

The internal walls or sides of the pelvis can be straight, convergent or divergent (Figure 4.1.13). Convergent sides are more often associated with a heart-shaped or anteroposterior oval inlet, where less rotation is generally required for the fetus to align itself with the widest diameter of the pelvic outlet. Again, however, all of these shapes can be altered by maternal position and pelvic mobility.

The pelvic outlet

The widest diameter of the pelvic outlet – the space bounded by the symphysis pubis, coccyx and ischial tuberosities – is generally the anteroposterior, which is why most babies are born facing their mother's back.

The size of this space is dictated by the subpubic angle, as a wider subpubic angle creates more space between the ischial tuberosities (Figure 4.1.14).

CHAPTER CHALLENGE

This chapter has given an overview of the pelvis that is very different to that found in many older textbooks. For almost a century, our understanding of the pelvis has been influenced by Caldwell and Moloy, who classified the female pelvis into four distinct types: gynaecoid, anthropoid, android and platypelloid. One of the main issues with these classifications is that the gynecoid pelvis came to be viewed as the 'best' and 'most suitable' for childbirth, and other

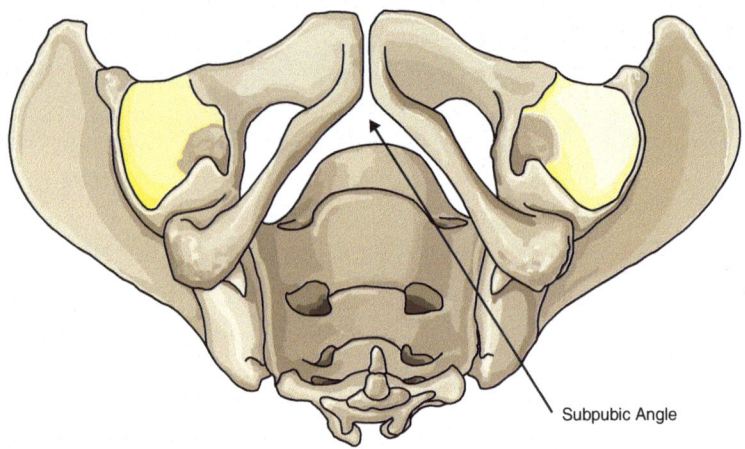

Subpubic Angle

Figure 4.1.14 The subpubic angle

shapes came to be viewed as inherently problematic. We now understand that individual pelvises do not conform so tidily to one of four categories, and to single out one shape as 'normal' and base our teaching and understanding on this is a great disservice to many women.

Have a look at the paper below, and think about how current practice might discriminate against some people, and how we might use our new understanding of the pelvis to practice more inclusively:

Betti L. Shaping birth: Variation in the birth canal and the importance of inclusive obstetric care. *Phil. Trans. R. Soc. B* [Internet] 2021, 376:20200024. doi:10.1098/rstb.2020.0024.

References

Betti L. Shaping birth: Variation in the birth canal and the importance of inclusive obstetric care. *Phil. Trans. R. Soc. B* [Internet] 2021, 376:20200024. doi:10.1098/rstb.2020.0024.

Gorman J., Roberts C. et al. Squatting, pelvic morphology and a reconsideration of childbirth difficulties. *Evol. Med. Public Health* 2015, 10(1):243–55.

Kuliukas A., Kuliukas L. Female pelvic shape: Distinct types or nebulous cloud? *Br. J. Midwifery* 2015, 23(7):490–6.

Physiology of the first stage of labour

Louise Hunter and Giada Giusmin

LEARNING OUTCOMES

▶ Understand the complexity of labour onset, and describe some factors thought to play a part in labour onset and amplification
▶ Describe the latent phase of labour
▶ Understand key physiological processes, and the interplay between these, during the established first stage of labour
▶ Describe transition, and outline signs which may indicate a woman is in transition

A deep understanding and trust in the physiology of birth is the cornerstone of midwifery practice. Knowledge confers confidence in the process of birth, enabling a midwife to use this knowledge to create an environment supportive of the physiology of labour and birth; while also recognising when physiology alone will not suffice, and greater intervention may be indicated.

The next three chapters outline the anatomy and physiology of birth, from the gradual escalation of uterine activity to the birth of the placenta and membranes. Although this is one continuous process, for ease of learning we have used the traditional three stage approach. This chapter discusses Stage 1: the opening up of the cervix. Chapters 4.3 and 4.4 outline the fetus' journey out of the uterus and into the world, and Chapter 4.5 details the birth of the placenta and membranes, and the control of uterine bleeding.

Definition and phases of the first stage of labour

In the first stage of labour, the cervix opens up to create a space for the baby to pass

DOI: 10.4324/9781003227571-22

through and be born. Traditionally, the first stage is said to commence with the onset of regular uterine contractions which **efface** (literally 'eliminate', but in labour this refers to a process of thinning out) and **dilate** ('open up') the cervix, and finish when the cervix has dilated enough to allow the fetus to pass through (fully dilated). Labour is not easily compartmentalised, however, and the first stage is further divided into three phases:

- ▶ **Latent phase**: For many women, labour begins with a period of **irregular contractions**. These have been termed 'latent' because, although they can be painful, initially they may not efface and dilate the cervix, or only do so very inefficiently. Over time, however, the contractions become more regular, and the cervix effaces and dilates up to around 4 cm.
- ▶ **Established phase**: When the cervix reaches around 4 cm dilation, **contractions become stronger, more regular (typically 3–5 minutes apart) and effective**. Established labour is measured from this point until the birth of the baby. Established first stage finishes when the cervix is fully dilated.
- ▶ **Transition**: This is the period when the cervix approaches full dilation and the baby starts to move down through the birth canal. It is characterised by increased anxiety, restlessness and sometimes fear in the birthing mother, as she starts to experience an urge to bear down.

It is difficult to assign a time span to each phase as this is individual to each woman. To do so is also to conform to a biomedical approach which sees time somewhat arbitrarily as demarcating physiological from pathological, rather than looking at the well-being of the mother and fetus. Most medical labour charts, or partograms, require a cervical dilation of 0.5 cm/hour.

Dilation rarely happens at a steady pace, however – it usually starts slowly and speeds up as contractions build in frequency, length and intensity. There is some evidence to suggest that women who are older, and women who have a raised body mass are more likely to have longer labours (Lundborg et al., 2021).

The onset of labour

It is perhaps strange to say that, at the present time, the exact trigger of labour onset is not fully understood. There is also very little consensus as to when exactly labour can be said to have started. Overall, the onset of labour is dependent on hormonal and mechanical factors and the interplay between the mother, the fetus and the placenta. Labour is generally expected to take place between 37–42 weeks of gestation, however, its timing is less accurate in humans than in other species.

Uterine quiescence in pregnancy

Progesterone, together with other hormones like human chorionic gonadotropin (hCG) and relaxin, is responsible for maintaining uterine quiescence (inactivity) in the first and second trimesters. These hormones modify the uterine myocytes and limit the formation of gap junctions between cells – this leads to reduced communication between cells. The uterus is never in a state of total quiescence, however, as very mild activity is present even outside pregnancy. As pregnancy continues, this mild activity becomes more noticeable, irregular and then more frequent and intense contractions. In labour, contractions are regular and intense, due to myometrial cells contracting synchronously as a result of **gap junction formation**.

From quiescence to activity

It is important to note that, unlike in many other species, progesterone levels do not fall towards the end of pregnancy in humans, causing labour to initiate; instead, there is a balance shift from progesterone dominance to **oestrogen dominance**. The exact mechanism of the switch is poorly understood, but it seems progesterone is either converted into oestrogen or metabolised into inactive compounds. Either way, progesterone levels remain high, but lose their sensitivity (called functional withdrawal). This change in the oestrogen/progesterone ratio is responsible for the increase in the production of uterotonics (substances that make the uterus contract), such as **prostaglandins** and **oxytocin**, essential for the activation of the myometrium and for the softening of the cervix.

Fetal input

To guarantee the survival of the species, it is imperative that the fetus is born only when able to survive outside the uterine environment. For this reason, the fetus has an input in determining the initiation of labour. It is suggested that fetal cortisol production is increased towards late pregnancy (see Phase 1 below), and this stimulates the placenta to metabolise progesterone into oestrogen, shifting the oestrogen/progesterone balance.

The myometrium in labour

The mild contractions that occur during late pregnancy **(Braxton-Hicks contractions)** do not generally have an effect on the cervix as the absence of sufficient gap junctions makes this uterine activity poorly coordinated. Before the beginning of labour, the myometrium becomes more excitable and responsive to uterotonics. At the same time, the formation of additional gap junctions enables the cells to act together. The pattern of contractions in labour is remarkably increased compared to pre-labour, and this can commence days before childbirth.

The processes thought to initiate the onset of labour have been divided into four phases (Lye, 1996):

▶ Phase 0: Quiescence
▶ Phase 1: Activation
▶ Phase 2: Stimulation
▶ Phase 3: Involution – not discussed in this chapter as it occurs in the postpartum period

Phases 0, 1 and 2 are discussed further below.

Phase 0, quiescence, is the state in which the myometrium is found for the majority of the pregnancy (approximately 95% of the time). During this time, progesterone, relaxin and other hormones inhibiting uterine contraction (uterotonic inhibitors) keep the uterus quiescent.

Phase 1, activation, is the phase in which uterotonic inhibitors are reduced and oestrogen increases. The transition from Phase 0 to Phase 1 is a slow and gradual process occurring a few weeks before childbirth:

▶ **Contraction-associated proteins (CAP)**, which include **gap junction proteins** enabling the transmission of signals between myometrial cells, **oxytocin** and **prostaglandin receptors**, and **calcium channels**, all increase. This might be coordinated by a **fetal inflammatory response** that takes place near the end of the pregnancy as a result of the fetus growing and stretching the uterine wall.
▶ This signal from the fetus also includes increased production of **placental corticotropin-releasing hormone (CRH)**, whose function is to stimulate fetal adrenal glands to produce steroids

(such as cortisol). Via a positive feedback loop, cortisol then stimulates placental CRH production. As the fetal hypothalamic-pituitary-adrenal system matures, both fetal and placental CRH increase, which enhances the production of **oestrogen**. This further alters the oestrogen/progesterone ratio, tipping the balance towards oestrogen.

▶ The above changes lead to increased myometrial excitability and response to uterotonics by stimulating gap junction formation and oxytocin and prostaglandin receptors. In this phase, myometrial contractions occur more often and are more intense.

Phase 2, stimulation: Only once the myometrium has been activated can it then react to the stimulation provided by uterotonic agents, in particular **oxytocin** and **prostaglandins**. Phases 1 and 2 combined activation and stimulation can initiate strong contractions in the myometrium, which dilate the cervix and deliver the unborn baby. Table 4.2.1 outlines the main hormones involved in this process.

INTERRUPTER

Complete the table in your workbook (or create your own) to embed knowledge of key hormones in latent and active first stage.

Anatomy of the first stage

The uterus

At the end of pregnancy, the uterus (Figure 4.2.1) is described as having two anatomically distinct segments. However, this can be misleading, as it is still one organ and functions as such, but this demarcation can help to explain how labour works.

▶ The **upper segment** is formed of the fundus and body of the uterus
▶ The **lower segment** is formed of the isthmus and cervix, and is about 8–10 cm long in length

The uterus is composed of three layers of smooth muscle cells: an outer longitudinal layer, a middle criss-cross or mesh-like layer, and an inner circular layer (Figure 4.2.2).

Table 4.2.1 Key hormones of the first stage

Hormone	Source and role
Oestrogen	Mainly produced by the placenta. Increases progressively during pregnancy. Promotes the production of prostaglandins and of prostaglandin and oxytocin receptors. Enhances gap junction formation between myometrial cells. All these changes are responsible for strong and synchronised myometrial contractions.
Prostaglandins	Produced by the placenta and membranes. Facilitates maternal cardiovascular adaptations in pregnancy, including enhancing uteroplacental blood flow. In labour, prostaglandins help the myometrium display oxytocin receptors and gap junctions. Prostaglandins also have an effect on cervical ripening. PGE2 (a type of prostaglandin) is essential to soften the cervix.
Oxytocin and oxytocin receptors	Oxytocin receptors increase in concentration toward the end of pregnancy (up to 100–200 times), meaning that oxytocin is more effective in generating contractions as pregnancy continues. Oxytocin is produced by the hypothalamus and secreted by the pituitary, but also by the myometrium, placenta and fetal membranes. Oxytocin stimulates myometrial contractions directly and by encouraging the release of prostaglandins.

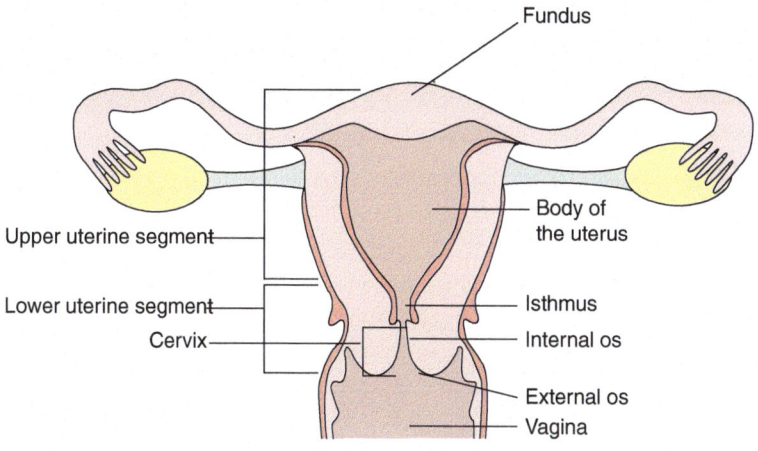

Figure 4.2.1 The uterus

4.2

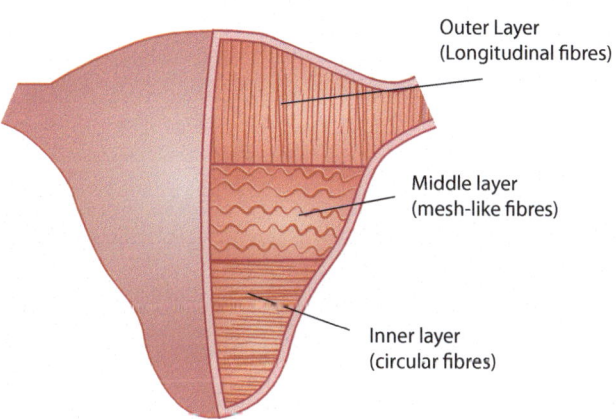

Figure 4.2.2 The uterine muscle layers

Smooth muscle is able to contract involuntarily, under the influence of oxytocin. It is composed of long, elastic filaments which shorten and thicken during a contraction. The proliferation of gap junctions between the uterine smooth muscle cells at term enables coordinated contraction activity. There is a higher density of smooth muscle and there are more oxytocin receptors in the upper uterine segment.

The cervix

The cervix is a rigid cylindrical structure about 4–7 cm long. Its rigidity is due to its high collagen content. It has an os, or opening, at each end – the internal os is adjacent to the uterus. Before labour, the cervix is closed and contains a small amount of gelatinous fluid – the **operculum**, or plug, – which helps to prevent pathogens entering the uterine cavity. The cervix of a multiparous woman may be shorter and the external os may feel more like a slit than a dimple (this is known as a **multips os**) – see Figure 5.1.3, Chapter 5.1.

Physiological processes in established labour

Contractions

Labour contractions are sometimes referred to as surges, or waves. They are **involuntary muscle tightenings**, meaning that they are not under conscious control – the uterus of an unconscious woman can contract, and uteri have been stimulated to contract outside of bodies altogether. That being said, birthing mammals possess a powerful **fight or flight** reflex – they react to external stressors (such as the

appearance of a predator, or being moved to a different environment) by producing adrenalin, which either stops early labour contractions (to give the birthing mammal time to escape) or intensifies late labour contractions (so that birth can be expedited prior to an escape).

During labour, uterine contractions are **coordinated**. They begin at the fundus, where smooth muscle is most densely concentrated. Electrical signals then pass over and down the uterus through the gap junctions in a wave, stimulating the rest of the smooth muscle to contract as they go. The contraction is strongest, and lasts for slightly longer, in the fundus. It builds to a peak and then subsides, seemingly fading from all areas simultaneously. This process is illustrated in Figure 4.2.3. The

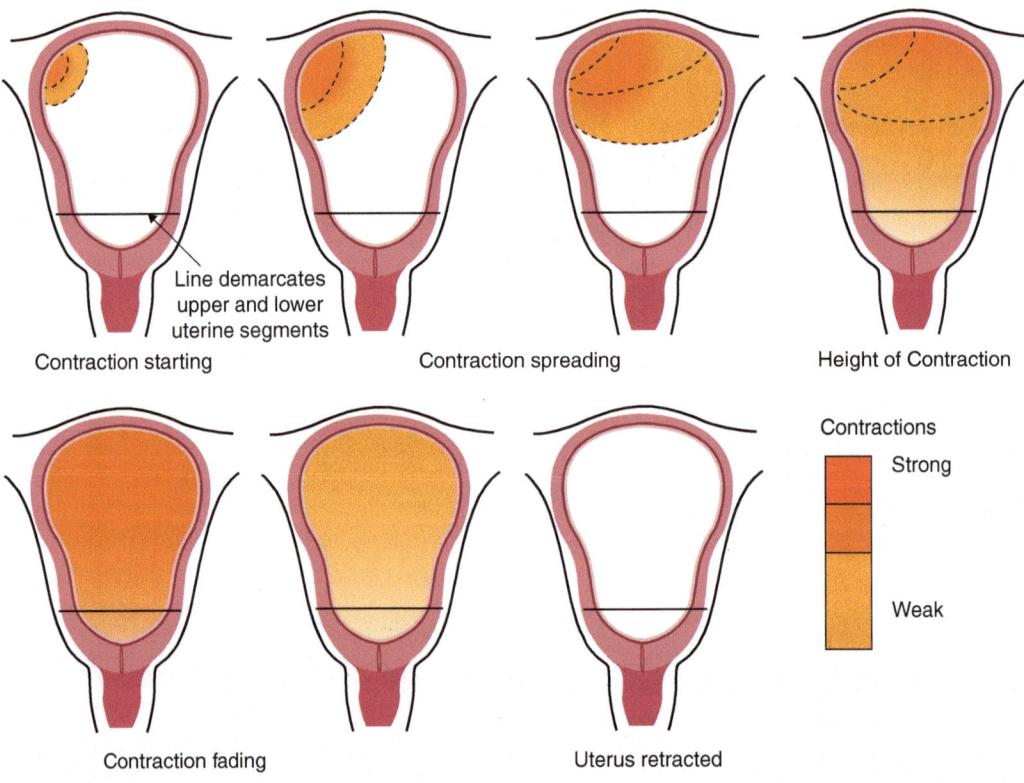

Line demarcates upper and lower uterine segments

Contraction starting

Contraction spreading

Height of Contraction

Contraction fading

Uterus retracted

Contractions

Strong

Weak

Figure 4.2.3 The path of a contraction

force of a contraction can be measured in mmHg, according to the pressure it exerts in the uterine cavity. In early labour, contractions can be irregular, with an intensity of around 20 mmHg, and typically last 20–30 seconds. As labour progresses, they become more regular, stronger, longer and more frequent. At the height of first stage they can have a peak intensity of 60 mmHg, last 45–60 seconds and occur every 2–3 minutes. Contractions are generally experienced as painful, most likely due to the tightening muscle fibres occluding blood supply. The pain can be felt in the lower abdomen, back or upper legs. They can sometimes be seen, and can also be felt, externally, as a muscle tightening under a hand placed on the abdomen.

Retraction and fundal dominance

Between contractions the uterus relaxes, but some of the shortening in the smooth muscle fibres is retained (Figure 4.2.4). This is known as **retraction**. As labour progresses, the muscle fibres gradually become shorter and thicker, reducing the size of the uterine cavity. Due to **fundal dominance**, with more smooth muscle cells being found in the fundus and less in the lower segment, this physically pulls the lower segment of the uterus up – causing effacement and dilatation of the cervix. During contractions, contents of the uterus (the fetus and amniotic fluid) are pushed down onto the cervix, also due to retraction and fundal dominance, which further aids the process of cervical dilation.

4.2

Polarity

Polarity refers to the coordinated activity of the upper and lower uterine segments. Muscle fibres in the upper segment contract and retract, pulling up the tissue in the lower uterine segment, which contains less contractile smooth muscle, and effacing and dilating the cervix. A ridge, or **retraction ring**, gradually forms between the two segments. In an obstructed labour (where strong contractions are unable to push the baby out of the uterus, usually due to the presenting part being larger than the maternal pelvis), this becomes visible above the symphysis pubis and is known as a **Bandl's ring**. This is a pathological sign and can presage uterine rupture. If the lower segment of the uterus contracts first, or more strongly, contractions will not dilate the cervix – this is known as 'incoordinate uterine activity'.

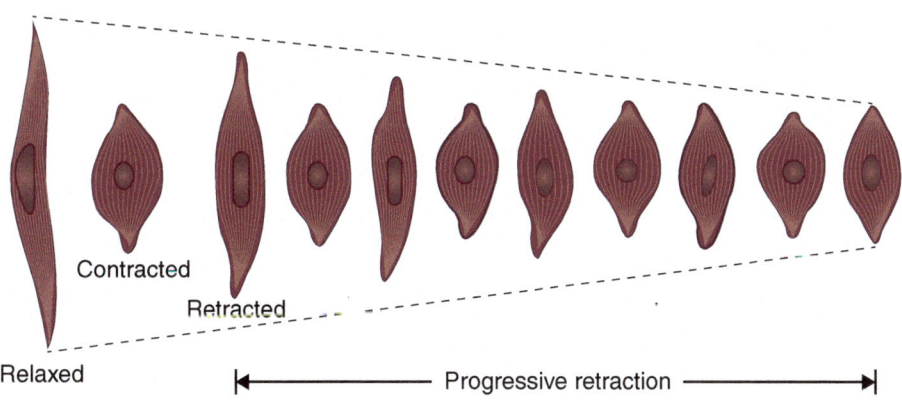

Contracted

Retracted

Relaxed

|← Progressive retraction →|

Figure 4.2.4 Contraction and retraction

Cervical dilatation

There are two stages to the dilation, or opening up, of the cervix:

Effacement

The thinning, or gradual elimination, of the cervix can start towards the end of pregnancy. Hormones including oestrogen, progesterone, relaxin, prolactin and prostaglandins act on the collagen in cervical tissue, causing the cervix to soften, or **ripen**, and lose its structural rigidity. An unripe cervix feels firm and rigid – a bit like the end of a nose. A ripe cervix feels soft and moist – like the inside of a cheek. Once ripened, the cervix starts to **thin** as it is drawn up into the lower uterine segment under the influence of early labour contractions (see Figure 4.2.5). This process happens from the bottom up – the outer tissue around the external os is pulled up first, while the internal os remains closed until dilation starts. As the external os is taken away, the operculum detaches and is expelled as a '**show**', often accompanied by a small amount of blood from the cervical wall.

Effacement can continue throughout the first stage, with the cervix becoming progressively thinner as it opens up. It is more common for effacement to precede dilation in a primiparous woman and occur simultaneously with dilation in subsequent labours. Effacement is sometimes expressed as a percentage – so a half-thinned cervix is said to be '50% effaced'.

Dilation

As contractions build and become regular, the cervix begins to open up, or dilate, as the smooth muscle fibres at the fundus exert pressure on it as they contract and retract. The space created by dilation is oval or circular, and is measured across its diameter in cm (see Figure 4.2.5). When this space is large enough to allow the passage of the fetus (this happens at around 10 cm dilation, and at this point no cervix will be felt in front of the presenting part) the cervix is said to be **fully dilated**.

APPLICATION TO PRACTICE

Midwives use different visual reference points to explain dilation to women (or even to judge it themselves). Below is a schematic using fruit (Figure 4.2.6) – you might like to come up with your own analogies that are relevant to you and the women in your care.

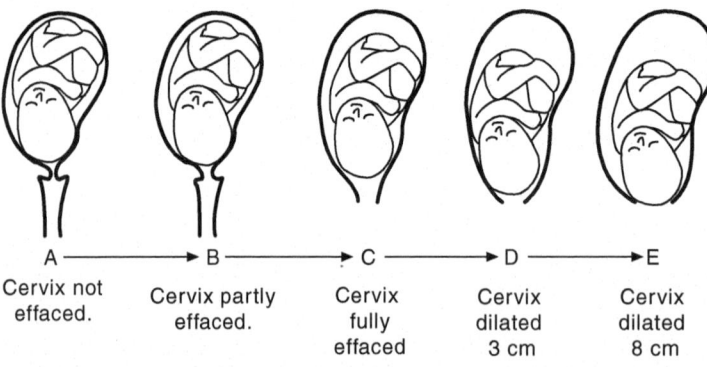

A ————▶ B ————▶ C ————▶ D ————▶ E

| Cervix not effaced. | Cervix partly effaced. | Cervix fully effaced | Cervix dilated 3 cm | Cervix dilated 8 cm |

Figure 4.2.5 Effacement and dilation

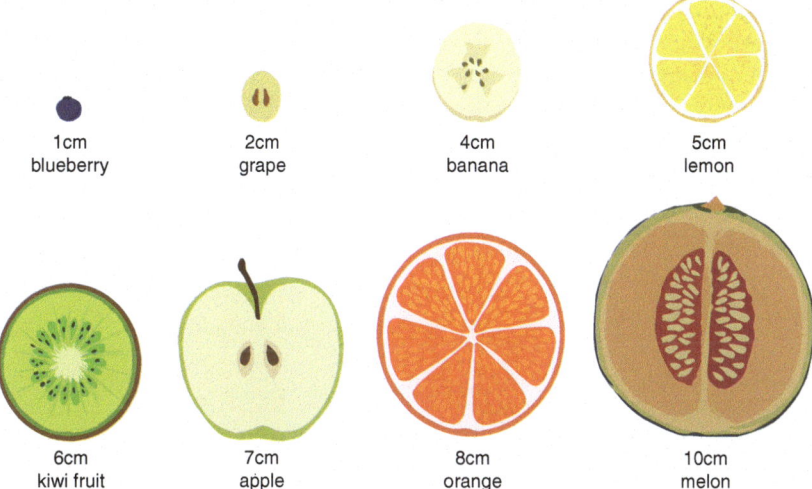

4.2

Figure 4.2.6 Cervical dilation fruit schematic

Formation of forewaters and membrane rupture

The cervix effectively dilates around the membranes, provided they are still intact. As the membranes are exposed by the retreating cervix, and the fetal head is pushed down into the maternal pelvis, a small amount of amniotic fluid usually becomes trapped in front of it. This is known as the **forewaters**. The waters behind the fetus's head are the **hindwaters** (Figure 4.2.7). As the pressure of the advancing fetal head increases, the membranes eventually give way and the waters break. This usually happens as the fetus starts to move through the birth canal in the second stage, but can also happen earlier in labour, or before the start of labour. Occasionally, the fetal head can be born with the membranes still intact. This is called being born **'en caul'**. As the membranes are attached to the placenta, they will break as the fetal body emerges. Membrane rupture is often conceptualised as a dramatic and sudden gush of fluid.

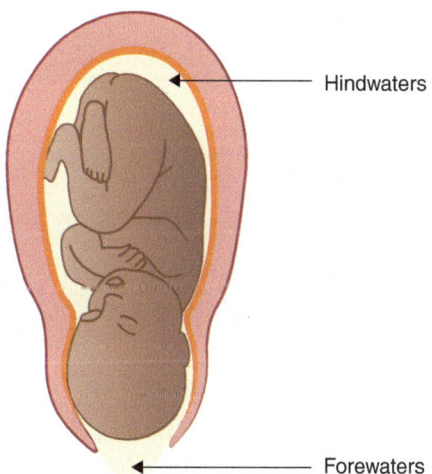

Figure 4.2.7 Forewaters and hindwaters

However, if the membranes break behind the fetus' head, the liquor may leak out gradually, resembling urine in all but smell.

General fluid pressure

The principle of general fluid pressure asserts that, while the membranes remain intact, the pressure of the uterine contractions is exerted on the amniotic fluid and, as fluid is **not compressible**, the pressure is equalised over the fetal body and placenta. In addition, the same amount of pressure will be applied onto and across the cervix, due to the pressure within the forewaters equalising, making it dilate evenly.

Once the waters have broken, general fluid pressure no longer applies – as there is a route out for the fluid. Therefore, pressure from contractions will no longer equalise across the fetus and placenta, which may lead to a reduction in oxygen supply during a contraction, and increased pressure on the fetal head. In addition, pressure no longer equalises over the cervix, as the head is now directly applied to it. Depending on how 'well' the fetal head is applied to the cervix, this may lead to uneven dilation of the cervix. However, direct pressure from the fetal head onto the cervix will increase stimulation and release of oxytocin, strengthening contractions. This is why labour can speed up once the waters have broken.

Ferguson reflex

The Ferguson reflex is an example of a **positive feedback loop**. In this case, it begins during the first stage of labour and continues until the birth of the baby, and even slightly beyond. In the first stage of labour, as the fetus descends, due to the processes described above, it applies pressure onto and stretches the cervix. This stretch triggers receptors, which send a message to the posterior pituitary to release oxytocin, which causes contractions to increase in length, strength and frequency. This causes the fetus to apply more pressure onto the cervix, which causes more stretch and more triggering of

receptors, which causes more oxytocin to be released – and so on.

Transition

The transition from contractions that pull the cervix up and open to contractions that push the baby out of the uterus can precipitate physical and psychological symptoms during labour, caused by a surge in catecholamines at this stage in the labour process. Some or all of the following symptoms may manifest:

▶ The woman appears worried, anxious, distressed and/or confused
▶ The rhythm of labour appears to be interrupted – pain management techniques that were working are no longer deemed helpful, the woman feels that they can no longer cope, and that they have lost control
▶ Nausea and vomiting
▶ Shaking
▶ Heavy show
▶ Urge to bear down
▶ Erratic contractions
▶ Contractions slow, or stop for a while

APPLICATION TO PRACTICE

The way women are cared for during labour directly impacts the physiology of birth:

▶ If women **feel safe**, understand what is happening to them and feel they have some control and agency over the process, their bodies are **less likely to produce adrenalin and stress hormones** which can inhibit oxytocin release, and more likely to produce endorphins, which help with coping and pain. Dim lighting, water, aromatherapy and music can all help women in labour to feel secure.

▶ Physiologically, humans are designed to birth in **upright and forward leaning positions**. The uterus contracts forwards, gravity assists the descent of the fetus, and the woman is able to move spontaneously to assist the fetus into the pelvis. Positions that require a woman to recline or lie on their back may provide a better view for the accoucheur but confer no benefit and may even cause harm to the mother and fetus. The weight of the fetus on major maternal blood vessels such as the vena cava can impede oxygenation to both mother and fetus, the contracting uterus and descending fetus are having to work against gravity, and the woman is less able to move. A Cochrane review found clear evidence that upright and walking positions in first stage shorten labour, lessen the perceived need for an epidural and result in fewer Caesarean sections, with no evidence of any adverse effect (Lawrence et al., 2013).

▶ Labour is a muscular activity that uses energy – **nutrition and hydration** at this time are therefore important. However, during labour digestion slows – it takes significantly longer for food to pass through the stomach (although interestingly, there is a small amount of evidence to suggest that this effect is much less marked in women who have epidural anaesthesia (Bouvet et al., 2022)). Concern over women potentially aspirating acidic stomach content into their lungs (Mendelson's syndrome) should a general anaesthetic be required has led to a long-running debate over whether women should eat solid food (see Chapter 4.7). It is unlikely, however, that someone in advanced labour will want to eat a large meal, and it should also be borne in mind that a stomach deprived of food will contain acidic bile.

▶ A **full bladder can impede the passage of the fetal head** into the pelvis and is more likely to be damaged by pressure from the advancing fetus. It can also make contractions more painful. It is therefore vital that women are encouraged to urinate at least every couple of hours.

▶ A **full bowel** can also impede the progress of the fetal head. Many women experience an urge to defecate in early labour (the bowel also contains smooth muscle and will contract under the influence of oxytocin), or at the beginning of second stage, as the muscles used for pushing are the same as those used to defecate.

4.2

References

Bouvet L., Schulz T. et al. Pregnancy and labor epidural effects on gastric emptying: A prospective comparative study. *Anesthesiology* [Internet] 2022, 136:542–50. https://pubs.asahq.org/anesthesiology/article/136/4/542/118338/Pregnancy-and-Labor-Epidural-Effects-on-Gastric.

Lawrence A., Lewis L. et al. Maternal positions and mobility during first stage labour. *Cochrane Database Syst. Rev.* [Internet] 2013. doi:10.1002/14651858.CD003934.pub4.

Lundborg L., Liu X. et al. Association of body mass index and maternal age with first stage duration of labour. *Sci. Rep.* [Internet] 2021, 11:13843. www.ncbi.nlm.nih.gov/pmc/articles/PMC8257589/.

Lye S. Initiation of parturition. *Anim. Reprod. Sci.* 1996, 42:495–503.

Further reading

Desseauve D., Fradet L. et al. Biomechanical comparison of squatting and "optimal" supine birth positions. *J. Biomechan.* [Internet] 2020, 105:109783. doi:10.1016/j.jbiomech.2020.109783.

Hanley G., Munro S. et al. Diagnosing onset of labor: A systematic review of definitions in the research literature. *BMC Pregnancy Childbirth* [Internet] 2016, 16(71). doi:10.1186/s12884-016-0857-4.

Leap N., Hunter B. *Supporting women for labour and birth*. Routledge; Abingdon, 2016.

CHAPTER 4.3

Physiology of the second stage of labour

Louise Hunter

As well as clearly describing the second stage of labour, this chapter takes a physiological lens to the evidence underpinning safe and supportive care during birth.

LEARNING OUTCOMES

▶ Define the second stage of labour
▶ Explain key concepts in the second stage of labour which aid the passage of the fetus through the birth canal
▶ Describe the Ferguson reflex as a positive feedback loop
▶ Describe the key stages of the passage through the pelvis for a cephalic fetus

Physiology of the second stage

The World Health Organization (WHO) defines the second stage of labour as the period of time between full cervical dilatation and the birth of the baby, during which the woman has an involuntary urge to bear down, as a result of expulsive uterine contractions (WHO, 2018). In first labours, the second stage is usually completed within three hours (it is generally much quicker but can also take longer). In subsequent labours, birth is usually completed within two hours of the commencement of second stage. These time lengths are widely integrated into practice, based on concerns about fetal hypoxia should second stage continue for longer.

DOI: 10.4324/9781003227571-23

The WHO definition is not without its difficulties: full dilatation of the cervix can only be confirmed by vaginal examination, and it is not always accompanied by an involuntary urge to bear down. Other authorities, such as NICE (2023), attribute a passive and an active phase to second stage labour, and enable it to be recognised by a range of possible physiological signs and events, not all of which require an invasive examination.

Passive second stage of labour recognises the possibility that the cervix may be found to be fully dilated before or in the absence of involuntary expulsive contractions (which are not initiated until the presenting part has descended to the pelvic floor). Passive second stage may last for up to two hours.

Active second stage can be diagnosed in a number of ways:

- ▶ The baby is visible at the introitus and/or
- ▶ The birthing woman is experiencing an involuntary urge to bear down (many women emit characteristic low grunting noises at this time) and
- ▶ Full dilatation of the cervix is confirmed by a vaginal examination where no cervix is felt and/or
- ▶ A visible rounded area in the lower back (known as the **rhombus of Michaelis**) is

seen when the woman is in an upright or all fours position. This is thought to be caused by the fetal head pushing the sacrum back as it descends

- ▶ A purple or dark/reddish line is visible on the skin over the sacrum, extending up the anal cleft from the anal margin (Figure 4.3.1). This is most likely due to the fetal head pressing on blood vessels in the sacral region. An observational study of 144 women (97% of whom were Caucasian) found that the mean length of this line at 9–10 cm cervical dilation was 9.6 cm (Shepherd et al., 2010)
- ▶ The anus appears flattened and dilated
- ▶ Women birthing without anaesthesia may report feeling their babies descend into the birth canal
- ▶ Women with an epidural may experience pressure above the level of the anaesthetic block, probably due to fetal descent
- ▶ Active pushing commences following a finding of full dilatation of the cervix but in the absence of an urge to bear down

Second stage events

Descent

Once the cervix is fully dilated, the fetus can descend through the birth canal and be born.

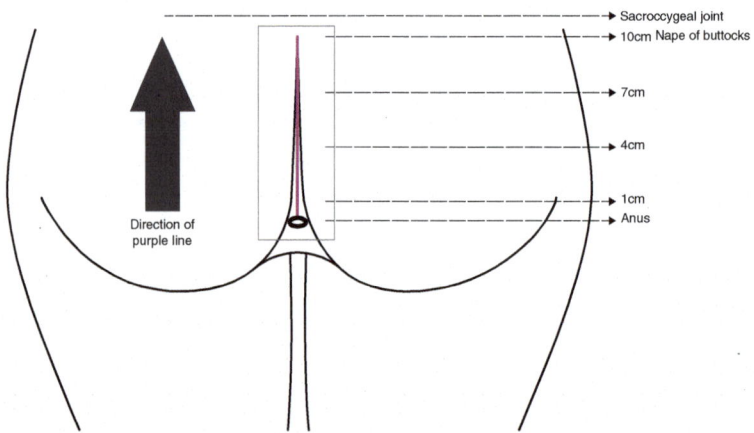

Figure 4.3.1 The trajectory of the purple line

In an unimpeded birth, descent happens with each contraction. The fetus will recede after the contraction ends, and then advance a little further with the next contraction. This allows for a **gradual displacement of soft tissues** and **stretching of the perineum**, and for the **fetal head to mould**, or shape itself, to fit through the available space. Moulding is possible as the fetal skull bones are not completely fused and can overlap. A moulded vertex will generally revert to its original shape in the first few days after birth. The pressure on the fetal head can also cause a swelling or **caput** over the occiput.

Hypoxia

Now that membranes are likely to have broken, general fluid pressure does not hold and the pressure exerted by contractions will reduce the oxygen supply to the fetus. A healthy, term fetus is able to withstand this and recover in between contractions. Close monitoring of the fetal heart is paramount at this time (see Chapter 4.4).

Fetal axis pressure

The force generated by the contracting uterus and maternal effort is transmitted down the fetal spine to its head. This process begins in first stage of labour but intensifies throughout labour – and particularly once the waters have broken, and when the fetus descends to the pelvic floor. Where the baby is in an occipito-anterior (OA) position (facing its mother's back), the pressure will be directed to the occiput, encouraging the head to flex. If a baby is occipito-posterior (OP) (facing its mother's front), the pressure can be directed to the chin, causing the head to extend (Figure 4.3.2). Although an OP position has historically been regarded as a problem, both scenarios ensure that the fetus is in an anatomically favourable position for birth (see *Passage of the fetus* below).

Ferguson reflex

As described in the previous chapter, the Ferguson reflex commences in first stage and continues through second, and into the third stage. During second stage, the fetus is no longer applying stretch to the cervix – which has disappeared. Instead, the fetus descends and stretches, distends and displaces the soft tissues of the pelvis and the pelvic floor. There are many more receptors here than in the cervix, and this causes a surge in signals

4.3

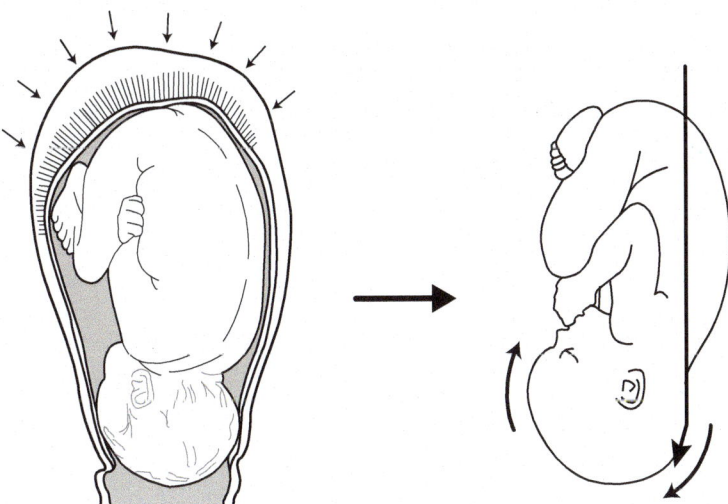

Figure 4.3.2 Fetal axis pressure

to the posterior pituitary to release oxytocin into the bloodstream. This causes an ever-increasing release of oxytocin, which further strengthens contractions, which causes further fetal descent and associated maternal soft tissue distention, which in turn causes more oxytocin to be released. While in the first stage this process was more controlled, in second stage the increase in receptors being triggered means that the process becomes increasingly overwhelming, bringing a maternal urge to push to 'help' the expulsive contractions.

The fetus is actively pushed through the birth canal by **uterine contractions**, but it is eventually aided in this process by **maternal pushing**. The Ferguson reflex ultimately causes an overwhelming urge to use the diaphragm and abdominal muscles to bear down during contractions. The action and feel are very similar to the urge to defecate, and it is not uncommon to see women actively clench their buttock muscles during contractions in an attempt to fight this urge as it starts to kick in. However, as the positive feedback loop continues, the ever-increasing urge to push becomes too overwhelming and the woman will use her secondary powers of expulsion to birth her baby.

INTERRUPTER

Use the space provided in your workbook to draw a diagram of the Ferguson reflex as a positive feedback loop. Try to include how the reflex differs in the first and second stages of labour.

Soft tissue displacement

As the fetus descends through the birth canal:

▶ the **pelvic floor** is displaced. Anteriorly, it is pushed up, taking the **bladder** into the abdomen. A full bladder may impede fetal descent, so regular voiding throughout the first stage of labour is paramount. Posteriorly, the pelvic floor is pushed down, and any faecal matter in the **rectum** will be pushed out as the rectum is flattened by the descending head.

▶ the **anus** will be stretched and appear flattened.

▶ the **perineum** bulges, stretches and becomes paper thin as the presenting part gradually becomes visible with each contraction.

Passage of the fetus

The fetal passage through the pelvis is perhaps best understood as happening in three phases:

▶ The entrance through the pelvic brim. This usually happens before (especially in a first birth) or at the beginning of labour (particularly in second or subsequent births)

▶ The arrival in the pelvic cavity, where the presenting part meets the pelvic floor and any necessary rotation will take place

▶ The exit through the pelvic outlet and perineum

Most fetuses enter the pelvis head first. However, whatever the presenting part and however it is aligned (see Chapter 4.4), the following will apply:

▶ A successful passage through the pelvis relies on the widest part of the fetus aligning with the widest part of the pelvic diameter at any given point. Where a woman's pelvic inlet is widest along the transverse or oblique diameter, and her pelvic outlet is widest along the anteroposterior diameter, the fetus must **rotate** as it advances (Figure 4.3.3). In a pelvis with an inlet that is widest in the anteroposterior diameter, rotation may not be necessary, as the fetal head will enter the pelvis facing directly forwards or backwards and be born in the same

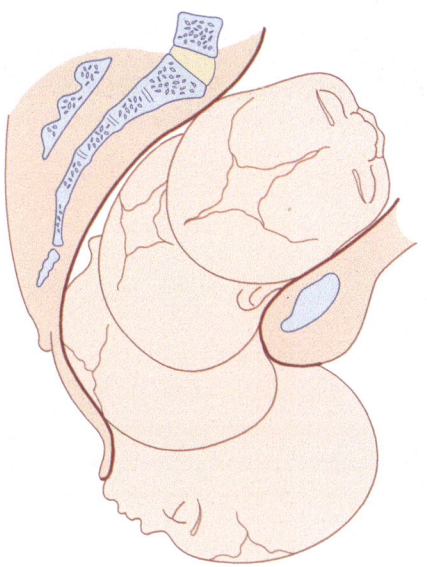
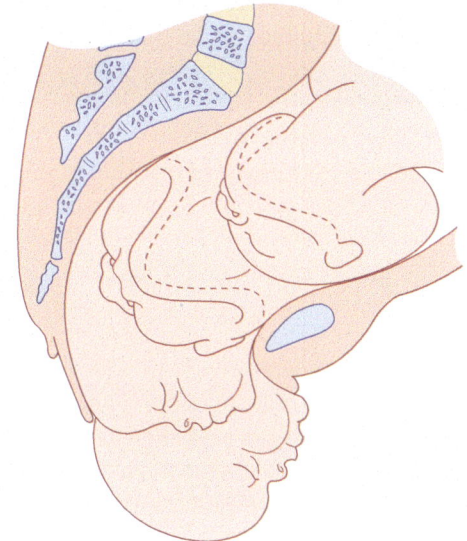

4.3

Figure 4.3.3 Descent and rotation of a fetal head entering the pelvis in a transverse or oblique position, first in an occipito-anterior position, second in an occipito-posterior position
Source: Figure 12.16, p.204 and Figure 12.26, p.216, Kenny and Myers (2017)

position. An element of rotation may be necessary, however, in order for the shoulders to enter the pelvic cavity.

▶ Rotation is aided by a combination of pressure from the fundus as the uterus contracts and the resistance provided by the **pelvic floor muscles**. On meeting the pelvic floor, and with the aid of fetal axis pressure, the presenting part will rotate and bend as it is pushed forwards under the pubic arch. Rotation in the pelvic cavity is sometimes referred to as **internal rotation**. Most (but not all) babies will rotate into an OA position at this point.

▶ In order to **exit** the pelvic cavity, the fetal head must pass **under the pubic arch**. A fetal head in the **OA position** bends upwards as it passes under the pubic arch, deflexing and extending as it stretches the skin around the perineum. The occiput will emerge through the perineum first. A fetal head that passes under the pubic arch in the **OP position**

will be forced to flex as it becomes visible at the perineum and will be born face first.

▶ While it negotiates its passage under the pubic arch, the fetus continues to advance and recede with contractions, and with each contraction more of the fetal head becomes visible at the introitus. When the widest part of the head is distending the perineum, the fetus will not recede, and is said to have **crowned**. The mother may feel an intense burning sensation at this point. The rest of the head will be born with the next contraction – it is usually helpful to advise the mother to take short, gentle breaths at this point so that the head advances slowly, minimising damage to the perineum.

▶ **Once the head is born, the shoulders will have entered the pelvic cavity**, and may also need to rotate to align themselves with the antero-posterior diameter of the pelvic outlet so that they, and the rest of the baby, can be born. As this happens, the head will rotate 90 degrees exteriorly to face the mother's right or left thigh. This is called **external rotation**. Some literature talks about **restitution** at this point, hypothesising that the head and shoulders may have become misaligned during the internal rotation and need to rectify this.

▶ The shoulders and body of the baby will generally be born with the contraction following external rotation. If the mother is in a semi-recumbent position, it is likely that the anterior shoulder will emerge first. If she is upright or on all fours, the posterior shoulder may be the first to emerge. The body will flex laterally as it passes under the pelvic arch and follow the curve of the mother's sacrum (the **Curve of Carus**).

Different cephalic presentations at the pelvic outlet

It is rare that a fetus cannot fit through a pelvis. Should this occur, it is likely to be because the presenting part is larger than the pelvis (due to injury or restricted growth of the pelvis, or uncontrolled maternal diabetes leading to fetal macrosomia), or because the presenting dimensions are too large to fit through either the pelvic inlet or outlet and the fetus does not rotate.

Fetuses, like pelvises, come in all sorts of shapes and sizes, but to give a rough idea of which presenting dimensions are prohibitive to a physiological birth, the generally agreed dimensions of the fetal skull are shown in Figure 4.3.4.

▶ In an **OA presentation with a well-flexed head**, the smallest diameter of the head – the **suboccipitobregmatic** (see Figure 4.3.5), measuring around

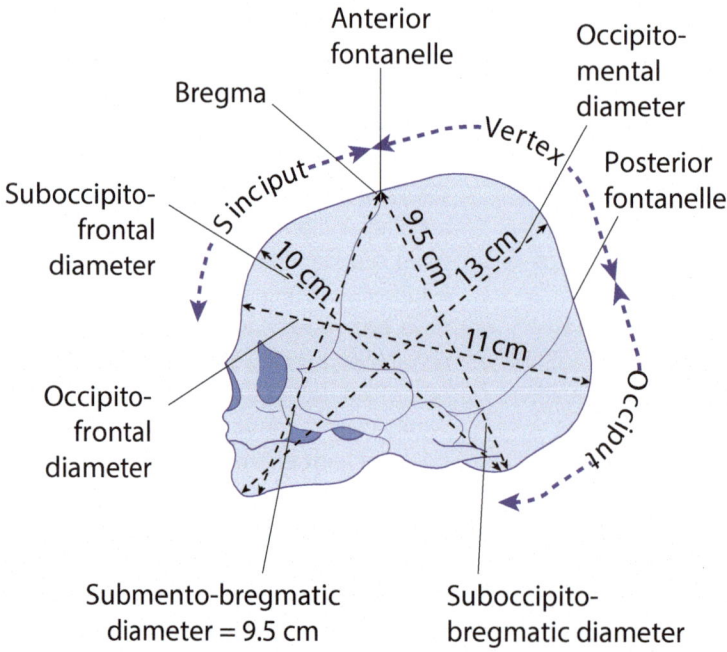

Figure 4.3.4 The approximate diameters of the fetal skull
Source: Figure 12.13, p.199, Kenny and Myers (2017)

	Flexed ➡️ Extended			
Attitude	Well flexed	Less well flexed (partially extended) or deflexed	Extended 'brow presentation'	Hyperextended 'face presentation'
Diameter	Suboccipito-bregmatic	Occipito-frontal	Occipito-mental	Submento-bregmatic
Measurement	9.5 cm	11.5 cm	13.0 cm	9.5 cm

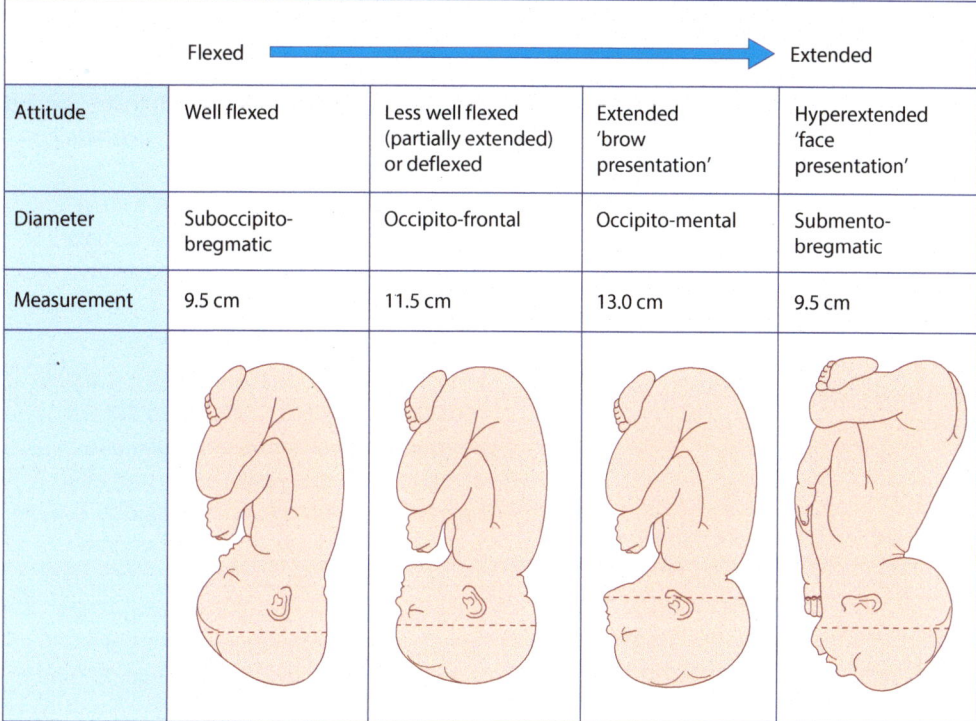

4.3

Figure 4.3.5 Presenting diameters of the fetal head
Source: Figure 12.14, p.200, Kenny and Myers (2017)

9.5 cm – will pass through the pelvis, stretch the perineum and be born first. The head is born as it uncurls from flexed to extended. This is the most common presentation at birth.

▶ Sometimes the fetus enters the pelvis in the **occipito-anterior or posterior position but with a deflexed head**, and fetal axis pressure does not cause the head to flex. In this instance, the presenting diameter at the pelvic outlet would be the **occipito-frontal** (approx. 11 cm).

▶ The fetus can also arrive at the pelvic outlet in an **OP position with a head that has been extended by fetal axis pressure**. In this instance, the head will be born by flexing from an extended position as it passes under the pubic arch. The **submentobregmatic diameter**

(also around 9.5 cm) will arrive first. This is known as a **face presentation**.

▶ The longest presenting diameter – the **occipito-mental** diameter (around 13 cm) – occurs when the fetus is in a **brow presentation**, with a partially extended head. This is usually the only presentation that cannot birth vaginally.

INTERRUPTER

There is really only one way to embed your understanding of the different ways a fetus might move through a pelvis – get physical!

Get your hands on a doll and pelvis and use the descriptions above to move the doll through the pelvic inlet, cavity and outlet. A soft, cloth pelvis is preferable as you can mould it into different shapes

(make it narrower at the top, perhaps, and see what effect this will have on the fetal journey)

Supporting physiology in the second stage

Good midwifery care supports and facilitates physiological processes to optimise health and well-being. It is therefore appropriate to examine common second stage interventions with both an evidence-based and physiological lens.

Charting progress

Watchful waiting is a crucial midwifery skill, and signs of progress such as cervical dilation, descent and rotation help to determine whether all is well. It is important to acknowledge, however, that much of our understanding of what constitutes 'acceptable' progress is based on the passage of a well-flexed, cephalic, OA fetal head that is well applied to the cervix through a pelvis that is wider laterally at the inlet. In this instance, descent and dilation occur simultaneously. Reed (2022) points out that when a baby is in the OP position, contractions are likely to be more irregular (as the head is less likely to be well applied to the cervix), and cervical dilation may be perceived as slower (as the head will not be pressing against the elastic cervix and keeping it fully stretched). Furthermore, descent, particularly when the maternal pelvic inlet is narrow, can happen after dilation. However, once the baby descends it will push through the cervix with comparative ease and can be born quickly.

Maternal position

The WHO (2018) recommends that women birthing with and without epidural analgesia should be encouraged to adopt any birthing position of their choice. Physiologically, an upright, forward leaning or all fours position will allow the woman's sacrum to tip back as the fetus passes through, creating more space in the pelvic cavity and at the pelvic outlet. Radiological studies have shown that squatting in particular increases the space available in the pelvic outlet (Gupta et al., 2017). Upright and forward leaning positions also prevent the fetus lying on and compressing major maternal blood vessels, reducing its own and its mother's oxygen supply.

A Cochrane review found that upright positions were associated with a possible reduction in duration of second stage, a reduction in assisted deliveries and episiotomies, and fewer abnormal fetal heart rate patterns (Gupta et al., 2017). A possible increase in second degree perineal tears was detected, but no clear difference for more substantive perineal damage. An increased incidence of estimated blood loss greater than 500 ml could be due to the loss being more likely to exit the vagina in upright positions.

INTERRUPTER

Again, you may understand the dynamic and mobile nature of the pelvis, and the effects of maternal position more clearly if you get physical and experiment.

Place one hand on your symphysis pubis and one on your sacrum. Try rocking and then bending forwards and backwards. Notice what happens to your hands. Is there more space between them?

How does sitting in a chair, sitting on the toilet, kneeling or placing one foot on a low stool affect the dimensions of your pelvic outlet?

Maternal pushing

A woman **pushing spontaneously** will typically take multiple breaths and push down more than once with each contraction. The **Valsalva manoeuvre**, where women are directed to take a deep breath, hold it, put their chin on their chest and push for up to 30 seconds, reduces blood flow to the uterus and is associated with a lower cord pH. It can also increase maternal fatigue, damage the pelvic floor and lead to impaired bladder function and increased perineal damage. Valsalva pushing also places additional demands on the maternal heart and is contraindicated in women with pre-existing cardiac conditions or severe anaemia. A Cochrane review comparing spontaneous versus directed pushing found no clear differences between the two approaches in duration of second stage, OASI, episiotomy, pushing duration or rate of physiological birth (Lemos et al., 2017).

'Hands on' or 'hands off' the birthing head

Debate continues to rage about whether or not midwives should place a hand on the fetal head as it is born. It is common practice in many medicalised settings for the attending midwife to put pressure on the advancing vertex in order to slow its advance and maintain an attitude of flexion. Together with placing a second hand on the perineum to prevent excessive stretching, this manoeuvre is designed to reduce perineal trauma. A Cochrane review (Aasheim et al., 2017) found no clear difference in the incidence of any perineal trauma using hands off (or poised) or hands on techniques. Hands on techniques may also interfere with the physiological processes of birth, which require a head in the OA position to be born by extension. A midwife may instead gently verbally coax a mother to birth her baby slowly.

Warm compresses

In a number of different cultural settings, warm compresses have been placed against the perineum as the fetal head becomes visible and starts to crown. The practice is hypothesised to lessen the risk of perineal tears by warming and softening the skin and enabling it to stretch, and to reduce pain by causing muscle relaxation and increased blood flow to the area due to vasodilation.

4.3

A randomised controlled trial in Saudi Arabia (Modoor et al., 2021) found that a gauze pad soaked in warm water and applied to the perineum during the second stage of labour reduced pain perception and the incidence of second- and third-degree tears. In a large randomised controlled trial in Portugal (Rodrigues et al., 2023), perineal massage in second stage labour, followed by the application of a warm compress during contractions, was compared to hands on delivery care alone and found to increase the incidence of intact perinea.

Fundal pressure

Although rarely used in the Global North, this procedure, which involves the accoucheur placing their hands at the top of the uterus and pushing down towards the birth canal, is routine practice in many under-resourced settings. The procedure aims to shorten the second stage. It can also be performed using an inflatable belt. A Cochrane review (Hofmeyr et al., 2017) found insufficient evidence of any benefit from fundal pressure, and there is concern that it is potentially painful and may damage the fetus or placenta.

Overall, it is perhaps worth remembering that although the passage of the fetus through the pelvis is a physical process, it is also a deeply human and personal event. Alongside adequate hydration, interventions that increase the likelihood of physiological birth include respectful care and continuous one-to-one support from a birth attendant (Wright et al., 2020).

CHAPTER CHALLENGE

There are a number of issues with research around reducing perineal trauma and pain during birth. Much of it treats the birthing woman as a passive participant in the process and assumes that babies are always born in the OA position. Look up and critique one of the studies mentioned in the warm compress section above. List the different factors that might have impacted the study outcome, and any factors that might mean that the trial is not completely generalisable to your practice setting.

Have a look at this medical expert review on methods used to prevent perineal trauma and use your knowledge of anatomy and physiology to critique each of the practices described:

Okiahialam N., Sultan A. et al. The prevention of perineal trauma during birth. *Am. J. Obstet. Gynecol.* [Internet] 2023, 37635056. https://pubmed.ncbi.nlm.nih.gov/37635056/.

References

Aasheim V., Nilsen A. et al. Perineal techniques during the second stage of labour for reducing perineal trauma. *Cochrane Database Syst. Rev.* [Internet] 2017. www.cochranelibrary.com/cdsr/doi/10.1002/14651858.CD006672.pub3/full.

Gupta J., Sood A. et al. Position in the second stage of labour for women without epidural anaesthesia. *Cochrane Database Syst. Rev.* [Internet] 2017. www.cochranelibrary.com/cdsr/doi/10.1002/14651858.CD002006.pub4/full.

Hofmeyr G., Vogel J. et al. Fundal pressure during the second stage of labour. *Cochrane Database Syst. Rev.* [Internet] 2017. www.cochranelibrary.com/cdsr/doi/10.1002/14651858.CD006672.pub3/full.

Lemos A., Amorim M. et al. Pushing/bearing down methods for the second stage of labour. *Cochrane Database Syst. Rev.* [Internet] 2017. www.cochranelibrary.com/cdsr/doi/10.1002/14651858.CD009124.pub3/full.

Modoor S., Fouly H. et al. The effect of warm compresses on perineal tear and pain intensity during the second stage of labor: A randomized controlled trial. *Belitung Nurs. J.* [Internet] 2021, 7(3):210–18. www.ncbi.nlm.nih.gov/pmc/articles/PMC10353617/.

NICE. Guideline NG235: Intrapartum Care [Internet]. 2023. www.nice.org.uk/guidance/ng235/chapter/Recommendations#second-stage-of-labour.

Reed, R. In celebration of the OP Baby. 2022. *Midwife Thinking* [Internet]. https://midwifethinking.com/2016/06/08/in-celebration-of-the-op-baby/ (last accessed 11.08.23).

Rodrigues S., Silva P. et al. Perineal massage and warm compresses – Randomised controlled trial for reduce perineal trauma during labor. *Midwifery* [Internet] 2023, 124:103763. www.sciencedirect.com/science/article/pii/S0266613823001663#bib0040.

Shepherd A., Cheyne H. et al. The purple line as a measure of labour progress: A longitudinal study. *BMC Pregnancy Childbirth* [Internet] 2010, 10:54. www.biomedcentral.com/1471-2393/10/54.

WHO. WHO Recommendations: Intrapartum Care for a Positive Childbirth Experience [Internet]. 2018. https://apps.who.int/iris/bitstream/handle/10665/272447/WHO-RHR-18.12-eng.pdf.

Wright A., Nassar A. et al. FIGO good clinical practice paper: Management of the second stage of labor. *Int. J. Gynecol. Obstet.* [Internet] 2020, 152(2):172–81. https://obgyn.onlinelibrary.wiley.com/doi/full/10.1002/ijgo.13552.

The fetus during labour

Jane Carpenter

LEARNING OUTCOMES

▶ Understand common presentations of the fetus at the onset of labour
▶ Understand key elements of the physiology of the fetal heart rate during labour, and apply these to the practice of fetal monitoring in labour

Fetal lie, presentation and position

During the preceding chapters of this section there was much discussion and exploration of the idea that during labour and birth, the fetus needs to make its way through the bony pelvis, often rotating and turning on its way in order to do so successfully. Historically, some texts referred to the 'power, passage and passenger' of labour – referring to the contractions (power), the birth canal (passage) and the fetus (passenger). This idea is largely rejected now, as it rather simplifies a highly complex process – and importantly it suggests that the fetus is merely 'a passenger' in the process of labour and birth. This is far from the case! As explored in Chapter 4.2, the fetal-placental unit may well have a key role to play in the onset of labour, but, in addition, the fetus is an active participant throughout labour and birth. The fetus actively moves in response to the contractions of labour, navigating its way through the particular shape of its mother's pelvis as required.

Given this, it can be useful to understand how the fetus is positioned at the start of labour, as this can help us to better understand how the fetus may make its journey through the pelvis and birth canal. However, the fetus is an active participant, and each woman's labour

DOI: 10.4324/9781003227571-24

and birth are individual, so knowing this information does not guarantee that labour will progress in one way or another, or that the fetus will behave in a particular way as it makes its way from inside to out. When exploring fetal position *in utero*, we consider the **fetal lie**, **fetal presentation** and **fetal position**. These are usually determined based on a thorough abdominal palpation, sometimes followed by a vaginal examination. Each of these is discussed in turn below. You will see some overlap with the previous chapters in this section. However, here the focus is on the fetus itself, rather than on its journey through the pelvis per se.

Fetal lie describes how the longest axis of the fetus (its spine) is situated compared to the maternal longitudinal axis (the maternal spine). The most common '**longitudinal lie**' describes where the longest axis of the fetus is positioned in line with the maternal longitudinal axis (Figure 4.4.1a and 4.4.1b). However, some fetuses may present **transverse**, where the longest axis of the fetus is situated perpendicular to the maternal longitudinal axis (Figure 4.4.1d). Rarely, a fetus may present in the **oblique** to the left or right, which means the long axis of the fetus is diagonal to the maternal longitudinal axis (Figure 4.4.1c).

Fetal presentation refers to the part of the fetus presenting at the maternal pelvic inlet at the onset of labour. A fetus is said to have a **cephalic** presentation if the head is leading at the pelvic inlet, and this is the most common fetal presentation. In this case, the fetal lie would be longitudinal. **Breech presentation**, where the buttocks or feet present at the pelvic inlet, is also possible with a longitudinal lie. **Shoulder presentation** is most likely to occur with an oblique or transverse lie. These are shown in Figure 4.4.1. A **compound presentation** is where another body part (such as a hand) presents alongside the fetal head.

It may help to revisit Chapter 2.5.4 here to refresh the key approximate diameters and key landmarks of the fetal skull before moving on in this chapter. Returning to our cephalic presentation, the fetal head could be flexed tightly (meaning the chin is pressed against the chest), or it may be less tightly flexed (neutral), extended or even hyper extended. How 'flexed' (or otherwise) the fetal head is will determine the angle at which the head enters and descends into the pelvis and therefore, which diameter of the fetal skull is presenting and moving through the pelvis and birth canal. Figure 4.4.2 shows how the degree of flexion can influence diameters presenting at the pelvic inlet giving rise to **vertex**, **brow** and **face presentations**. However, labour is dynamic and the fetus is an active participant, therefore it is important to remember that it does not necessarily follow that a deflexed head early in labour will remain so throughout. Nonetheless, a brow presentation will give rise to a fetal skull diameter which is likely to be wider than the pelvic diameter – this presentation may be impossible to birth vaginally, as described in Chapter 4.3.

Fetal position refers to how exactly the fetus is positioned in relation to the maternal pelvic inlet. Although other presentations are possible, as described above, here we are assuming a vertex presentation.

Figure 4.4.3 shows the possible ways in which to describe the relationship between the maternal pelvis and the fetal skull. Concentrating on the occiput of the fetus, we can describe whether this is presenting to the left or right of the maternal pelvis, and to the anterior or posterior of the maternal pelvis. We note this by stating direction first (left, right or direct), the presenting part (in this case occiput) and then finally, whether presenting to the anterior aspect or posterior aspect of the pelvis. Understanding this relationship

4.4

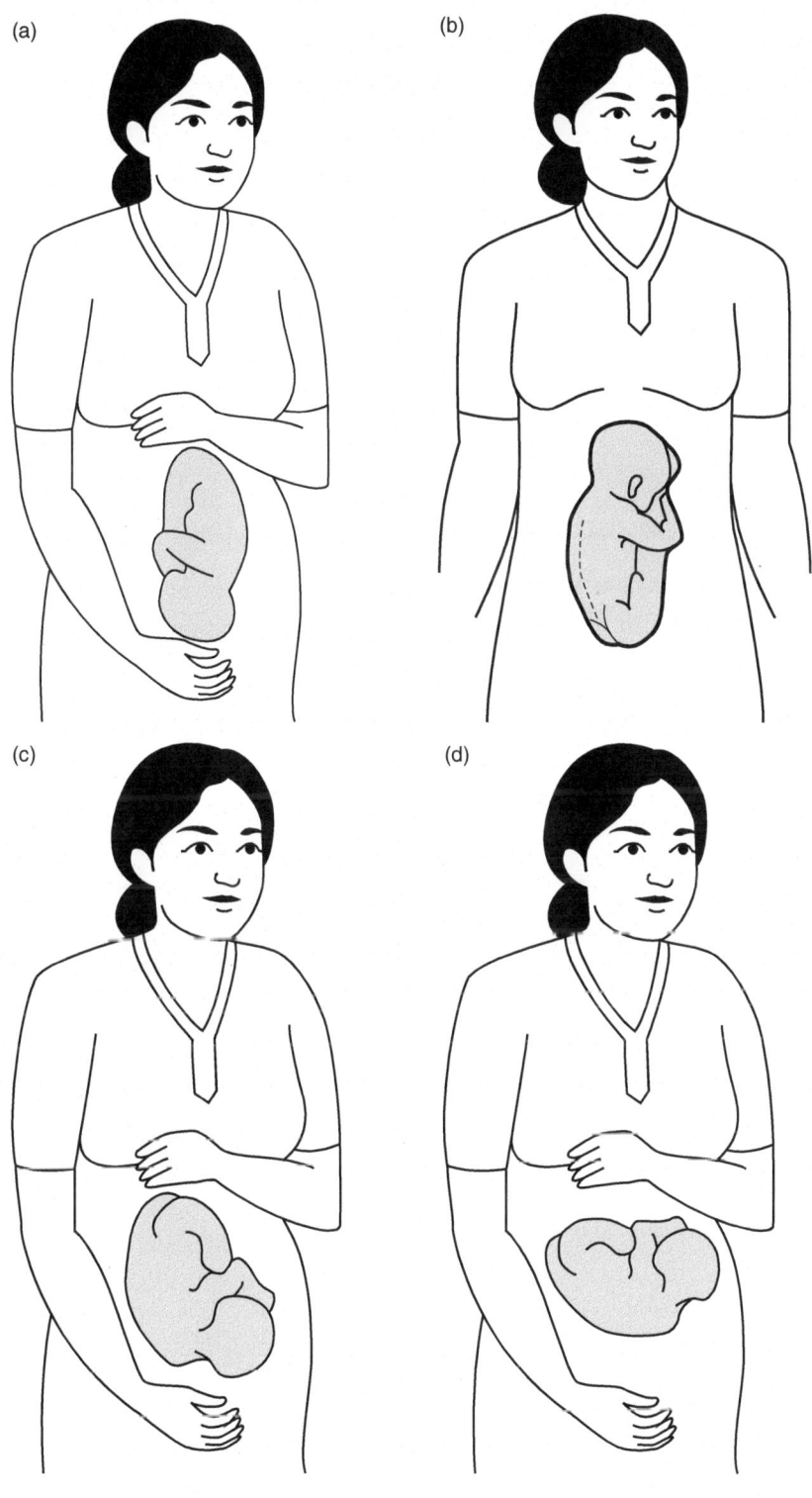

Figure 4.4.1 Fetal lie and presentation. a) Longitudinal lie, cephalic presentation, b) Longitudinal lie, breech presentation, c) Oblique lie, shoulder presentation and d) Transverse lie

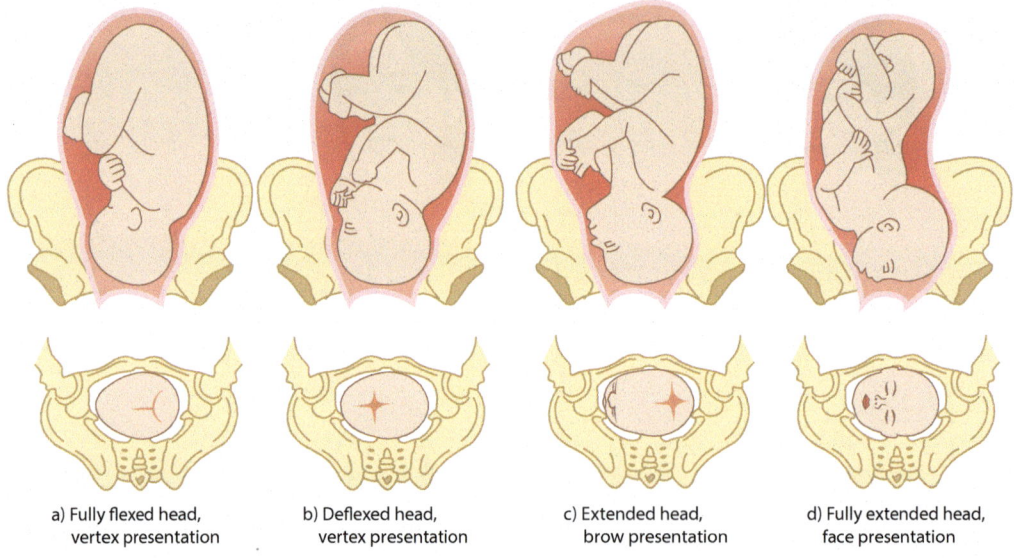

a) Fully flexed head, vertex presentation

b) Deflexed head, vertex presentation

c) Extended head, brow presentation

d) Fully extended head, face presentation

Figure 4.4.2 The degree of flexion and influence on diameters presenting at the pelvic inlet

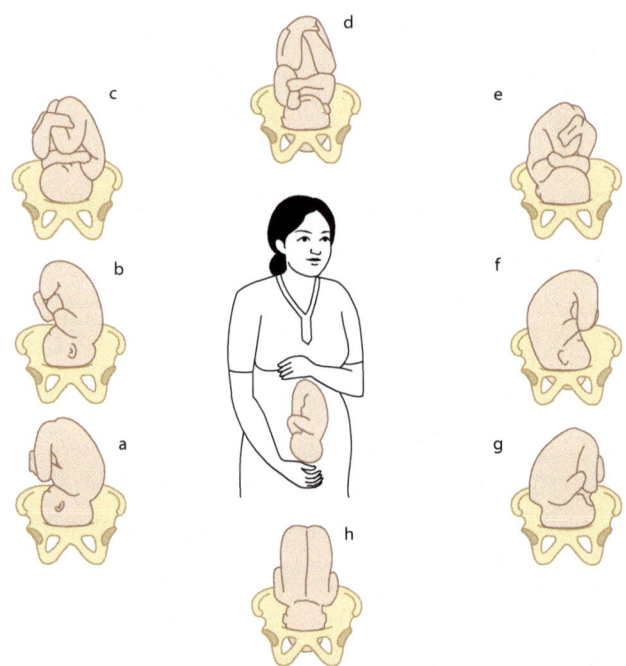

Figure 4.4.3 Describing fetal position: a) Left occipito anterior (LOA), b) Left occipito lateral (LOL), c) Left occipito posterior (LOP), d) Direct occipito posterior (OP), e) Right occipito posterior (ROP), f) Right occipito lateral (ROL), g) Right occipito anterior (ROA), h) Direct occipito anterio (OA)

between the fetal skull and maternal pelvis can give an indication of how the fetus may need to rotate in order for labour to progress. Again, though, this is dependent on a number of factors and not just how the fetus is presenting at the onset of labour.

INTERRUPTER

There is really only one way to embed your understanding of fetal lie, presentation and position – and that is to, again, get physical!

Get your hands on a doll and pelvis, and use the descriptions above to try out the different combinations of fetal lie, presentation and position. As you are doing this, carefully consider how these would influence the passage of the fetus through the pelvis during labour.

Fetal heart rate during labour

As described in the preceding chapters, labour is physically demanding, and requires active participation from the fetus. For a physiological birth with a healthy, term fetus this is unlikely to cause any problem. However, where things deviate from normal physiology, or where the fetus is preterm or unwell, the fetus may be less able to cope with the demands of labour over time. In addition, the situation can change as labour progresses, and the health of the woman will also directly influence the process of labour.

All of this means that the ability to accurately monitor the health of the fetus during labour has long been sought after. We are not there yet and thus, instead we rely on the tools we do have to help us try to understand the health of the fetus during labour. Currently, monitoring of fetal health relies largely on observation

of the fetal heart, alongside thorough consideration of the wider clinical picture. Two key ways exist of doing this, either listening directly via a Pinard stethoscope or sonic aid, or use of a cardiotocograph, which records the fetal heart rate pattern over a period of time. Both of these tools have their limitations, and thorough understanding of the appropriate use of these techniques is important for anyone undertaking intrapartum fetal monitoring. Detailed consideration of these techniques, and how to implement them, is outside the scope of this textbook. It is important to explore and understand the key aspects of fetal heart function, however, in order to support appropriate use of these tools when undertaking clinical care. This is what we will explore now.

Sympathetic vs parasympathetic control of fetal heart rate

The function of the fetal heart is regulated by both the somatic and autonomic components of the nervous system. The somatic nervous system functions to control conscious, or voluntary, actions. When the fetus moves *in utero*, this is controlled via the somatic nervous system, and as a result of such movement a 'spike' in fetal heart rate will be recorded, known as an **acceleration**. These accelerations are taken to be a sign of health, as a fetus which is moving has the energy to do so. Loss of accelerations *may* be a sign that the fetus is trying to conserve its energy due to stress of some form.

The autonomic control of fetal heart occurs via the parasympathetic and sympathetic nervous system. As described in Chapter 3.3, the parasympathetic nervous system is in ascendance when the body is at rest – often referred to as the rest and digest state. Conversely,

4.4

253

Table 4.4.1 Explanation of the core components of fetal heart rate

Component	Explanation
Baseline rate	The resting heart rate. This should be determined outside of a contraction, excluding any marked variability during that time. A normal baseline rate for a term fetus is between 110–160 beats per minute.
Baseline variability	Fluctuations, or minor oscillations, in the baseline heart rate that are irregular in amplitude and frequency, caused by the reactivity between the parasympathetic and sympathetic control of the fetal heart rate. Normal variability is between 5–25 beats per minute, although this may be reduced during periods of sleep. Absence of variability is not normal and should be further investigated.
Acceleration	Transient increase in fetal heart rate of 15 beats a minute or more, lasting 15 seconds or more.
Deceleration	Transient episodes where the heart rate dips to more than 15 beats per minute below the baseline rate for at least 15 seconds. It is important to differentiate between baroreceptor and chemoreceptor mediated decelerations in order to determine the likelihood of hypoxic injury/metabolic acidosis.

the sympathetic nervous system will be activated in response to stress, the so-called 'fight or flight' response. Therefore, the parasympathetic system will reduce the fetal heart rate, whereas the sympathetic system will increase the fetal heart rate.

In a healthy state, these two systems constantly interact with each other in terms of the fetal heart, and thereby slightly decrease and increase the heart rate continuously. The 'agreement' reached between these two systems is known as the **baseline heart rate**. The constant fluctuation between the two is known as the **baseline variability**. Table 4.4.1 defines each of the core components of fetal heart rate.

Parasympathetic control

Whilst the fetus is *in utero*, it is of course unable to access atmospheric oxygen. It must obtain all of its oxygen requirements from the maternal supply, via the placenta. It does this via adaptation across cardiovascular, metabolic and haematological systems to enable adequate oxygenation to body systems. However, should the fetus be exposed to **hypoxic stress** (inadequate supply of oxygen), it will

always aim to safeguard the myocardium of the heart – as this is the all-important pump which can then maintain oxygen perfusion to other areas.

The fetus will do this via reducing the fetal heart rate, conserving energy (losing fetal movements and hence, accelerations) and the release of catecholamines (see below). Reduction of, or **deceleration** of, the fetal heart rate is controlled by the parasympathetic system mediated by two different kinds of receptor: **baroreceptors** and **chemoreceptors**.

Baroreceptors are stretch receptors found in the carotid sinus and in the arch of the aorta. As labour progresses, and particularly once the waters have broken, the fetal head and the umbilical cord may undergo repeated compression during uterine contractions. This can cause baroreceptor mediated decelerations as follows:

▶ Compression causes occlusion of the umbilical artery which in turn leads to an increase in fetal systemic blood pressure
▶ This causes stretch and thereby stimulation of the baroreceptors
▶ Stimulation causes activation of the parasympathetic cardiac inhibitory centre

This will trigger the atrioventricular node in the heart to slow down the heart rate

Baroreceptor stimulation also causes a decrease in sympathetic stimulation of the heart

Baroreceptor mediated decelerations are usually short-lasting and directly related to uterine contractions. As the contraction dissipates, the stretch on the baroreceptor is also removed, meaning the slowing of the fetal heart rate is no longer triggered. The fetal heart will return to normal baseline. This means that the fetus will not usually be exposed to hypoxic injury from baroreceptor mediated decelerations.

Chemoreceptors are found peripherally on the aortic arch and carotid arteries, and centrally in the brain. Chemoreceptors, as the name suggests, are stimulated by changes in biochemical composition of the blood and are sensitive to changes in pH and oxygen saturation. During labour, activation of chemoreceptors will stimulate the parasympathetic nervous system and, as described above, this will cause a decrease in the fetal heart rate. Unlike baroreceptor mediated decelerations, chemoreceptor mediated decelerations are slow to return to the baseline. This is because the chemoreceptors will continue to be activated until fresh oxygenated blood reaches them, removing the stimulus. These decelerations are more often associated with fetal **metabolic acidosis** (where the fetus receives inadequate oxygen to maintain normal metabolism).

Sympathetic control

If the fetus is subjected to ongoing, persistent hypoxic stress, the sympathetic nervous system will trigger the release of catecholamines (adrenaline and noradrenaline). These catecholamines will cause:

An increase in placental circulation

Peripheral vasoconstriction to selectively perfuse vital organs and increase glucose availability

A slow and progressive increase in baseline fetal heart rate.

Therefore, it is important to keep a careful eye on the baseline heart rate of the fetus throughout labour to enable recognition of a gradually evolving hypoxic stress.

4.4

Overall pattern of response to hypoxic stress

Taking all of this into consideration, usually, during labour the fetal heart will have a stable baseline rate between 110 and 160 bpm, with good variability. Accelerations are likely to be present, and any decelerations will be baroreceptor mediated.

If hypoxia were to develop during labour, the initial response will be **compensatory** (the fetus will aim to compensate for the hypoxic stress):

Decelerations will become deeper and wider, becoming chemoreceptor mediated

The fetus will reduce its movements to conserve energy, meaning accelerations may disappear

Catecholamine release will cause a slow rise of the baseline rate

If the cause of the hypoxic stress is not addressed, the fetus will eventually **decompensate**, leading to:

Loss of baseline variability

Myocardial hypoxia and acidosis will lead to a progressive fall in baseline rate, ultimately culminating in a terminal fetal bradycardia

Types of fetal hypoxia

Intrapartum fetal hypoxia could have a number of causes, classically split into four types: acute, subacute, gradually evolving and chronic hypoxia. We will briefly discuss each in turn – although an in-depth consideration of these is outside the scope of this book.

Acute hypoxia

This is sudden onset of a prolonged deceleration, leading to a sudden drop in baseline heart rate to less than 80 bpm which lasts for at least three minutes. Such hypoxia is often secondary to an intrapartum accident such as placental abruption, cord prolapse or uterine rupture – and in these cases will rapidly lead to the onset of metabolic acidosis.

Subacute hypoxia

If the fetus spends more time below the baseline than at the baseline, this is said to be subacute hypoxia. This occurs because the fetus is protecting the heart during the deceleration and returns to baseline for just one third of the time in order to exchange gases and to protect the brain. If not rectified, the shortage of sufficient time for oxygenation will lead to metabolic acidosis.

Gradually evolving hypoxia

This type of hypoxia will lead to the compensatory mechanisms outlined above, such as a gradually increasing baseline rate, and if these are insufficient, to decompensation. This will lead to reduced oxygenation in the brain leading to loss of baseline variability.

Chronic hypoxia

Often caused by chronic utero-placental insufficiency due to, for example, pre-eclampsia, this hypoxia can persist for days or even weeks leading up to labour and birth. The fetus will have compensated for the hypoxia, as outlined above and therefore, at the onset of labour will have vastly reduced 'reserves'. Instead, such fetuses are at risk of rapid decompensation, meaning quick intervention is indicated.

Summary

Of course, in the normal, physiological process of labour and birth the term fetus will cope well with the demands of labour, and such hypoxia will not be evident. Nonetheless, it is important that all midwives and other professionals involved in intrapartum care have sound understanding of the underpinning physiology of the fetal heart during labour, so that if and when deviations from normal physiology do occur, these are identified, escalated and addressed as appropriate.

APPLICATION TO PRACTICE

Next time you have the opportunity to review a cardiotocograph (CTG), have a look for the features described throughout this chapter. If you can, look at several CTGs from different stages of labour.

If the CTG has decelerations, try to determine whether they are more likely to be baroreceptor or chemoreceptor mediated. How will you come to this decision? Would any other information help you to make your decision?

CHAPTER CHALLENGE

Read the Cochrane Review by Alfirevic et al. (2017):

Summarise the findings of this review in your own words. What key information would you want to include when having an informed discussion with a woman around the appropriate use of fetal monitoring in labour? How would this conversation differ if the woman had no intrapartum 'risk factors' compared to a woman with pre-eclampsia?

Reference

Alfirevic Z., Gyte G. et al. Continuous cardiotocography (CTG) as a form of electronic fetal monitoring (EFM) for fetal assessment during labour. *Cochrane Database Syst. Rev.* [Internet] 2017. www.cochranelibrary.com/cdsr/doi/10.1002/14651858.CD006066.pub3/full.

Further reading

Chandraharan E. (Ed). *Handbook of CTG interpretation: From patterns to physiology* (12th edition). Cambridge: Cambridge University Press, 2021.

Pereira S., Chandraharan E. Recognition of chronic hypoxia and pre-existing foetal injury on the cardiotocograph (CTG): Urgent need to think beyond the guidelines. *Porto Biomed. J.* [Internet] 2017, 2(4):124–9. https://pubmed.ncbi.nlm.nih.gov/32258602/.

4.4

The third stage of labour

Kirsten Baker

LEARNING OUTCOMES

- ▶ Define the third stage of labour, including its three phases
- ▶ Describe clinical signs of placental detachment
- ▶ Describe processes involved in achieving haemostasis
- ▶ Understand the methods used to manage the third stage
- ▶ Recognise normal and abnormal blood loss, and combine blood loss assessment with other physiological markers to build a clinical picture to inform care

Physiology of the third stage

The third stage of labour commences once the baby is born, and comprises the birth of the placenta and membranes, and control of uterine bleeding.

Birth of the placenta and membranes

Before the placenta and membranes can be expelled from the body, the placenta needs to detach from the uterine wall. This detachment is widely described as occurring in three phases, described below, as the uterus continues to contract and retract after the birth of the baby.

Latent phase

This is the time from the birth of the baby until the placenta starts to separate. This is a short phase, during which uterine contractions continue to cause retraction of smooth muscle, causing the now empty uterus to shrink in size. The retraction causes the uterine wall to thicken, but there is minimal thickening over the placenta (as the placenta is applying some resistance).

DOI: 10.4324/9781003227571-25

Detachment phase

This includes the separation and detachment of the placenta and membranes from the uterine wall. As retraction of smooth muscle continues, the area over the placenta is also forced to contract. Unlike the uterus, the placenta is not an elastic organ – it cannot shrink. The uterine wall therefore starts to shear off the placenta, most likely from around the outside edge (the area of least resistance) towards the middle. Imagining a postage stamp stuck to the inside of a deflating balloon may help conjure the image of separation. It has also been hypothesised that placental separation may begin at the centre of the placenta, as bleeding vessels from the retracting uterus or blood forced out of the constricting placenta cause a clot to be formed between the placenta and the uterine wall which then effectively pushes the placenta away. Support for this theory is, however, waning, and physiologically there is no reason why any such clot would form at the centre of the placenta.

Continuing contractions and gravity cause the separated placenta to fall to the bottom of the uterus, and as it falls it peels the membranes from the uterine wall.

Expulsion phase

This is the period from complete separation of the placenta to the birth of the placenta and membranes. The placenta and membranes can be birthed by maternal effort or delivered by gentle manual traction from an accoucheur (see below). Two differing methods of placental presentation have been identified and are commonly named after nineteenth century obstetricians. More often than not, the placenta will present centrally, at the point of cord insertion, fetal surface first ('**Schulze**' presentation). Although this presentation has been attributed to central placental separation aided by a clot, it seems more likely that it is aided by the downward

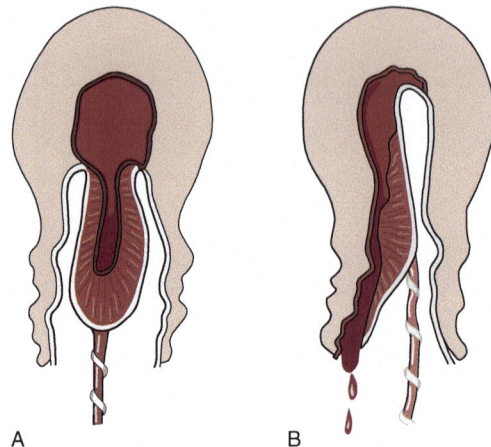

A= Schulz. B= Matthews Duncan.

Figure 4.5.1 The Schultz and Matthews Duncan placental presentations

force of uterine contractions and external traction on the cord, particularly if this occurs before the membranes are fully separated. In a Shulze presentation, blood loss can be contained behind the placenta, and it generally clots prior to exiting the vagina. Less commonly, the placenta will present sideways, and the blood loss will be more immediate and visible. This is known as a '**Matthews Duncan**' presentation and is more likely if the placenta implanted at the side of the uterus. The Schulz and Matthews Duncan placental separations are illustrated in Figure 4.5.1.

Clinical signs of placental detachment

There are several clinical signs that the placenta has detached from the uterine wall:

▶ As the muscle fibres retract and its surface area decreases, the uterine wall thickens. This bulkiness can be felt as a high hard fundus at the level of the umbilicus.
▶ Once the placenta detaches, the fundus rises as the side walls of the uterus move towards the centre (see Figure 4.5.2).

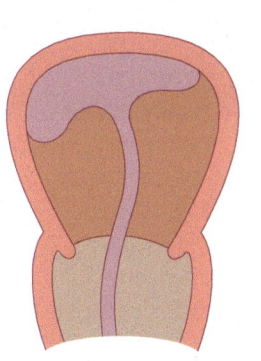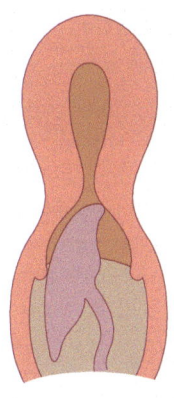

Figure 4.5.2 Separation and descent of the placenta
Source: Figure 12.20, p.212, Kenny and Myers (2017)

▶ As the placenta separates from the uterus, there may be some trickling blood visible at the introitus, often referred to as a **separation bleed**.

▶ As the placenta moves into the lower part of the uterus, the cord visible at the introitus can lengthen.

Control of uterine bleeding

Uterine blood flow and the fetoplacental unit

Over the course of a pregnancy, uterine blood flow adapts to meet the needs of the developing embryo/fetus. A network of villi ensures a large surface area for exchange between maternal and fetal blood via the placenta. At term, blood flow through the uterine arteries is approximately 500 ml per minute – and as this is maternal arterial supply it is circulating at high pressure. As long as the placenta remains attached to the uterine wall, the cord continues to pulsate, sustaining the fetus during the initial transition to extrauterine life. If, after the separation of the placenta, the maternal placental blood supply is not quickly controlled, rapid maternal exsanguination will ensue.

Control of bleeding

There are a number of key mechanisms which promote haemostasis:

▶ Once the placenta has been birthed, the retraction of smooth muscle continues under the influence of contractions. It is hypothesised that the walls of the uterus are brought into apposition at this point, effectively applying pressure to the placental site (see Figure 4.5.2). Until it has left the uterus, the placenta's bulk will prevent these contractions from being fully effective and the risk of bleeding remains high.

▶ The maternal spiral arteries, which 'spiral' their way through the smooth muscle fibres, are occluded by the ongoing retraction of those muscles via '**living ligatures**' (Figure 4.5.3), which constrict the torn vessels.

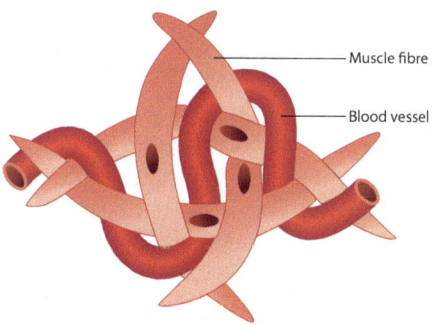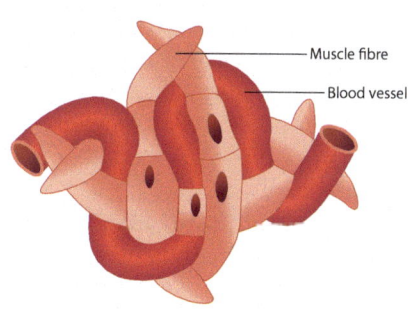

Figure 4.5.3 Living ligatures

▶ Pregnancy is a hypercoagulable state – women have an increased capacity for clotting, and there is a further transient rise during labour in preparation for birthing the placenta. Usual clotting processes commence, and the placental site is quickly covered in a fibrin mesh.

▶ Skin-to-skin contact with her baby at birth further stimulates maternal oxytocin production, which is further enhanced when neonates start to breastfeed, encouraging ongoing uterine contractions. A baby in skin-to-skin contact who starts to crawl towards the breast will also kick down on its mother's belly, further strengthening her contractions.

INTERRUPTER

Practical task

Blow up a balloon but do not put a knot in it (hold the end with your finger and thumb, or use a freezer clip as a temporary seal). With a marker pen, draw a crisscross of lines on it, as if playing noughts and crosses. Imagine these are uterine muscle fibres, and a uterine artery passes through each square. Finally, stick a sticker or attach a small piece of paper onto the balloon with Sellotape. Slowly let the air out of the balloon.

This, with a bit of imagination, roughly illustrates placental separation and the function of the living ligatures. As the surface to which it is attached shrinks, the sticker shears off. At the same time, the muscle fibres move closer together, effectively occluding the blood vessels thereby causing blood flow to abate and then cease. Effective uterine contractions are key to both of these.

Management of the third stage

Women's experiences of birthing the placenta vary, influenced largely by the attitudes and actions of care givers. This varies from watchful waiting, called '**expectant management**' to '**active management**' by drug administration, cord clamping and 'controlled cord traction'. The socio-economic context of maternity care is of course a significant factor in what practice is appropriate. Women can of course choose between active and expectant management of the third stage of labour. However, for some women with particular clinical conditions, impaired physiology may strongly indicate that active management is a safer option and they should be informed of this. In other instances where physiology has been altered due to events in labour – for example, where synthetic oxytocin has been administered to induce or increase contractions prior to birth – women may similarly be advised that the use of a uterotonic to aid uterine contraction reduces their risk of excessive blood loss.

Expectant management

Expectant management involves facilitating a physiological third stage and birth of the placenta and membranes by maternal effort. Monitoring requires a delicate balance between leaving a woman and her baby uninterrupted to enhance oxytocin production, thereby facilitating uterine contractions, while ensuring that the living ligatures are doing their job and the placenta separates before the mother bears down to expel it. As well as observing signs of separation (see above) and watching and hearing the mother's experience of any contractions, the shearing of the placenta from the uterine wall can be palpated by putting a hand on the fundus which will feel hard, contracted and at or above the umbilicus. In expectant management, the cord is not clamped or cut until it has stopped pulsating. Some mothers choose not to clamp the cord or separate their baby from the placenta at all. This is called a **lotus birth**, and entails preserving the still-attached placenta using salt and herbs until the cord falls off naturally.

Leaving the new mother undisturbed, warm and in dim light will facilitate oxytocin production as the parasympathetic system remains dominant. Skin-to-skin contact, especially if the baby massages and licks the nipple, will also help. It is important that the mother's bladder is empty to ensure contractions are effective. It is likely that the mother's stomach muscles will have been over-distended and weakened during pregnancy and while birthing the baby. Therefore, once the placenta has separated, upright positions, gentle coughing or grunting, or sometimes a hand placed gently on the lower abdomen, may help the mother to birth it.

Active management

This describes a series of extrinsic interventions to enable the separation and birth of the placenta and the maintenance of haemostasis. It is the practice recommended by the World Health Organization (2018) to reduce the incidence of **postpartum haemorrhage (PPH)**, a leading cause of maternal death globally. PPH is a blood loss of over 500 ml. If it occurs within 24 hours of giving birth it is described as a primary PPH. After 24 hours it is known as a secondary PPH. The volume of blood lost can also be less than 500 ml if it nevertheless causes symptoms of severe haemorrhage (such as maternal collapse). The burden of PPH and maternal death is heavily skewed towards resource-poor (often previously colonised) countries, particularly in Northern Africa and Eastern Asia where skilled birth attendants

are sparse, and underlying pathologies such as malnutrition and malaria are common. Routine active management of the third stage is, however, widely contested in the Global North where health-care systems are well established and the underlying health of women is generally better.

The core elements of Active Management of the Third Stage of Labour (AMTSL) are as follows:

- ▶ Administration of a uterotonic drug to induce uterine contractions
- ▶ Clamping and cutting the umbilical cord
- ▶ Observing signs of placental separation
- ▶ Controlled cord traction
- ▶ The placenta being extracted by the care giver with little or no maternal effort

Administration of a uterotonic

A uterotonic is administered as or shortly after the baby is born. This practice became widespread in the 1950s when oxytocin was first synthesised, while randomised controlled trials to examine its effectiveness did not take place until the 1980s. The recommended uterotonic is (synthetic) **oxytocin**, though in some instances where cold storage or skilled birth attendants are not available **misoprostol tablets** may be the best option. Synthetic oxytocin, sometimes referred to as Syntocinon, is generally administered intramuscularly as an injection, but can also be given intravenously. **Ergometrine** is a second line uterotonic, which, although more effective, causes significant side effects such as vasoconstriction, raised blood pressure, nausea and vomiting. It is not suitable for people with raised blood pressure, cardiac conditions or vascular disease. Ergometrine also inhibits prolactin secretion and can therefore reduce breastmilk production. **Syntometrine**, a first line uterotonic combining synthetic oxytocin and ergometrine, is not widely used in many European countries due to the side effects of ergometrine described above.

Actions of synthetic oxytocin and ergometrine

Synthetic oxytocin acts on the smooth muscle of the uterus, stimulating contractions and causing the fibres to contract and retract; it is used as part of the management of induction or augmentation of labour, and may be continued or initiated as part of the management of the third stage of labour. It takes effect within three to seven minutes (it will work more quickly if given intravenously rather than intramuscularly) and works for between 30 minutes and an hour. Ergometrine acts more slowly, becoming effective after five to seven minutes, but produces a more sustained contraction which can last for up to three hours.

For healthy women at low risk of bleeding, the disadvantages of AMTSL may outweigh the benefits. Discussion in this area is however hampered by what a Cochrane review (Begley et al., 2019) calls 'low or very low' quality evidence: placental birth is undoubtedly an arena where more well focussed research is needed.

Clamping and cutting the umbilical cord

Originally, as part of AMTSL, the cord was clamped and cut immediately after birth. However, clamping the cord while blood is still flowing (palpable as a pulse in the cord) leaves fetal blood within the placenta and cord. This means the neonate does not receive all of its own supply, and also leaves the placenta bulkier than it needs to be. It is now known that **optimal cord clamping** (sometimes called delayed cord clamping) is beneficial for neonates, not least because this allows the neonate to receive more of its own blood before the cord stops pulsating naturally. With active third stage, it is now usual to leave the cord to pulsate for at least one minute before clamping and cutting.

Controlled cord traction

Controlled cord traction is performed 2–3 minutes after the administration of the uterotonic drug, once signs of placental separation have been observed. Evidence suggests that it makes very little difference to the risk of severe haemorrhage (Gülmezoglu et al., 2012).

APPLICATION TO PRACTICE

Controlled cord traction

Controlled cord traction involves the mother lying on her back or semi-reclining while the accoucheur holds the cord in one hand and places their other hand just above the woman's pubic bone. When the mother next experiences a contraction, gentle downward traction is applied to the cord while exerting counter-pressure to the abdomen (Figure 4.5.4). When the placenta is visible at the introitus, a slight upwards pressure will facilitate its delivery, which should be controlled and steady to avoid leaving any placenta or membranes behind.

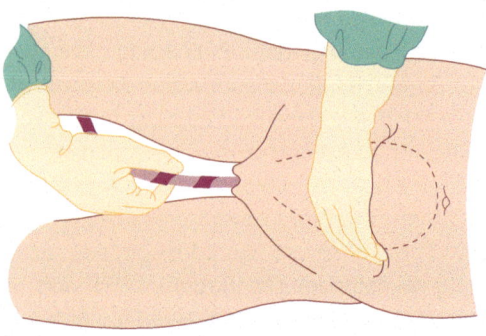

Figure 4.5.4 Controlled cord traction
Source: Figure 12.21, p.212, Kenny and Myers (2017)

Confirming completion of third stage

Both expectant and active management include careful examination of the cord, placenta and membranes, and an estimation of blood loss. The third stage is not considered complete until haemostasis (stabilisation of blood loss) has been achieved; so, careful monitoring of blood loss is an essential component, along with confirming that the placenta has been birthed in full.

Estimating blood loss

It is worth noting that as the woman's circulating blood volume increases during pregnancy, to a degree blood loss is very sustainable and indeed beneficial for her. In addition, due to the haemodilution which occurs during pregnancy, losing a volume of blood does not represent the same loss of haemoglobin as would be the case in a woman who has not just given birth; it will be proportionally less.

It is generally agreed that the upper limit of normal blood loss is 500 ml. However, it is of course self-evident that the same amount of blood loss will have different effects on different women due, amongst other things, to their size and underlying health. A tall healthy woman may for example withstand a loss of 1000 ml, whereas a petite woman or one who has malaria may be compromised by a much smaller loss. An important part of the midwife's role is recognising a loss which compromises the woman's well-being, bearing in mind that in some instances this may be below the estimated 500 ml.

Accurate estimation of blood loss is notoriously difficult, with decreasing levels of accuracy with increasing amounts of blood loss. Visual estimates can only ever be an approximation, and weighing blood-soaked items and then subtracting their dry weight (each 1 g of blood equates to 1 ml of loss) is hampered by the possible presence of amniotic fluid and urine in the mix (approximations though, are given in Table 4.5.1). It is also significant that blood loss following placental birth is usually assessed and recorded within one or two hours. When a uterotonic has been given and the uterus has contracted as a result of the drug action, blood loss during this short time frame may be low compared with a physiologically contracting uterus as Sara

4.5

Table 4.5.1 A guide to visual estimation of blood loss

Item	Description	Approximate blood loss
Soiled sanitary towel	Blood-soaked area covers around ⅔ of towel	30 ml
Soaked small swab	10 cm × 10 cm gauze swab completely soaked in blood	60 ml
Soaked sanitary towel	Towel completely soaked in blood	100 ml
Soaked incontinence sheet	Blood-soaked area covers around ½ of the sheet	250 ml
Soaked large swab	45 cm × 45 cm gauze swab completely soaked in blood	350 ml
Kidney dish	Blood in dish reaches the inner rim (approx. 1 cm from top)	500 ml
Soaked bed sheet	Blood covers around ¾ area of sheet, but has not spilled onto the floor	1000 ml
Soaked bed sheet with blood spilling onto floor	As above, but blood pooling and dripping onto floor	2000 ml

Wickham (2018) suggests. However, further blood loss may ensue once the action of the uterotonic wears off.

PPH can be classified as 'minor' (500–1000 ml), 'moderate' (1000–2000 ml) or 'severe' (above 2000 ml) – although variations in these classifications exist. Aside from an insufficiently contracted uterus, other causes of excessive bleeding after birth are **trauma** (bleeding from a tear or an episiotomy), **thrombin** (clotting disorders) or **tissue** (retained products, making it difficult for the uterus to contract). Together with **tone** (lack of uterine tone, called atony) these are known as the '4Ts'. The most common cause of PPH is the latter (at about 70% globally), though it is important not to disregard the others.

Systematic examination of the placenta, membranes and cord

However it is delivered, systematic examination of the placenta, membranes and cord needs to be undertaken in a good light, and on a surface where the placenta can be spread out to its full extent. The main purpose of this thorough examination is to ascertain that all has been completely expelled, as any residue correlates to a risk of PPH and uterine infection. In addition, information from a visual inspection can detect abnormalities or deviations from the norm which might in turn warrant further examination such as histology and can also inform neonatal care.

It is helpful to first lay the placenta out with the fetal surface uppermost, lifting the cord to ascertain how it is inserted into the placenta, its length, thickness and any knots. The **placenta** is a discoid organ of approximately 20 cm in diameter, with the membrane sac emanating from it and with the cord inserted into it. The **position of the cord insertion**

varies. Most commonly, this is central with the sides of the placenta sloping away, covered in the chorion and amnion which give it a shiny greyish appearance. There should be three **umbilical vessels** evident at the point where the cord has been cut: if these are not easily visible, an extra cut can be made. Fewer than three vessels may indicate a congenital abnormality: the baby needs a paediatric referral and a sample of cord blood taken (see below). The cord is surrounded by **Whartons jelly**, some irregularities in this may give the appearance of a **'false knot'**. On rare occasions, a **'true knot'** may be present: this is usually loose but if pulled tight can cause occlusion of the umbilical vessels and fetal distress.

Variations in placental construction and cord insertion (Figure 4.5.5) include:

- ▶ **Battledore insertion** – cord inserted at the edge of the placenta
- ▶ **Velamentous insertion** – cord inserted into membranes outside the placental boundary
- ▶ **Succenturiate lobe** – a separate placental lobe linked by a blood vessel to the main body
- ▶ **Circumvallate placenta** – fetal membranes fold backwards over the edges of the placenta
- ▶ **Bi (or tri)partite placenta** – placenta divided into two (or three) discrete lobes

Lifting the placenta by the cord allows the **chorion and amnion** to be viewed, including the rupture in these through which the baby was born. The chorion and amnion can be separated, and examined for completeness.

Turning the placenta over positions the maternal side uppermost. This is dark red, though it may have some **white fibrous patches** in areas where the blood supply has been insufficient: these are common in

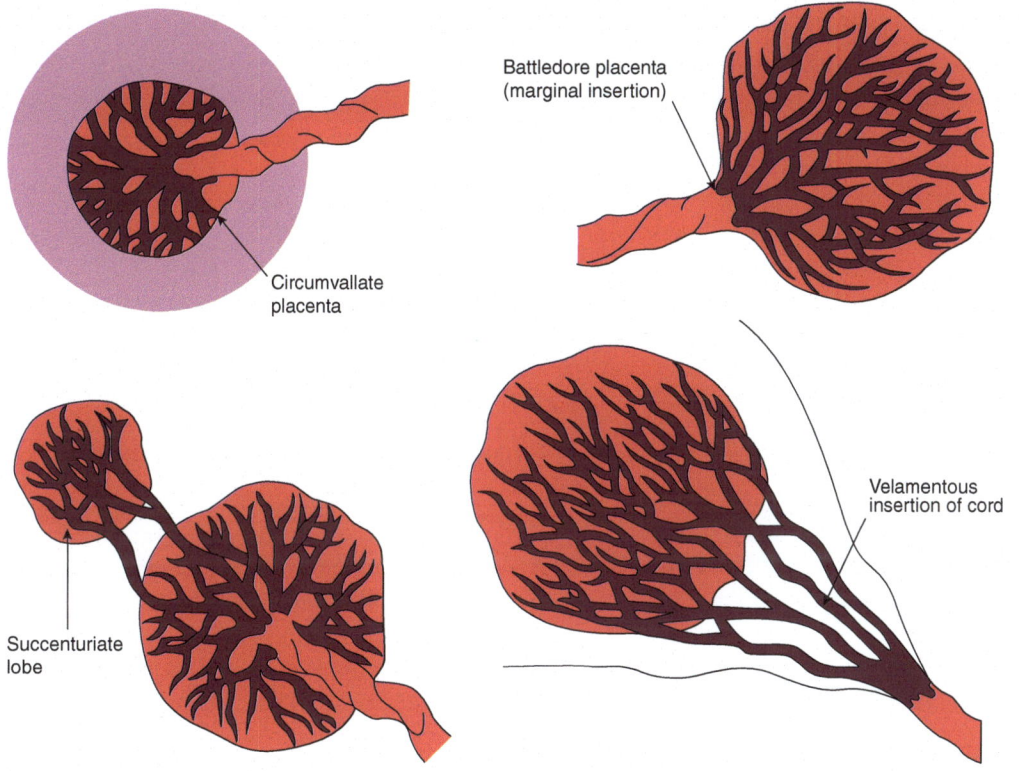

4.5

Figure 4.5.5 Placental variations

women who smoke or have hypertension. Some small whitish gritty patches may be seen and felt, particularly if the pregnancy was prolonged. The appearance is mainly of **15–20 cotyledons**, roundish sections of the placenta grouped closely together and separated by septa. Again, these structures must be examined closely to ascertain completeness.

If there is any uncertainty about the completeness of the placenta and membranes, the woman and her midwife need to be vigilant about any offensive discharge, uterine pain or fever as this may indicate an infection necessitating antibiotics. If it seems that any remains have not been expelled, or these are clearly missing during the initial inspection, these need to be removed in theatre.

APPLICATION TO PRACTICE

Next time you have the opportunity, conduct your own systematic examination of the placenta, cord and membranes, noting all the features described here.

INTERRUPTER

What to do with a placenta?

It is estimated that a hefty 50 million kg of placenta is produced globally each year (Yoshizawa and Hird, 2020). How these are used or disposed of varies enormously. Some contexts lean into placentae being clinical waste to be incinerated; some bestow symbolic value and bury it in their land of origin; some women eat it either in its original form or encapsulated (processed into pill capsules). This latter practice seems to have gained purchase in the Global North in recent years. In some settings, placentae may be used to train detection dogs in smelling human remains; or make their way into a laboratory for a range of investigations.

Printmaking and other art representing placentae are increasingly popular. Have a look at some online. How do you feel about this practice and those listed above? What presuppositions are informing your reaction? Think about how you would facilitate choices that might appear strange to you.

Final thoughts

It can be complicated to maintain a healthy respect for a physiological process such as birthing the placenta, while holding an emergency mindset in readiness if needed. This mental balancing act pervades many aspects of maternity care and is perhaps part of the beauty of the profession. Nowhere is this fine balancing act more in evidence than during placental birth.

References

Begley C., Gyte G. et al. Active versus expectant management for women in the third stage of labour. *Cochrane Database Syst. Rev.* [Internet] 2019. Available from www.cochranelibrary.com/cdsr/doi/10.1002/14651858.CD007412.pub5/full.

Gülmezoglu A., Lumbiganon P., et al. Active management of the third stage of labour with and without controlled cord traction: A randomised, controlled, non-inferiority trial. *Lancet* 2012, 379(9827):1721–7.

Wickham S. Further Thoughts on the Third Stage [Internet] 2018. Available from www.sarawickham.com/articles-2/further-thoughts-on-the-third-stage/.

World Health Organization. WHO Recommendations: Intrapartum Care for a Positive Childbirth Experience [Internet]. 2018. Available from www.who.int/publications/i/item/9789241550215.

Yoshizawa R., Hird M. Schrodinger's placenta: Determining placentas as not/waste. *EPE Nat. Space* 2020, 3(1):246–62.

Pelvic floor and perineum

Katherine Palles-Dimmock, Claire Smith and Louise Hunter

LEARNING OUTCOMES

▶ Understand the structure and function of the pelvic floor
▶ Describe the categories of perineal trauma which can occur during childbirth
▶ Understand the reasons for perineal repair

Pelvic floor and perineum function and structure

The pelvic floor and the perineum are a complex structure of muscles, fascia (sheets or bands of connective tissue that attach, stabilise and enclose organs, muscles, blood vessels and nerves) and ligaments that surround the pelvic outlet.

They form a sling or hammock that supports the pelvic organs, holds them in place and assists them to function (for example, by maintaining continence). In females, the pelvic floor and perineum surround and support three outlets: the urethra, vagina and rectum (Figure 4.6.1).

The perineum

The **perineum** extends from the skin to the inferior surface of the pelvic floor. It is bounded anteriorly by the pubic arch, posteriorly by the apex of the coccyx and laterally by the ischial tuberosities. The perineum can be divided into two triangular parts by drawing an imaginary line transversely between the ischial tuberosities (see below). The anterior triangle – the **urogenital triangle** – tilts down and back, and the

DOI: 10.4324/9781003227571-26

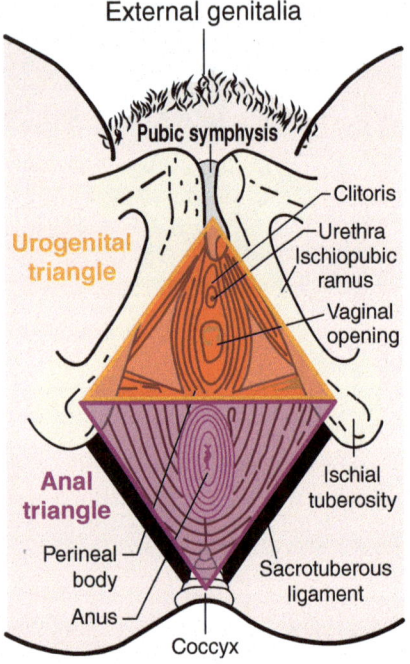

External genitalia

Pubic symphysis

Urogenital triangle

Clitoris
Urethra
Ischiopubic ramus
Vaginal opening

Anal triangle

Ischial tuberosity

Perineal body

Anus

Sacrotuberous ligament

Coccyx

Figure 4.6.1 The perineum

posterior triangle – the **anal triangle** – tilts down and forwards (Figure 4.6.1).

The **urogenital triangle** is composed of a number of fascial layers and contains the clitoris, vaginal opening and external genitalia, part of the urethra and the external urethral sphincter (a voluntary muscle controlling urine flow).

The **anal triangle** contains the anal aperture (opening of the anus), the **external anal sphincter (EAS)** muscle (a voluntary muscle responsible for opening and closing the anus) and two ischioanal fossae – one either side of the anus. The ischioanal fossae contain fat and connective tissue, and allow for expansion of the anal canal during defecation.

Between the urogenital hiatus and the anal canal lies a fibrous node known as the **perineal body**, which joins the pelvic floor to the perineum and acts as a point of attachment for muscle fibres. The perineal

body is liable to sustain damage during vaginal birth (see below).

The elasticity of the perineal skin is influenced by the amount of collagen in the underlying connective tissue. There is evidence that perineal massage, undertaken from 34 to 35 weeks of pregnancy, increases the elasticity of perineal tissue, reducing the likelihood of perineal trauma (particularly for those having their first baby) and ongoing perineal pain (Beckmann and Stock, 2013).

Functions of the perineum

▶ The perineum essentially forms the outer surface of the pelvic cavity
▶ It supports the pelvic floor muscles
▶ It stretches to enable birth, and also controls the passage of urine and faeces
▶ Its rich nerve supply and erectile tissue make it a focus for sexual pleasure

APPLICATION TO PRACTICE

Perineal massage explained – information to share with pregnant women

Dr Ethel Burns

Perineal massage can be done by you or your partner. It can be best performed after a bath or shower, when the blood vessels in the area are more dilated and you are feeling warm and relaxed.

Technique:

▶ Wash your hands.
▶ Assume a comfortable position such as standing with one leg on a stool, sitting on the toilet or reclining on a bed or sofa with your knees bent out and supported.
▶ Use a small amount of unscented, organic oil such as olive, sunflower or grapeseed to lubricate your thumbs and the perineal area.

- Place one or both thumbs on and just within the back wall of your vagina, resting one or both forefingers on your buttocks. You may prefer to use only one hand (see Figure 4.6.2).
- Pressing down a little towards your rectum (back passage), gently massage by moving your thumb(s) and forefinger(s) together upwards and outwards then back again, in a rhythmic 'U' shaped movement. You are aiming to massage the area inside your vagina, rather than just the skin on the outside.
- Perineal massage should be comfortable but you will also feel a stretching sensation. This is similar to how your perineum will open up as you give birth to your baby.
- Focus on relaxing your perineum as much as possible during the massage.
- The massage can last as long as you wish but aim for around five minutes at a time.
- With time and practice, as your perineum becomes more elastic, you will increase your ability to relax and can increase the pressure towards your rectum. Being able to relax through this feeling of increased

pressure will help you to relax as you feel the pressure in labour and your baby's head is about to be born.
- Repeat as often as you wish. For most benefit, aim for a massage every day or every other day.

4.6

Do not do perineal massage if you have:

- Vaginal herpes
- Thrush or any other vaginal infection

If you feel pain at any point, stop and try again another time. If you continue to find this painful, speak with your midwife or GP and they will help you to check your technique.

The pelvic floor

The muscles and ligaments that form the **pelvic floor** span the base of the pelvis, separating the pelvic cavity from the perineum. They extend front to back from the pubic bone to the coccyx, side to side between the ischial tuberosities and around the openings of the anal canal, urethra and vagina. Pelvic floor muscles are under voluntary as well as involuntary control and can be strengthened at will.

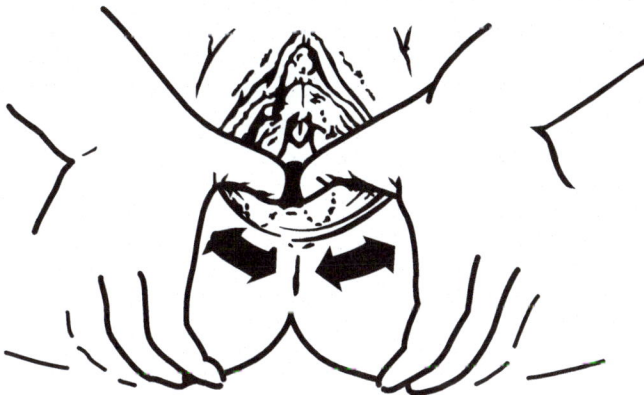

Figure 4.6.2 Perineal massage

They are excitable, contractile, extensible and elastic.

Functions

Functions of the pelvic floor can be summarised under four headings:

- **Support the pelvic organs**: the bladder, vagina, uterus and rectum, protecting against the effects of gravity. Along with the abdominal muscles, pelvic floor muscles provide **resistance** to increases in intra-pelvic/abdominal pressure during activities such as lifting, coughing, straining and bending. They are a key component of the '**core**' muscles which help the hips and spine to move, provide spinal and pelvic stability and help to maintain posture.
- Maintain **urinary and faecal continence**: Pelvic floor muscles facilitate voluntary control of the opening of the bladder and rectum as they relax and lengthen, allowing micturition and defecation. They maintain sphincter pressure and the colorectal angle (see below), and respond to an increase in intra-abdominal pressure by contracting around the urethra and anus to prevent leakage.
- Support **sexual function and satisfaction**: Sufficient strength of the pelvic floor muscles is necessary for orgasm and the voluntary and involuntary contraction of the muscles contributes to sexual arousal and sensation.
- **Support for the growing uterus** during **pregnancy** and facilitation of **childbirth** through providing resistance, assisting the rotation of the descending presenting part (see Chapter 4.3).

Muscles of the pelvic floor

Pelvic floor muscles are traditionally divided into superficial (closer to the skin) and deep muscles, although recently three layers of muscle slings have been described (Baramee et al., 2020).

Deep pelvic floor muscles

The **levator ani** and **coccygeus** muscles form the funnel-shaped structure of the deep pelvic floor (Figure 4.6.3).

The **levator ani** are a broad, thin group of muscles composed of three separate, paired muscles: **pubococcygeus**, **puborectalis** and **iliococcygeus**, which are situated on either side of the pelvis. The names of the muscles describe where they sit – for example, the pubococcygeus runs from the pubis to the coccyx. Each pair of muscles meets in the middle of the pelvis to form the **perineal body**. The levator ani form the greater part of the pelvic floor and have both a supportive and protective function. They are composed of striated muscle fibres, with differing degrees of fast-twitch (30%) and slow-twitch (70%) fibres. The fast-twitch fibres exert more force and tire more quickly than the slow-twitch fibres, which can sustain a muscle contraction for a longer period of time. Tightening the levator ani muscles enhances the effectiveness of the sphincter muscles around the anus and urethra, helping to maintain continence. This is especially important when intra-abdominal pressure is raised, for example during exercise, sneezing, coughing, laughing, lifting and straining. The levator ani contract rhythmically during orgasm and are the target of pelvic floor exercises.

The **pubococcygeus** is the largest muscle of the levator ani. It stabilises and supports the pelvic and abdominal organs. The **puborectalis** muscle is a 'U shaped sling' under the pubococcygeus muscle and around the anus. Its tonic contraction bends the anal canal anteriorly, creating the **anorectal angle** (90°) between the anus and the rectum. This supports faecal

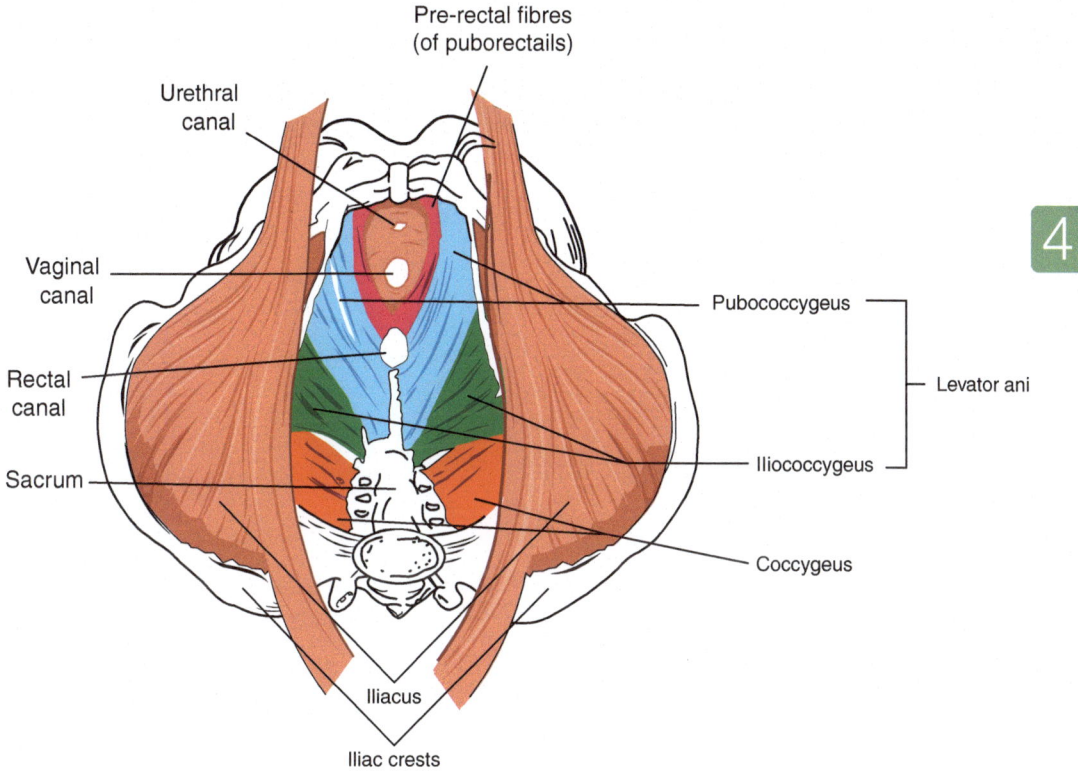

Figure 4.6.3 Deep pelvic floor muscles

continence. The puborectalis relaxes during defecation, creating an anorectal angle of 135° and facilitating stool passage. Some of the puborectalis muscle fibres (sometimes called the **pre-rectal fibres** or the pubovaginalis) encircle the urethra and vagina, aiding in narrowing the vaginal entrance and maintaining urinary continence. These muscle fibres can also contribute to sexual pleasure.

The **iliococcygeus** is a thin muscle layer that spans from one side of the pelvis to the other with thin slow-twitch muscle fibres. These maintain muscle tone and are highly resistant to tiring, providing a supportive base across the pelvic floor. This part of the levator ani is the actual 'levator', as its action elevates the pelvic floor and the anorectal canal.

The **coccygeus** is the smaller and most posterior part of the pelvic floor. It originates from the ischial spines and travels to the lateral aspect of the sacrum and coccyx, along the sacrospinous ligament. Its function is to stabilise the sacroiliac and sacrococcygeal joints, holding the coccyx in a flexed position.

Superficial pelvic floor muscles

The **superficial transverse perineal muscle** along with the **bulbocavernosus muscle** and the **ischiocavernosus muscle** (Figure 4.6.4) support and anchor the deep muscles of the pelvic girdle and assist in initiating and maintaining clitoral erection, vaginal contractions and orgasm during sexual activity.

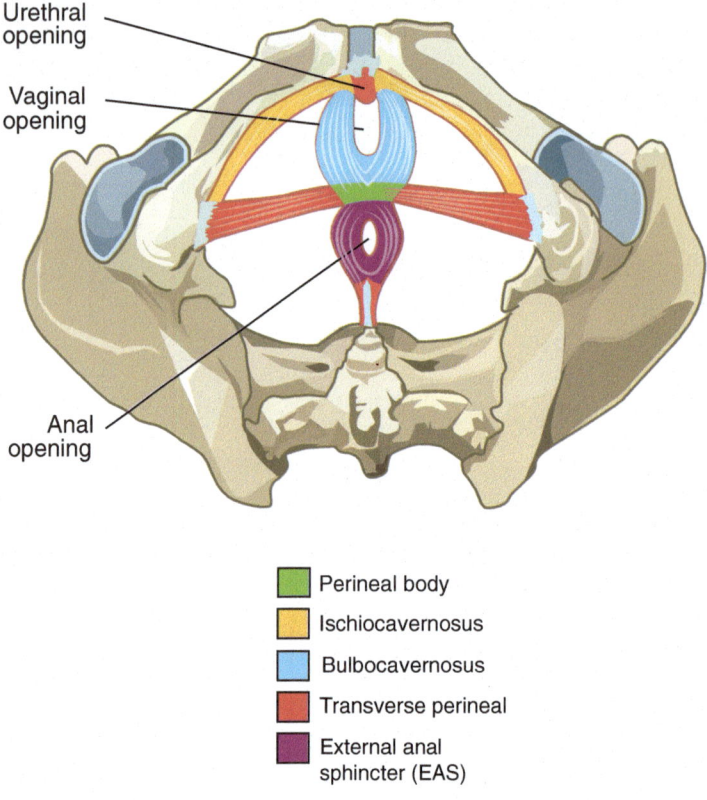

Urethral opening

Vaginal opening

Anal opening

■ Perineal body
■ Ischiocavernosus
■ Bulbocavernosus
■ Transverse perineal
■ External anal sphincter (EAS)

Figure 4.6.4 Superficial pelvic floor muscles

The **superficial transverse perineal muscles** interlink to support the perineal body. The **bulbocavernosus muscle** effectively forms a sphincter around the vagina meaning it is slightly contracted at rest. The **ischiocavernosus muscle** helps to maintain clitoral erection during sexual arousal by pushing blood to the tip of the clitoris and restricting venous outflow.

The anal sphincter complex

The anal sphincter complex sits within the pelvic floor and perineum. It is important that midwives are familiar with its anatomy as it can be damaged in severe perineal trauma (see below). It is composed of the internal and external anal sphincters (Figure 4.6.5).

The **internal anal sphincter (IAS)** is a continuation of inner rectal muscle which has thickened, circular fibres, up to 5 mm thick and 3–4 cm long. It is composed of visceral muscle. The EAS is composed of skeletal muscle and is categorised into deep, superficial and subcutaneous parts:

▶ The **deep EAS** is made up of circular muscle fibres, blends with the puborectalis part of the levator ani and is called the anorectal ring. It is palpable on rectal examination.

▶ The **superficial EAS** is made up of elliptical muscle fibres and extends from the tip of the coccyx posteriorly to the perineal body anteriorly.

▶ The **subcutaneous EAS** is made of circular muscle fibres, the lower ends curve inwards and lie below the end of

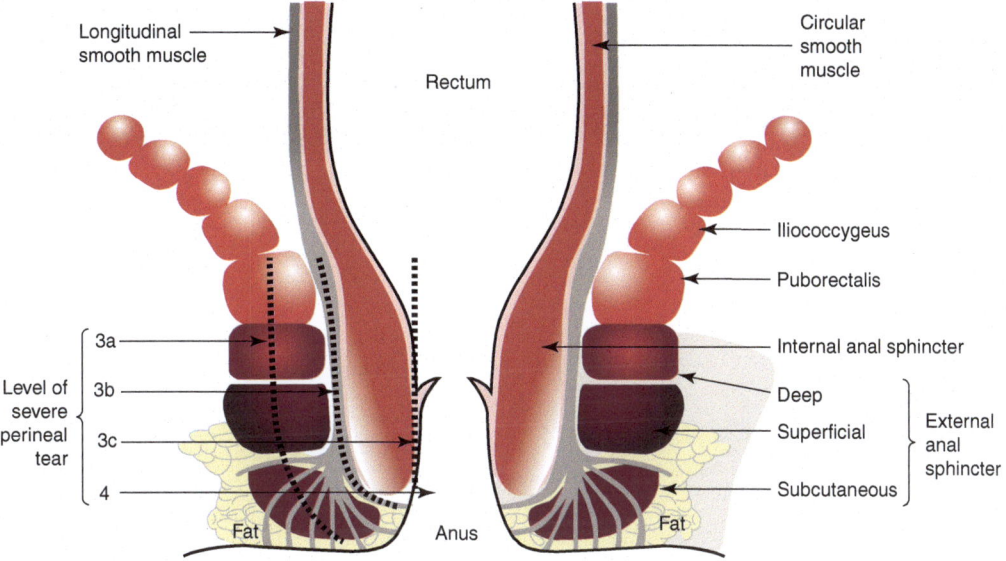

Figure 4.6.5 The anal sphincter complex

4.6

the IAS. The inter-sphincter groove that results is palpable on examination.

Ligaments

There are three sets of ligaments in the pelvic floor: the **transverse** or cardinal, **uterosacral** and **pubocervical** (Figure 4.6.6). They play an important role in maintaining support of the uterus and anchoring the cervix. Overstretching of these ligaments may result in pelvic organ prolapse.

Neurovascular supply to the pelvic floor and perineum

The **pelvic floor** is innervated by the **pudendal nerve**, apart from the levator ani muscles, which are innervated directly from the **pelvic nerves**. Blood reaches the area via the **internal iliac arteries** (Figure 4.6.7).

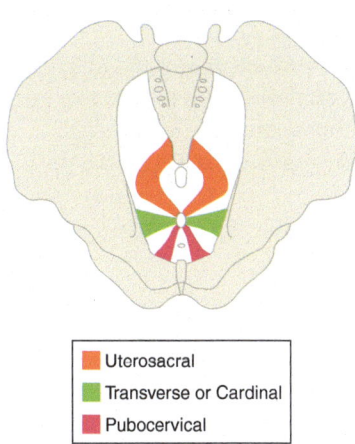

■ Uterosacral
■ Transverse or Cardinal
■ Pubocervical

Figure 4.6.6 Pelvic floor ligaments

> **INTERRUPTER**
>
> Label the diagrams of the pelvic floor muscles in your workbook.

Pelvic floor dysfunction

Pelvic floor pain or dysfunction can originate in any of the pelvic floor muscles. Its causes are generally multifactorial and may include:

▶ Increasing age
▶ Obesity

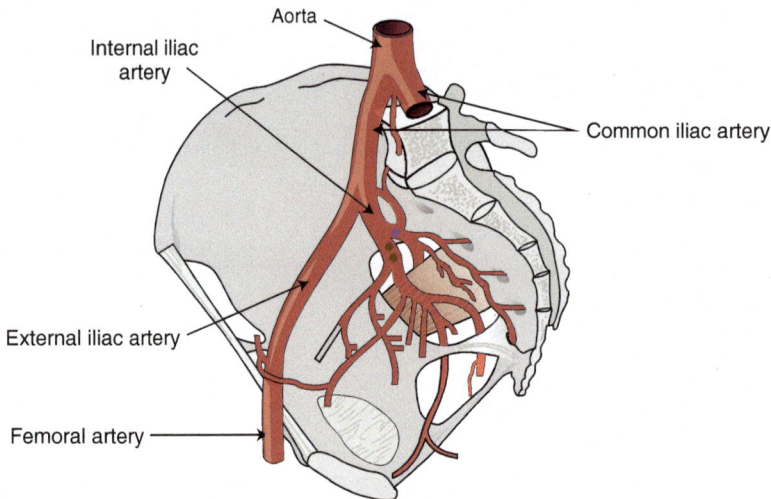

Figure 4.6.7 Blood supply to the pelvis

- Pregnancy and childbirth
- After gynaecological or urologic procedures
- Chronic straining
- After repetitive minor trauma from activities such as horse riding or gymnastics
- After sexual abuse
- As a result of hormonal changes during the menopause

Increased parity, prolonged second stage of labour and operative vaginal birth may increase the likelihood of pelvic floor dysfunction following birth, and third- and fourth-degree perineal lacerations (see below and figure 4.6.5) are a risk factor for faecal incontinence.

Pelvic floor dysfunction will present with a range of signs and symptoms relating to the abnormal functioning of the pelvic floor muscles and the weakening of the structural support of the urethra, vagina and anal canal. These include:

- Urinary and/or faecal incontinence
- Genitourinary prolapse
- Pelvic pain
- Sexual dysfunction

Pelvic floor exercises

Pelvic floor exercises are a set of exercises designed to increase strength, endurance and maintain normal functional control of the pelvic floor muscles. Pelvic floor exercises are particularly important during and after pregnancy and birth, both of which can subject the area to considerable stress and damage. When carried out regularly, they can reduce the incidence of pelvic floor disorders, such as stress incontinence and pelvic organ prolapse in pregnancy, the puerperium and in later life (the muscles will become further weakened during the menopause). Improved muscle tone is also likely to increase sexual pleasure.

APPLICATION TO PRACTICE

Pelvic floor exercises

Pelvic floor exercises are an essential part of a healthy lifestyle for all women, but particularly those who are pregnant or have given birth. They should be performed throughout pregnancy, although women may find that they become more challenging as pregnancy progresses. They can be resumed shortly after giving birth and continued as a lifestyle habit. The exercises should be performed more often if urinary incontinence is experienced. Additionally, women should be counselled to tighten and lift their pelvic floor muscles before coughing or sneezing, laughing, lifting anything or performing any other activity that places the muscles under stress.

An ability to explain how to perform pelvic floor exercises is a key part of a midwife's role. Use the links and instructions below to help you perform your own pelvic floor exercises and pass this important skill to women and birthing people:

Squeezy App: www.youtube.com/watch?v=zWbLbUy0cDk

A video by Oxford University Hospitals NHS Trust Physiotherapy Team: www.youtube.com/watch?v=KdN2gQX2280

1. Sit up straight and lean forward slightly towards the edge of a chair. Your feet should be flat on the floor and about hip width apart, your knees should be soft, and your hands should be resting on your knees.
2. Imagine that you are trying to stop yourself from passing wind and urine. You need to first tighten the muscles around the vagina and rectum, and then lift them up. Some people find it helps to visualise drawing a tampon up the vagina.
3. It is important only to tighten and lift the pelvic floor muscles, so make sure you are not clenching your buttocks or legs, engaging your abdominal muscles or holding your breath. Your

face, hands and knees should also stay soft and relaxed.
4. Once you have isolated, tightened and lifted the correct muscles, hold the lift for a second or two, and then let go. You should be able to feel both the tightening and the relaxing sensations. Rest for 1–2 seconds. Repeat this tighten, hold, release, rest cycle about ten times.
5. It is also important to perform longer pelvic floor holds. In addition to performing 1–2 second holds, you should aim to be able to hold ten pelvic floor tightenings for ten seconds each before releasing them. Start with whatever you can manage and build up to this.
6. Repeat three times a day. Some people find that it helps to link pelvic floor exercises with a regular activity, so that they become instinctive. You could do them while you brush your teeth, boil the kettle or turn on your computer.

Perineal trauma in childbirth

Around 85% of women will sustain some form of perineal injury during vaginal birth. This can range from minor cuts and grazes to deep and extensive damage (see Figure 4.6.8). Perineal trauma is often classified as follows:

Superficial: Minor grazes to the skin

Tears:

▶ **First-degree tear**: These tears will involve the skin but not the underlying muscle, are often small and heal quickly, with no requirement for suturing (stitches) or intervention. Labial tears, though, can fuse together and therefore are often sutured to prevent adhesion.
▶ **Second-degree tear**: A second-degree tear involves the muscle layers of the

4.6

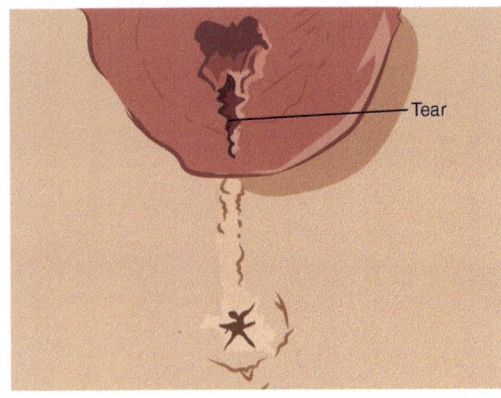

First degree perineal tear

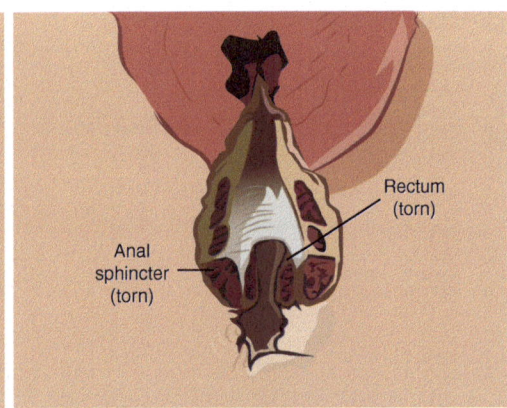

Second degree perineal tear

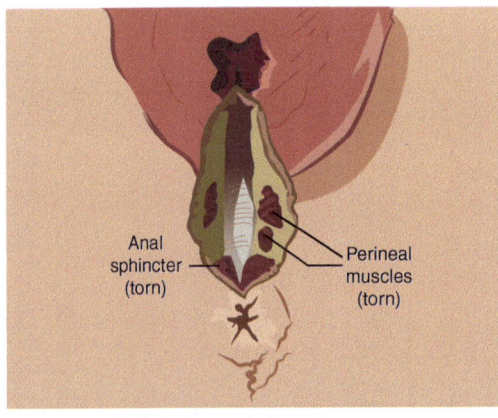
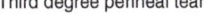

Third degree perineal tear

Fourth degree perineal tear

Figure 4.6.8 Perineal tears

perineum. Close inspection is required in order to determine whether a repair is indicated. Some second-degree tears can be complex and involve a considerable amount of muscle damage.

▶ **Third-degree tears**: This type of tear involves the muscles of the anal sphincter. They are sometimes further classified into:

  ▶ 3A – where less than 50% of the EAS is torn

  ▶ 3B – where over 50% of the EAS is torn

  ▶ 3C – where the external and internal anal sphincters are torn

Midwives should seek assistance from an obstetrician, who, with maternal consent, will repair the damage while maintaining the integrity of faecal continence.

▶ **Fourth-degree tear**: This tear extends through the anal sphincter to the rectal mucosa. Action and advice may be required from gynaecologists and colorectal surgeons. Surgical repair will be necessary to maintain the integrity of the pelvic floor and bowel function.

Perineal repair

The purpose of suturing is to achieve both **haemostasis** and **alignment**. In terms of haemostasis, the aim is to ensure active bleeding points are ligated. This will minimise blood loss and also reduce the likelihood of potential complications such as infection or a haematoma. Suturing also aims to bring torn tissues back into alignment. This will aid healing and the aim is for the healed area to return to near pre-tear condition. If the tear is left gaping, or suturing does not bring alignment, then although the tear will heal this may cause scar tissue.

Third- and fourth-degree tears, often referred to as severe perineal trauma or obstetric anal sphincter injury **(OASI)**, require specialist treatment due to their severity and hence, potential for significant complication. Around 3 women in 100 will experience this type of perineal injury, although certain 'risk factors' may increase a woman's risk of OASI. OASI is associated with faecal incontinence and pain. Therefore, careful confirmation of a lack of OASI is required when examining the perineum post birth by rectal examination. If OASI is confirmed, suturing will ideally need to be performed in theatre to ensure good position, lighting and pain relief. This enables the careful repair which is required to reduce ongoing effects of the trauma.

4.6

References

Baramee P., Muro S. et al. Three muscle slings of the pelvic floor in women: An anatomic study. *Anat. Sci. Int.* 2020, 95(1):47–53.

Beckmann M., Stock O. Antenatal perineal massage for reducing perineal trauma. *Cochrane Database Syst. Rev.* [Internet] 2013. Available from www.cochranelibr ary.com/cdsr/doi/10.1002/14651858. CD005123.pub3/abstract.

CHAPTER 4.7

Changes to body systems in labour and birth

Giada Giusmin

LEARNING OUTCOME

▶ Understand the key changes which occur to the maternal body systems during labour and apply this to practice

In the previous section, we explored some of the changes to key body systems during pregnancy. In this chapter, we will focus on how these body systems work and adapt during labour and birth.

Blood and cardiovascular system

Blood parameters

In Chapter 3.1, we introduced physiological anaemia (low haemoglobin) of pregnancy, which results from a mismatch between a 50% plasma volume increase and only a 20–30% red blood cell rise. In labour, however, we may observe a **higher haemoglobin** level due to **haemoconcentration**, the opposite of the haemodilution that occurs in pregnancy. Haemoconcentration in labour and birth occurs predominantly because of two factors, dehydration and the increased erythropoiesis taking place as a stress response.

White cell count (WCC) is already increased in pregnancy compared to non-pregnant levels. During labour and birth, WCC level, especially neutrophils, **rises even further** as a stress response. Although this is a physiological process, it can be mistaken for a bacterial infection,

DOI: 10.4324/9781003227571-27

especially in the presence of maternal dehydration, tachycardia and mild pyrexia.

Pregnancy is known as a state of **hypercoagulability**, and during the intrapartum period it is intensified further – this helps to protect the birthing woman from bleeding excessively by ensuring prompt haemostasis after the placenta has separated. During labour and birth, increased levels of clotting factors can be observed, with peak activity after placental separation. Furthermore, fibrinolytic activity is reduced to encourage clot formation when the placenta separates – this ensures the formation of a haemostatic fibrin mesh on the now-exposed placental wound. Following the third stage, some levels, like fibrinogen, can be reduced due to increased consumption. As a result of these events, women in the immediate postpartum are at higher risk for thromboembolic events.

Cardiovascular system

As discussed in Chapter 3.1, a significant change occurring in pregnancy is an increase in cardiac output. In labour, **cardiac output increases** by a further 10–15% during the first stage of labour and by up to 50% during the second stage, with a surge immediately after childbirth. The cardiac output increase is more marked during contractions, but still present in between. This is because uterine contractions in labour are responsible for the auto-transfusion of 300–500 ml of blood back into the maternal circulation. So, the cardiac output increase is mostly due to the increased stroke volume, rather than heart rate. However, during contractions, together with the increased circulating volume, transient tachycardia can be observed. There are a number of factors that can affect cardiac output increase, like epidural analgesia and maternal position. Epidural analgesia can limit the cardiac output rise during labour and birth. Regarding positions,

the supine position can be responsible for lowering cardiac output and stroke volume, however, this then generates a compensatory heart rate increase.

Blood pressure generally decreases slightly in pregnancy. In labour, especially when the woman experiences pain and anxiety, **blood pressure can rise**. This rise in blood pressure is particularly marked during contractions, whereas in between contractions, it returns to baseline. In the first stage of labour, systolic blood pressure can rise by around 35 mmHg, whereas the diastolic blood pressure can rise by around 25 mmHg. Both systolic and diastolic blood pressure rise even further during the second stage of labour. Some women might have transiently raised blood pressure after childbirth while the vascular tone returns to normal.

The birth of the baby and the expulsion of the placenta and membranes cause significant cardiovascular changes due to blood loss and other changes. It takes approximately one hour from the birth of the baby for the cardiac parameters to return back to the pregnancy state and around two months for the parameters to return back to the non-pregnant state.

Respiratory system

During labour and birth, the main factor affecting the respiratory system is the **increased expenditure of energy** necessary to support the muscular work required in childbirth. This can result in two different states that the woman can present, maternal acidosis and alkalosis, depending on the changes in ventilation and pH.

Maternal alkalosis

Due to pain and anxiety, birthing women have a tendency to hyperventilate by increasing the number of breaths (respiratory rate) and the tidal volume (the amount of air entering and exiting the lungs in one breath, which has already risen in pregnancy). This is further amplified in the second stage of labour, especially during directed pushing, when the woman holds her breath during the expulsive efforts and then hyperventilates when the contraction has eased off.

During the intrapartum period, oxygen consumption and intake increase by around 40–60%, and this peaks even more during contractions. The increased oxygenation because of hyperventilation will lead to a decline in CO_2 level in the blood ($PaCO_2$), causing a state of respiratory alkalosis and a marginal rise in pH level.

Maternal acidosis

In labour, with the increasing uterine muscle activity, the requirement for oxygen grows concurrently. It is essential for there to be spaces between contractions, to allow sufficient time for the oxygen to reach the uterine muscle in between contractions. If the time between contractions is reduced, this can cause a significant reduction in oxygen levels in the uterine muscle and subsequent tissue hypoxia. If this persists, it can lead to metabolic acidosis – an increased hydrogen ion concentration in the blood that reduces the pH to below 7.35 with a low bicarbonate level. Metabolic acidosis also increases pain perception for the birthing mother. Moreover, if maternal metabolic acidosis occurs due to intense and too frequent contractions, the blood flow to the fetus is also compromised, causing a build-up of CO_2 in the fetus and a drop in fetal pH. This occurs because the fetus cannot effectively perform gas exchange at the placental site and accumulates CO_2. Maternal acidosis is worsened during active second stage due to the additional effort of pushing.

Respiratory alkalosis and metabolic acidosis are two different states that can coexist during labour and birth. For example, respiratory alkalosis in isolation can be typical of the first stage, whereas towards the end of the first stage and throughout the second stage of labour, respiratory alkalosis attempts to compensate for the metabolic acidosis. It is important to note that both metabolic and respiratory changes can be influenced by a number of factors, such as labour induction or augmentation, or pharmacological and non-pharmacological analgesia.

Gastrointestinal system and nutrition

Similar to pregnancy, **gastric motility is reduced** during labour and birth, albeit more significantly. Some analgesia, like opioids, can exacerbate this. When this is combined with an already relaxed lower oesophageal sphincter and increased gastric acidity, normal in pregnancy, the **risk of aspiration** (where stomach contents are regurgitated into the mouth and then enter the lungs) during general anaesthesia increases. However, in recent years, only a small proportion of women require general anaesthesia and anaesthetic procedures are more sophisticated. In labour, birthing women use between 700–1100 calories per hour. Available glucose is soon depleted, especially when oral intake is limited. In order to continue to sustain the energy demands of labour, lipolysis (breakdown of body fat) occurs. This results in ketones being produced, which in turn, could lower fetal pH. Moreover, the use of anaerobic metabolism (see Chapter 3.2) causes the maternal pH to drop because of an excess of lactate (metabolic acidosis). Women are, therefore, recommended to eat a light diet when in labour, and possibly withhold food if at high risk for general anaesthesia.

4.7

Regarding laboratory tests, it is important to note that aspartate aminotransferase (AST), alanine transaminase (ALT) and lactate dehydrogenase (LDH) can double in the intrapartum period due to the stress induced by labour.

APPLICATION TO PRACTICE

Eating and drinking in labour

The very small risk of aspiration in labour needs to be balanced against the very real need for additional energy at this time, especially since fasting is not a guarantee of a less acidic or empty stomach. Research in this area is limited, but no benefits or harms of restricting food and fluids in labour to women at low risk of needing anaesthesia have been identified (Singata et al., 2013).

There is widespread agreement that women should be enabled to eat and drink as they wish in labour. Carbohydrate and sugar-rich foods such as honey may satisfy the body's need for glucose at this time, while food rich in fat or fibre may delay gastric emptying. Isotonic drinks, which have a similar osmolarity, or concentration of carbohydrates, sugar and salt, as blood, are quickly absorbed, replace constituents lost through metabolism and sweat, and may be more beneficial than water.

Antacids in labour are not recommended routinely, however, they should be given with consent in case of opioid administration or if the woman is at high risk for Caesarean section.

There is more information about gastric aspiration and food and fluid in labour, and a very interesting discussion, in this blog post: https://evidencebasedbirth.com/evidence-eating-drinking-labor/

Renal system

During the intrapartum period, both maternal and fetal **renin-angiotensin systems see increased levels,** and this is thought to have an impact on the reduction of uterine blood flow after the birth of the baby. Pregnant women, especially during labour and birth, are at **higher risk of hyponatraemia** (also referred to as water intoxication), when sodium is below the normal level. This occurs because, in pregnancy, the sodium level is slightly lower (lower range moved from 135 to 130 mmol) and in the third trimester there is a predisposition to retain water, which in turn further dilutes sodium levels (dilutional hyponatraemia). During the intrapartum period, this can be seen to a greater extent as oxytocin, both endogenous and synthetic, has an antidiuretic effect. If synthetic oxytocin is combined with intravenous administration of fluids, it greatly increases the risk of hyponatraemia. For this reason, it is vital to maintain a neutral fluid balance by carefully monitoring intake and output. Women with pre-eclampsia, due to their impaired renal function, are at higher risk for hyponatraemia.

Anatomically, the bladder moves upwards towards the abdomen to prevent damage during labour. However, trauma and oedema to the bladder and urethra can occur during second stage due to the increased pressure exercised during expulsive pushes, especially if for a prolonged period of time. This could lead to issues with passing urine after birth. Moreover, a full bladder could slow down labour progress as it can prevent the fetal head descending further down the birth canal, this in turn can cause effective contractions and progressive dilatation to slow down. A full bladder could cause delays in the third stage and excessive blood loss as it prevents the uterus from contracting effectively.

Nervous system

Pain is a highly complex, individual and subjective phenomenon that can be impacted by physical, psychological, cultural and spiritual factors. A full consideration of pain is well outside the scope of this book. However, the importance of pain in labour and birth means it is appropriate to briefly address the topic.

Pain influences some of the other body systems discussed in this chapter, for example, pain stimulates the release of catecholamines, which increase heart and respiratory rates. There are two types of pain that birthing women can experience, somatic and visceral. **Somatic pain** is generally localised and specific to different sensations, such as pressure, hot/cold. During childbirth, somatic pain manifests during the end of first stage and throughout second stage due to the pressure of the fetal presenting part on the birth canal and

perineum. **Visceral pain** is poorly defined pain emanating from the internal thoracic, pelvic or abdominal organs. It occurs in labour because of reduced blood flow in the uterine muscle during contractions and because of the cervix stretching. Visceral pain is predominant in the first stage of labour and more generalised as it can extend towards the back, the buttocks and upper thighs. This occurs because visceral pain, during the first stage of labour, is transmitted via nerve fibres arriving between T10 and T12 (T = thoracic vertebrae) and L1 (L = lumbar vertebrae). As the spinal cord neurons stimulated by the uterus and cervix also innervate the abdomen, birthing women can experience 'referred pain' which is more generalised. Somatic pain in second stage, which originates from the stretching of the cervix and perineum, sends impulses through the pudendal nerves to S2 to S4 (S = sacral vertebrae) (see Figure 4.7.1).

It is thought that the majority of pain experienced during childbirth originates from the cervix, as it is more densely

4.7

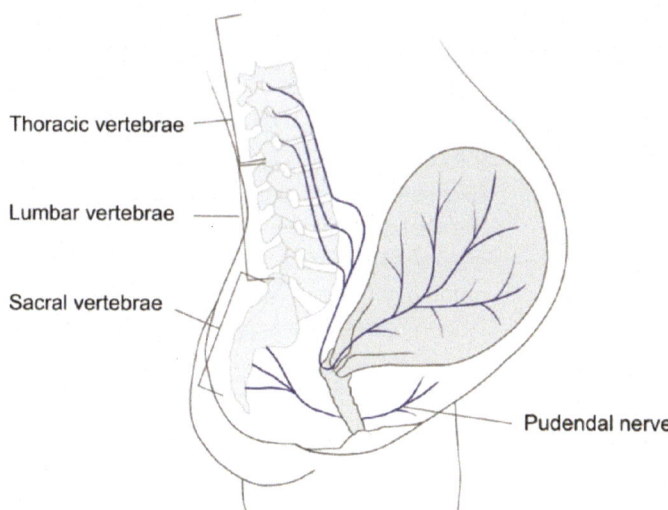

Thoracic vertebrae

Lumbar vertebrae

Sacral vertebrae

Pudendal nerve

Figure 4.7.1 Nerves responsible for visceral and somatic pain during childbirth

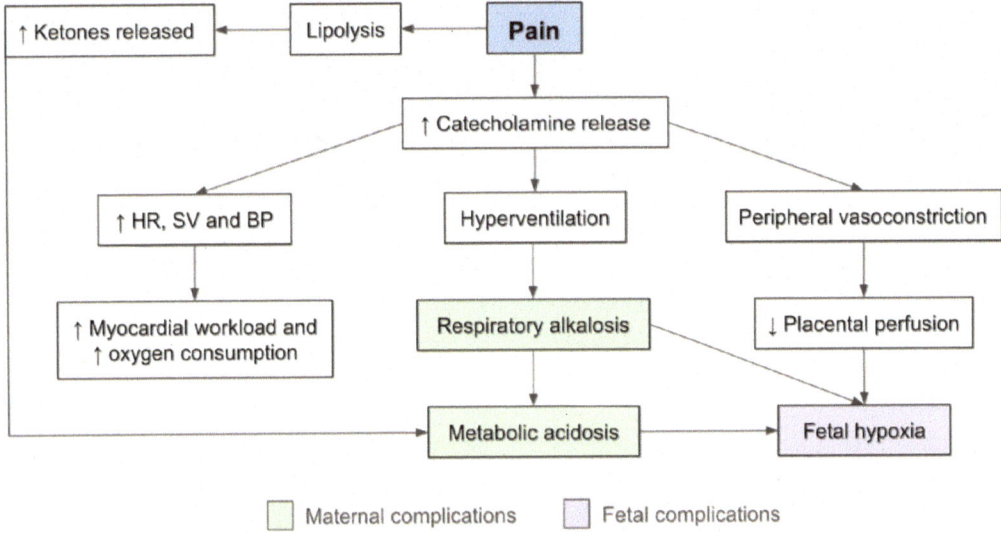

Figure 4.7.2 Overview of maternal and fetal complications that can occur because of excessive contractions in labour

innervated than the uterus at term. However, during late pregnancy, the number of nerve endings in the area of the spinal cord linked to the cervix is reduced. This, together with higher levels of beta-endorphins (these attenuate pain perception), is thought to induce 'pregnancy-induced analgesia', which is an increased maternal threshold to pain. This higher pain threshold predominantly occurs between 36 weeks and 24 hours after birth.

Pain in labour can instigate anxiety in the birthing woman. This in turn can cause a number of physical responses such as hyperventilation and release of catecholamines, leading to increased cardiac output, blood pressure, respiratory rate, metabolic rate and oxygen consumption. It is also responsible for delaying gastric emptying, potentially leading to vomiting, and delayed bladder emptying.

Pain can be modulated in different ways during labour and birth, with the use of

pharmacological methods, like epidural or opioids, or non-pharmacological interventions such as hypnobirthing, movement, massage, water immersion, music and transcutaneous electrical nerve stimulation (TENS).

The **gate-control theory** of pain is explored in detail in Chapter 3.3 and so is not covered again here – but is an important mechanism for use of certain pain-relieving processes which may be implemented during labour.

Excessive contractions in labour, either due to over-use of labour-stimulating drugs or as a physiological response to an underlying pathology (for example, an obstructed labour) can lead to a number of maternal and fetal complications, as outlined in Figure 4.7.2.

References

Singata M., Tranmer J. et al. Restricting oral fluid and food intake during labour. *Cochrane Database Syst. Rev.*

[Internet] 2013. www.cochranelibr
ary.com/cdsr/doi/10.1002/14651858.
CD003930.pub3/full.

Further reading

Soma-Pillay P., Nelson-Piercy C. et al.
Physiological changes in pregnancy.
Cardiovasc. J. Afr. 2016, 27(2):89–94.

www.ncbi.nlm.nih.gov/pmc/articles/
PMC4928162/.
Verma A., Roach P. The interpretation
of arterial blood gases. *Australian
Prescriber* [Internet] 2010, 33(4).
www.nps.org.au/assets/AP/pdf/
The-interpretation-of-arterial-blood-
gases.pdf.

4.7

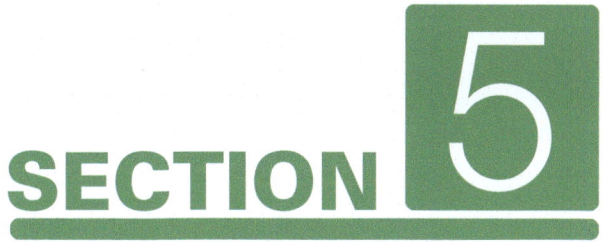

SECTION 5

The Puerperium

Claire Smith, Sarah Fleming and Kirsten Baker

The woman has given birth, and now we come to the period after birth – referred to as the puerperium. Having conceived, then nurtured and developed the embryo and then fetus, undergone a myriad of changes and adaptations across all body systems, the mother has then laboured and the fetus has made its journey from in utero *to being born, along with the placenta. Now, comes the all-important task of her body returning close to its pre-pregnancy state, while the fetus transitions to life outside the uterus. Again, each and every body system must undergo change now that the woman is no longer pregnant, while the fetus must learn to regulate its own body systems for itself. The puerperium is a period of huge change, physically, socially and psychologically, as woman and newborn adapt to this new world.*

DOI: 10.4324/9781003227571-28

Maternal postnatal physiology

Claire Smith

Traditionally known as the 'lying in period', the World Health Organization (WHO) defines the postnatal period as being from the first hour of post-placenta delivery until the sixth week (42 days) following the birth of the infant (WHO, 2022). The puerperium is a time of physical and psychological adjustment for all members of a new family.

Physically, the body needs to recover from birth, and the changes and adaptations made to support the growing fetus need to be reversed. Psychologically, many new parents need support and reassurance as they adapt to their new roles.

Concerns have been raised across the Global North by both mothers and midwives regarding the erosion of postnatal care due to reduced staffing and service provision, well documented in contemporary literature. Furthermore, there is minimal input from obstetricians around this time, yet the puerperium is associated with

DOI: 10.4324/9781003227571-29

high levels of maternal morbidity and mortality; 86% of women who die during pregnancy and childbirth in the UK do so in the postnatal period (MBRRACE-UK, 2023). As lead practitioners during this time, midwives support mothers' recovery from childbirth, promoting physiological transitions and identifying potential associated complications.

Changes to body systems in the puerperium

Almost all body systems adapt over the course of pregnancy to support the growing fetus, so it stands to reason that they are all affected post pregnancy, as the body adapts to the new status quo. The systemic changes are outlined in Table 5.1.1.

Table 5.1.1 Physiological changes in the puerperium

System/component	Physiological influences	Outcome
Cardiac	Initial increase in circulating blood volume as the uterus contracts post birth	An initial increase in stroke volume and heart rate rapidly declines, and the heart returns to pre-pregnancy function within 2 weeks
	Reduced levels of progesterone and oestrogen (which caused vasodilation)	Vascular resistance reverts to normal
Haematological	Blood loss during birth	Level of white blood cells returns to normal within 4 weeks postnatally
	Haemoconcentration	Haemoglobin levels return to normal within 4–6 months
Coagulation	Hypercoagulation	Platelets rise in the first 48 hours following birth, reducing the risk of haemorrhage but increasing the risk of thrombosis
		This state gradually decreases over 8–12 weeks
Renal	Increased serum levels of atrial natriuretic peptide promote urinary sodium excretion	A brisk diuresis can continue for up to 2 weeks. The glomerular filtration rate returns to its pre-pregnancy functioning by 8 weeks postnatally
	Diuresis: fluid shifts from the extravascular to the intravascular space	Bladder – possible loss of sensation and incontinence
	Lower progesterone levels should increase bladder tone, but bladder damage can occur due to overdistention, stress and trauma during labour	Kidneys – return to normal size after 6 months
Respiratory	Reduction of progesterone	Respiratory rate reduces from 15 to 20 breaths per minute back to 12
		Tidal volume returns to normal
		Bronchioles regain tension
		Less nasal congestion and epistaxis
		Full inhalation/exhalation is enabled
		Diaphragm returns to pre-pregnancy location

(Continued)

Table 5.1.1 (Continued)

System/component	Physiological influences	Outcome
Gastrointestinal	Decrease in progesterone Bowel emptying during second stage of labour	Oesophageal sphincter tone improves, resolving acid reflux and associated symptoms within a week Gastrointestinal transit time decreases during labour. Normal bowel movements should resume 2–3 days post birth
Thyroid	Human chorionic gonadotropin levels fall dramatically (this mimics thyroid stimulating hormone)	Metabolic alterations in thyroid processes gradually reverse over 4–6 weeks, but can persist for 6–12 weeks Transient disorders of thyroid function are seen in some postnatal women Around 5% will develop postnatal thyroiditis, where the thyroid is attacked by antithyroid antibodies; this can result in weight loss, anxiety, a rapid heart rate and excessive hair loss in the first 6 months after birth, followed by symptoms such as weight gain, fatigue, depression, and feeling cold thereafter Postnatal thyroiditis is more common in women with type 1 diabetes or a history of thyroid dysfunction
Endocrine	Decreased levels of oestrogen, progesterone and cortisol Rise in prolactin	Elevated prolactin levels while the mother is breastfeeding inhibit ovulation In the absence of breastfeeding, menstrual function resumes within 6–8 weeks Ovulation can occur in tandem with breastfeeding, and will precede menstruation This means that the absence of periods is not a guarantee that pregnancy will not occur Increased production of breastmilk
Uterus	Involution	Returns to pre-pregnant state (see below)
Breasts	Decrease in progesterone levels enables a rise in prolactin	Lactation (see Section 6)
Vagina	Decrease in oestrogen level Vaginal muscles may be weakened by a long second stage, episiotomy or tears	Epithelium thins, reduction in vaginal lubrication Increased likelihood of incontinence and prolapse (see below)
Abdomen	Stretching during pregnancy Strain during labour Mechanical stretching during Caesarean birth	Tone and elasticity should return within 6–8 weeks Divarification (separation) of the rectus abdominus muscles may result, causing lower back pain and pelvic dysfunction which may require physiotherapy input (see Chapter 3.5) Stretch marks become less visible but may remain over abdomen and legs
Miscellaneous		Hair loss can be a concern following birth with regrowth occurring after a few months Skin pigmentations such as melanoma fade

5.1

INTERRUPTER

Fill in the gaps in the physiological changes table in your workbook to help embed this knowledge.

Postnatal physiology and care

Uterine involution

Involution is the returning of the uterus to its pre-pregnant state. The uterus gains approximately 900 g during pregnancy

Table 5.1.2 Postnatal changes in uterine structure, weight and cervical changes

Postnatal stage	Approximate weight of uterus (g)	Approximate size/consistency of cervical opening
3rd stage	1000	Open, soft
After 1 week	500	2cm
After 2 weeks	300	1cm
End of 6 weeks	60	A 1cm slit

and can reduce back to its normal 60 g size (see Table 5.1.2 and Figure 5.1.1). By six weeks it is no longer palpable abdominally.

The process of involution begins immediately on expulsion of the placenta and membranes. Rapid destruction of the uterine tissue results in over 50% of its mass being lost within the first 24 hours. This physiological event is brought about by a process known as **autolysis**, which is the digestion of muscle fibres by proteolytic enzymes (enzymes which break down protein). Waste products of autolysis are then removed by macrophages in the blood and lymphatic systems.

Involution is also assisted by **oxytocin**, which causes the muscles within the myometrium to continue to contract and act as living ligatures on the uterine blood vessels, thereby reducing the uterine blood supply (see Chapter 4.5). Breastfeeding stimulates oxytocin secretion, further assisting the process of involution.

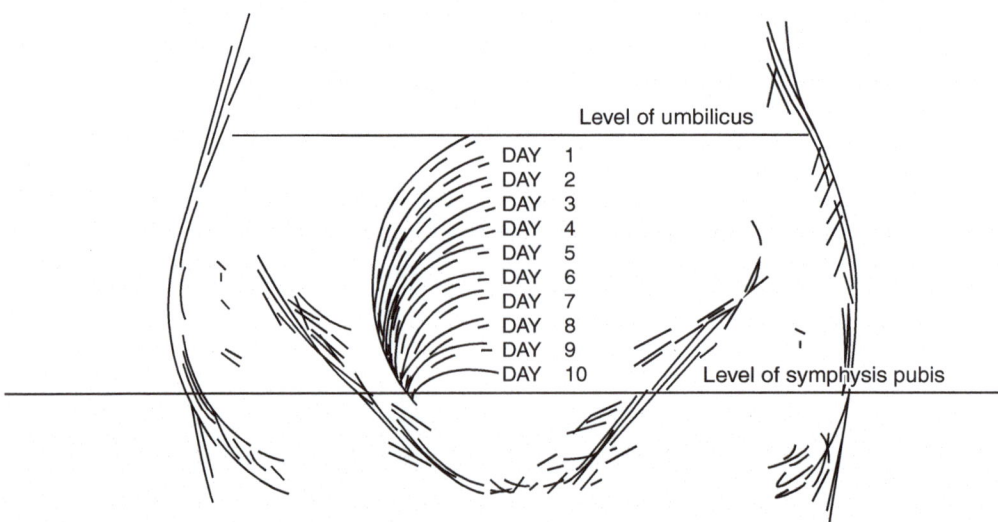

Figure 5.1.1 Stages of uterine involution

APPLICATION TO PRACTICE

Abdominal palpation

The technique of palpation has remained the same for over a century. It involves sinking the hand, palm to pubis into the abdomen above the navel, and walking it down until it is checked by the fundus (see Figure 5.1.2).

Although palpation has been a cornerstone of postnatal care for many years, there is in fact little evidence to support this practice – it is unlikely to yield any additional information to questions concerning the consistency, volume and smell of blood loss, and maternal well-being.

Involution occurs rapidly over the first ten days at approximately 1 cm a day following a vaginal birth. On palpation, the uterus should feel hard, round and central, and is often described as being 'like a cricket ball'.

Involution following a lower segment Caesarean section is a slower, more uneven process but should be completed as with vaginal birth by six weeks. Involution may also be slower when there has been overdistention of the uterus, in the presence of multiple pregnancy, polyhydramnios or a macrosomic fetus.

Delayed involution

The uterus may feel 'boggy' and tender to touch due to retained products of conception, such as fragments of membranes and placental tissue, inhibiting effective uterine contraction; this may also indicate uterine infection.

Cervical changes

In tandem with involution, the cervix recovers from its initial bruising and damage within the first week following a vaginal delivery. Although the cervix heals, it will not return to its original shape (Figure 5.1.3a) – the external os will resemble a slit (Figure 5.1.3b), as opposed to the nulliparous dimple.

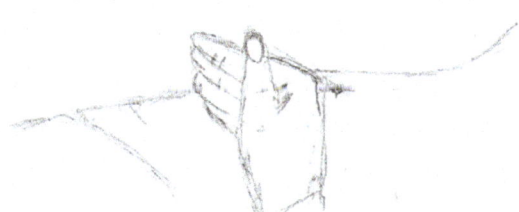

Figure 5.1.2 A cupped hand approach to assessing involution
Source: Image from Claire Smith

(a)

(b)

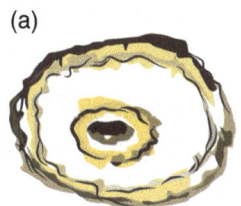
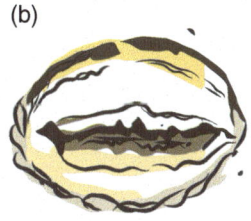

Figure 5.1.3 The nulliparous and parous cervix
Source: Image from Claire Smith

Table 5.1.3 Stages of lochial loss

Name	Day	State of lochia
Lochia rubra	1–4	Red. Thick mucoid consistency. Decidual tissue which is initially sterile until colonisation occurs from vaginal flora
Lochia serosa	5–c.10	Dark red/pink/brown. Watery. Contains leucocytes, mucus, vaginal epithelial cells, necrotic decidua, non-pathological bacteria
Lochia alba	10 onward	Yellow-white discharge. Mostly serous fluid and leucocytes, plus some cervical mucus and microorganisms

Blood loss

Haemostasis

A certain amount of maternal blood loss after birth is part of a normal adjustment post pregnancy, as maternal blood volume will have increased antenatally to support the growing fetus. The body's mechanisms for stemming blood loss (haemostasis) in the postnatal period are outlined in Chapter 4.5.

The rough, bleeding surface left by the placenta regenerates after two weeks due to the reforming of the epithelium. However, it takes six weeks to heal fully and during this time has the potential for development of infections. The residual uterine fibrous tissue created in the healing process increases with each pregnancy.

Lochia

Postnatal blood and other vaginal loss is known as **lochia**. It is made up of blood from the placental site, dead cells (including white blood cells) and decidual sloughing caused by autolysis and ischaemia. Initially, lochia can be heavy and is often compared to a heavy period. For those women who have never experienced heavy menstrual flow it can be quite alarming, especially as the blood flow is often accompanied by 'after pains' and occasional clots. Lochial loss also increases as a hormonal response to breastfeeding, which stimulates uterine contractions. Lochia has a characteristic musty odour, due to its alkaline pH, which is essential for the avoidance of ascending infection.

The appearance of lochia changes as involution progresses – see Table 5.1.3. Initially the flow is thick, sometimes with small clots and bright red in colour; progressively darkening and then lightening and becoming less viscous.

There will be less lochial loss following Caesarean section, as the obstetric surgeons clear the uterus of the placenta and membranes during surgery; nonetheless there will be some loss, which can persist up to six weeks.

Sanitary pads should be changed every 2–3 hours while lochia is at its heaviest, then less often as the loss diminishes. Tampons are contra-indicated until six weeks postnatally, as inserting internal products may increase the possibility of uterine infection while the placental site is still healing.

After pains

Lochia is often accompanied by uterine cramps, often referred to as 'after pains', small contractions or 'period pains' The act of breastfeeding stimulates uterine contractions which can be experienced as painful during the first 48 hours. They are more common for multiparous women. The typical management of these pains includes the use of pain relief such as paracetamol, ibuprofen, naproxen or codeine, warm compresses, wheat bags, hot water bottles (not too hot) and transcutaneous nerve stimulation (TENS).

Abnormal lochia

If the lochia is offensive – a definite odour not attributed to the usual metallic smell of blood – then a high vaginal swab should be taken to identify vaginal microbiology and treat with appropriate antibiotics. A pelvic ultrasound may be performed to exclude retained products of conception, but this can prove unreliable. The most common site for sepsis, the third most likely cause of maternal death in the perinatal period in the UK (MBRRACE-UK, 2023), is in the genital tract and in particular the uterus.

Postpartum haemorrhage

Excessive bleeding within 24 hours of birth is referred to as **primary postpartum haemorrhage –** see Chapter 4.5. Excessive bleeding more than 24 hours after birth is called a **secondary postpartum haemorrhage**.

Secondary postpartum haemorrhage (sometimes referred to as late or delayed) can occur between 24 hours and 12 weeks following birth and is usually the result of **infection** and/or **retained products of conception** within the uterine cavity. These may need to be evacuated either by the use of uterotonics or surgery. Blood loss can be brisk and severe (over 2000 ml), or present as a persistent heavy flow which is red, viscous and contains clots. Urgent medical aid should be sought in the event of a sudden brisk blood loss which can lead to hypovolemic shock and maternal collapse. Risk factors include Caesarean section, premature rupture of membranes and long labours, those women with pre-existing blood disorders and women taking anticoagulant therapy. In addition to blood loss, secondary postpartum haemorrhage can be preceded or accompanied by offensive smelling lochia and a high, tender uterus which feels 'boggy' to palpate.

APPLICATION TO PRACTICE

Ritualistic postnatal practices

It is interesting to consider to what extent cultural practices around the puerperium are influenced by beliefs about the uncleanliness of birth and blood loss, and to what extent they celebrate or undermine the feminine power of birth. Consider the following examples of cultural practices from Dennis et al. (2007) (and any others of which you are aware) and think about the underlying messages they may be conveying:

▶ Excluding new mothers from community life until postnatal bleeding ceases
▶ The ancient British tradition of churching: the ritual of cleansing and purifying women after childbirth by allowing them back into the temple or church after six weeks have passed
▶ In Japan, women are traditionally sent to stay with their mothers from late pregnancy until eight weeks postnatally – a practice known as *Satogaeri bunben*
▶ In Fiji, postnatal women are encouraged not to take part in activities perceived to be potentially harmful to the mother or the infant such as sitting up, physical exertion, combing their hair or exposing themselves to the sun

Perineal healing

Perineal damage

It is likely that damage will occur to the genital tract during childbirth, the severity of which can vary from superficial to

5.1

intense, requiring surgical intervention (see Chapter 4.6). An understanding of wound healing is essential in order for midwives to be able to recognise deviations from normal and provide appropriate advice.

Stages of perineal healing

Often, perineal damage will be sutured to aid healing. Wounds that are not sutured will heal by **secondary intention** – from the bottom up. As with any wound, perineal lacerations heal in four stages:

▶ **Haemostasis** – see Chapter 3.1. Blood flow ceases and a scab can form over the wound.

▶ **Inflammation** – The damaged vessels leak transudate (a fluid containing water, salt and protein), causing localised swelling. This encourages neutrophils to rush to the wound site to destroy pathogenic bacteria and remove debris. Their numbers peak around 48 hours after the injury. As they retreat, macrophages arrive and spend 4–6 days continuing to clear debris and secreting growth factors and proteins which attract immune system cells to the site to facilitate tissue repair. During this time, wounds can appear swollen, inflamed, hot and painful. See Chapter 3.8 for further information on this process.

▶ **Proliferation** – The now clean wound bed is filled with collagen (a process also referred to as **granulation**), and new blood vessels are formed. Myofibroblasts then grip the wound margins and contract, pulling the wound closed. Finally, epithelial cells arising from the wound bed or margins resurface the wound. This can take from four to 24 days, and happens faster if wounds are moist and hydrated.

▶ **Maturation** – Collagen laid down in the proliferation stage is generally disorganised and thick. During maturation, the collagen is aligned along lines of tension and the new tissue gradually gains strength and flexibility. Repair cells that are no longer required are removed by apoptosis (programmed cell death) and excess water is removed. Healed skin will generally only have 80% of the tensile strength of unwounded skin.

Particularly if their perineum has been sutured, women can experience discomfort and fear around urinating and opening their bowels in the early postnatal period. Urine can cause open wounds or grazes to sting, particularly if it is concentrated. Women can be advised to use a jug or a squirty bottle to pour water over their perineum as they urinate, in order to dilute the urine's acidity. Running water from a tap may help them start to release the flow. Holding a clean pad against the perineum may lessen fears of wounds opening during defecation.

Wounds generally heal in 4–6 weeks. Healing can be delayed in women with diabetes, who smoke and those who are malnourished. Table 5.1.4 outlines some of the signs of compromised healing.

Pelvic organ prolapse

During examination of the perineum, a midwife may observe a protrusion at the entrance to the introitus. This can be a sign of pelvic organ prolapse. Prolapse occurs due to weakness of the pelvic floor or connective tissue which results in the cervix, uterus or vaginal walls descending from the confines of their usual structures. The bladder and/or bowel can also weaken and bulge or sag into the vaginal space. The incidence of prolapse after childbirth increases with a prolonged second stage of labour, large babies and instrumental deliveries. Symptoms may include a heavy dragging feeling in the lower pelvis,

Table 5.1.4 Signs of compromised healing

Issue	Signs and symptoms	Management
Infection	Swelling of perineum Inflammation Heat Pain (especially if worsening) Pus-like, offensive discharge	Symptoms can be physiological in first 24–48 hours Keep the wound clean and moist Keep mother hydrated Anti-inflammatory pain relief If symptoms persist refer to GP for perineal swab to identify causative organism and prescribe antibiotics
Haematoma (a large collection of blood within the tissues of the peritoneum, usually due to birth trauma or a ruptured broad ligament)	Pain in buttock or extreme pain around perineal bruising	Although superficial bruising is normal, a haematoma may require surgical drainage Conservative management may include bed rest, analgesia and the judicial use of ice packs or ice gel packs Ice packs should always be covered and not applied directly to the skin as this can cause damage to the tissues Although ice can relieve the discomfort of perineal pain, prolonged application will prevent blood flow, which is necessary for healing, to the affected area
Wound breakdown Breakdown of perineum	Skin edges parting Deep muscle layer visible Increase in pain New bleeding or discharge Signs and symptoms of sepsis	Refer to GP/Obstetrician for swab and antibiotics Anti-inflammatory pain relief Wound may need to be resutured after the infection has been treated If signs and symptoms of sepsis are present, immediate hospital admission and IV antibiotics will be required

5.1

particularly at the end of the day, pain and backache. Visualising the perineum and asking a woman to cough or gently push may reveal a prolapse if these symptoms are present. Pelvic floor exercises and physiotherapy are recommended. Where symptoms persist, referral to a gynaecologist may be necessary.

Bladder and bowel function

Both the bladder and bowel are affected by hormonal changes in pregnancy and can undergo stress and sustain damage during labour. Checking that voiding and bowel function are returning to a normal pattern is paramount, as is encouraging pelvic floor exercises which are preventative of, and the first line of management for, many bladder and bowel problems.

Bladder

The stretching and pressure exerted on the perineum during the late stages of pregnancy and labour can deplete the strength of the pelvic floor, affecting urinary voiding capabilities. In labour, the bladder is at risk of overdistention and bruising of the urethra is not uncommon, plus potential temporary nerve damage and a loss of muscle tone. Furthermore, damage to the urethral sphincter can occur. The risk factors, signs and symptoms, and

Table 5.1.5 Postnatal bladder complications

Issue	Risk factors	Signs and symptoms	Management
Weakened or damaged pelvic floor muscles	According to a large Australian cohort study (Durnea et al., 2017), risk factors in primiparous women include: Pre-pregnancy symptoms Recurrent urinary tract infections Larger hip circumference/ raised BMI Smoking Depression Vigorous exercise Induction of labour Forceps delivery	Stress incontinence (urinary urgency and/or a loss of small amounts of urine associated with coughing, laughing or exercise) Bladder prolapse	Pelvic floor exercises Adequate hydration (avoiding caffeine, citrus and carbonated drinks and alcohol)
Infection	Catheterisation Long labour Recurrent urinary tract infections in pregnancy	Sharp or burning pain, especially on urinating Urinary frequency Voiding very small amounts Cloudy or foul-smelling urine	Take mid-stream urine sample to identify pathogen Treat with antibiotics Adequate hydration (avoiding caffeine, citrus and carbonated drinks and alcohol)
Urinary retention (can be due to nerve damage and may resolve spontaneously)	A systematic review (Qiaomeng and Xiao, 2020) found that independent risk factors for urinary retention included: Episiotomy Epidural analgesia Instrumental delivery Primiparity Prolonged second stage	Inability to empty bladder fully No urge to pass urine Low abdominal pain Passing only small amounts of urine Urinary frequency Urinary incontinence	Adequate hydration (avoiding caffeine, citrus and carbonated drinks and alcohol) Pain relief Urinary catheter to empty and 'rest' bladder Refer to urogynaecology nurse if problem persists
Damage to urethral sphincter	Instrumental birth	Persistent stress incontinence, despite good pelvic muscle tone	Refer to urogynaecology specialists

management of these issues is outlined in Table 5.1.5.

A natural diuresis (expelling of fluid) occurs in the early postnatal period as levels of oestrogen decline and the body gets rid of the additional fluid accumulated in pregnancy. The bladder is therefore likely to fill rapidly and larger than normal amounts of urine are often passed for the first 2–3 days.

Bowels

The risk factors, signs, symptoms and management of postnatal bowel complications are outlined in Table 5.1.6.

Table 5.1.6 Postnatal bowel complications

Issue	Risk factors	Signs and symptoms	Management
Constipation	Severe perineal damage Poor diet Dehydration	Infrequent passing of stools Difficulty passing stools Lumpy, large, hard stools	Keep hydrated – drink at least 1.5 litres of water per day, and avoid caffeine and alcohol Eat a high fibre diet with plenty of fruit and vegetables Gentle exercise such as going for a walk Experiment with sitting on the toilet differently – e.g. raising feet or leaning back Laxatives can be used if self-help measures are insufficient
Haemorrhoids	Pre-pregnancy haemorrhoids Prolonged pushing Constipation	Tense, itchy, painful swellings around the anal opening – can be around the size of a pea or a grape Can be internal or external Rectal bleeding following a bowel movement	Can resolve spontaneously Avoid straining to pass stools Keep clean Soak in warm water (such as in a bath) to soothe pain and irritation Use a cold pack to lessen swelling Topical creams and suppositories can be applied. Care should be taken to avoid contact with any perineal damage if using haemorrhoid creams, as this could create a suitable environment for infection
Faecal urgency or incontinence	Weakened pelvic floor	Inability to control passage of stools, or experiencing urgency to defecate	Pelvic floor exercises Refer to physiotherapist or other specialist service if persists
Excessive gas/ flatus	Weakened pelvic floor Caesarean section Constipation	Inability to control passage of wind/ excessive wind Abdominal pain	Pelvic floor exercises Yoga poses to aid digestion Gentle exercise Peppermint capsules or peppermint tea

5.1

APPLICATION TO PRACTICE

Obstetric fistula

An obstetric fistula is a hole which forms between the genital tract and either the bladder (vesico-vaginal fistula) or rectum (recto-vaginal fistula). Although uncommon in the Global North, the United Nations Population Fund (UNFPA) estimates that half a million women and girls in sub-Saharan Africa, Asia, the Arab States region, Latin America and the Caribbean are living with this condition (UNFPA, 2022). Fistulas can develop during long, obstructed labours, when the soft tissue in the pelvis is compressed between the fetal head and the maternal pelvic bones and is therefore starved of blood and oxygen. When labour extends over several days, the tissue dies and a hole develops, leaving the mother with chronic incontinence. Long, obstructed labours also almost inevitably result in stillbirths. Obstetric fistulas, which in many settings result in already impoverished women and girls being ostracised by their communities, are entirely preventable with timely medical support.

Thrombosis and thromboembolic disorders

Postnatal hypercoagulability, particularly in the first 48 hours following birth, increases the risk of thrombosis and thromboembolic disorders (VTE), which include deep vein thrombosis (DVT) and pulmonary embolism (PE). DVT is the formation of a blood clot in a deep vein, usually in the lower leg or thigh. A PE can ensue if the clot breaks loose and travels through the bloodstream to the lungs, obstructing oxygen supply. Clots can also travel towards the heart, causing myocardial infarction, or to the brain, causing a stroke. Thromboembolism is the leading direct cause of maternal mortality during and up to six weeks postnatally in the UK (MBRRACE-UK, 2023).

Additional risk factors for DVT

- Immobility leads to reduced blood flow and increased risk of clots forming
- Caesarean section and other obstetric procedures such as instrumental delivery
- Postnatal complications such as infection
- Severe obesity
- Smoking
- Blood clotting disorders

- A family history of DVT, or previous DVT
- Health conditions such as diabetes, Crohn's, heart or lung disease
- There is some evidence to suggest that women over the age of 25 are more at risk postnatally

Presenting symptoms

DVT:

- Throbbing or cramping pain in one leg (usually in the calf)
- Swelling in one leg (rarely, it can be both)
- Painful area feels warm and surrounding skin may appear darkened
- Swollen veins that are hard and/or sore
- Localised itchiness

Pulmonary embolism:

- Pain (particularly chest pain)
- Shortness of breath or difficulty breathing
- Irregular or rapid heart rate
- Numbness or weakness on one side of the body
- Sudden change in mental state
- Collapse

APPLICATION TO PRACTICE

Prevention of DVT

- **Low molecular weight heparins (LMWH)** such as dalteparin and enoxaparin are anticoagulant drugs used in the prophylaxis and treatment of blood clots. Rather than 'thinning the blood', the active agent antithrombin prevents the formation of a clot by inhibiting the final common pathway of the coagulation cascade.

▶ **Anti-embolic stockings** providing a calf pressure of 14–15 mmHg. Stockings should be properly applied, of appropriate size and provide graduated compression. They should be worn day and night and removed for 30 minutes each day in order to wash and check underlying skin for any damage.

▶ **Flotron boots** are often used when mobilisation is hindered, or early LMWH is not suitable, for example, major obstetric haemorrhage. The legs are encased in boots which have an inflatable sleeve that exerts intermittent pressure. This activity increases blood flow to the legs thus reducing the potential for DVT.

Further guidance from The Royal College of Obstetricians and Gynaecologists can be found at www.rcog.org.uk/media/qejfhcaj/gtg-37a.pdf

General well-being

Headaches

Blood pressure should be checked if high blood pressure or other signs and symptoms of pre-eclampsia were experienced antenatally, particularly if ongoing headaches are accompanied by blurred vision, stomach pains, shortness of breath, swelling and/or feeling nauseous. Eclampsia is a leading cause of maternal death globally, and up to a third of cases occur in the first week after birth.

Energy levels

It is not unusual for new mothers to have bursts of energy and then experience extreme fatigue. Persistent fatigue can be a sign of anaemia or depression.

Maternal anaemia

Postnatal anaemia is defined as a haemoglobin level below 100 g/L. Haemoglobin levels should be checked if women describe feeling breathless on exertion (dyspnoea), dizzy, experience palpitations and appear pale and tired or lethargic. Women who are identified as anaemic in the postnatal period are often prescribed treatment such as 100–200 mg elemental iron for three months (Hunter et al., 2021).

5.1

Mental well-being

Transient or ongoing mental health issues are a common feature postnatally. In the UK, depression and anxiety affect 15–20% of women in the first year following childbirth (NICE, 2020), and suicide is a leading cause of maternal death in the first year after giving birth (MBRRACE-UK, 2023). Poor postnatal mental well-being is often exacerbated by sleep deprivation. There is a spectrum of postnatal psychiatric disorders experienced by mothers ranging from anxiety to puerperal psychosis (see Table 5.1.7 and Figure 5.1.4).

APPLICATION TO PRACTICE

Identifying postnatal mental health issues

Conversations about mental well-being obviously need to be initiated sensitively and without judgement. There are a number of tools that can be used, such as the Whooley Questions (Whooley et al., 1997) recommended by NICE (2020) in the UK:

▶ During the past month have you been feeling down, depressed or helpless?

► During the last month, have you often been bothered by having little interest or pleasure in doing things?

If women answer either question in the affirmative, midwives should work with appropriate members of the multidisciplinary team to ensure that they receive help and support tailored to their needs. Support and treatment options range from self-help measures such as relaxation and Mindfulness exercises, to listening visits, Cognitive Behavioural Therapy and medication.

Table 5.1.7 Postnatal mental health conditions

Condition	Risk factors	Presentation
General anxiety disorder: Common long-term condition where anxiety is non-specific and relates to a large range of situations	Linked to panic disorders and depression	Persistent anxiety over many days for at least 6 months often with a history of panic attacks Excessive worrying, difficulty managing these worries Considerable variation in presentation
'Baby Blues' Temporary mental impairment associated with low mood after childbirth	A study in France (M'Balilara et al., 2005) found links to psychological factors, low self-esteem, type of birth and high level of stress	Unexpected irritability, stress, crying Predictive risk factor for postnatal depression (Moyo and Djoda, 2020)
Persistent insomnia		Sleep latency – frequent waking, early morning wakefulness Strong correlation between sleep deprivation and postnatal depressive symptoms (Poeira and Zngao, 2022)
Postnatal depression	Socio-economic deprivation Identified depression in the antenatal period Family history of depression	Symptoms may present in a similar way to 'baby blues' but they persist and commonly present 4–6 months following birth Irritability, sleep disturbance, anxiety, tearfulness, difficulty with concentration, negative thoughts
Post-traumatic stress disorder	Associated with perceived birth trauma Exacerbated by pre-existing relationship difficulties and known health problems	Inability/difficulty in expressing emotion (alexithymia) Avoidance, anger, guilt and helplessness
Puerperal psychosis: Postnatal psychosis is sudden in onset and affects 1–2 in 1000 people who give birth (NICE, 2020)	Women with previous history of puerperal psychosis History of bipolar disorder	Hallucinations, delusional thoughts Mania – low and high moods Irrational behaviour Acting 'out of character' Extreme lethargy Restlessness

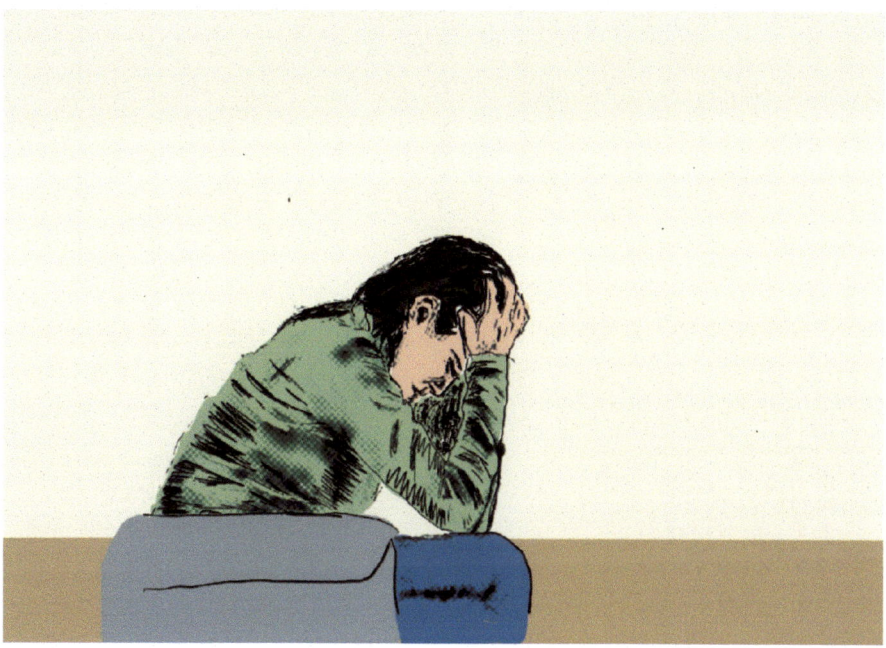

5.1

Figure 5.1.4 Postnatal blues
Source: Image from Claire Smith

Contraception

The World Health Organization recommends that comprehensive and evidence-based information regarding contraception should be offered to all postnatal women and couples (WHO, 2022). Closely spaced pregnancies are associated with preterm birth, low birth weight, stillbirth and neonatal death, while women who have more than four children are at increased risk of maternal mortality. Contraceptive options and their physiological mechanisms are listed in Table 5.1.8.

CHAPTER CHALLENGE

We started this chapter highlighting widespread concern about the level of postnatal care offered to women.

Think about the postnatal care services local to you. Now that you have a greater understanding of the physiology occurring over this period, what do you think is good about the care that is offered, and what needs improving? As a future care organiser and leader, how would you ensure that the physiological well-being of families is supported and enabled? Search for some recent research on postnatal care to inform your thinking.

Table 5.1.8 Contraceptive methods

Type	Method	Physiology	Suitability	Risks/caution
Progesterone only contraception	1. Pill – take daily 2. Progesterone only injection – lasts 8–13 weeks 3. Levonorgestrel and etonogestrel implant – small flexible rod placed under skin of upper arm Lasts 3 years	Thickens cervical mucosa and thins the lining of the uterus; thus, preventing implantation of the fertilised egg	No adverse effects on lactation Minimal effect on coagulation factors, blood pressure or lipid levels	Remembering to take the pill
Combined hormonal contraception	1. Pill: Monophasic – taken for 21 days and then a break for 7 days Phasic – taken daily in a specified order 2. Transdermal patch – placed on skin and replaced weekly Not worn every 4th week to allow menstrual bleed to occur 3. Vaginal ring – small, soft plastic ring placed inside the vagina Left *in situ* for 21 days; 7-day gap after removal to allow menstrual bleed to occur	Synthetic version of oestrogen and progesterone altering menstrual cycle Oestrogen prevents ovulation, progesterone thickens the mucus lining at the entrance of the uterus making fertilisation difficult	Uncomplicated medical history Risk assess for VTE	Not suitable for breastfeeding women If started too early post delivery, increased risk of VTE due to increased clotting factors Caution for women with a history of hypertension, women aged over 35, women who smoke, or women with BMI >35 Remembering to take the pill
Intra uterine devices (IUC)	A small, T-shaped plastic and copper device is inserted into the uterus Effective for 5–10 years	Copper changes cervical mucus, preventing sperm reaching egg and surviving Also stops any fertilised eggs implanting	Can be used within 10 minutes after 3rd stage following a vaginal delivery, or within 48 hours following an uncomplicated LSCS	Early insertion not advised with a history of prolonged rupture of membranes, unresolved sepsis and persistent haemorrhage Occasional expulsion of IUC device (4.6%)

5.1

Barrier methods	Female condom/diaphragm (cap) – a small silicone cup placed over the cervix before intercourse More effective if used with spermicidal cream Male condom – a thin latex sheath placed over an erect penis to 'catch' sperm	Physical barrier which prevents sperm from reaching eggs; thus, prevents fertilisation	Safe to use for those at risk of sexually transmitted diseases (STD)	Wait 6 weeks after birth before using female device to allow for full involution of the uterus (size and shape may change) High risk of unintended pregnancy
Permanent methods of contraception	Sterilisation	Female: fallopian tubes are blocked or sealed to prevent eggs reaching sperm Male: Vasectomy –Vas deferens (tubes that carry sperm from the testicles to the penis) cut or sealed	Effective method of permanent contraception Rates of pregnancy after 1 year low	Early tubal ligation may be associated with regret
Fertility awareness methods	Focusing on signs of fertility such as changes with vaginal discharge		For all – linked to some cultural and religious beliefs	High risk of pregnancy Difficult to assess ovarian function if fully breastfeeding

References

Dennis C., Fung K. et al. Traditional postnatal practices and rituals: A qualitative systematic review. *Women's Health* 2007, 3(4):487–502.

Durnea C., Khashan A. et al. What is to blame for postnatal pelvic floor dysfunction in primiparous women-pre-pregnancy or intrapartum risk factors? *Eur. J. Obstet. Gynecol. Reprod. Biol.* 2017, 214:36–43.

Hunter L., Carpenter J. et al. Anaemia in pregnancy. *Midwives – The Magazine of the Royal College of Midwives* 2021, Jan:46–8.

MBRRACE-UK. MBRRACE-UK Saving Lives Improving Mothers' Care – Lessons learned to inform maternity care from the UK and Ireland Confidential Enquiries into Maternal Deaths and Morbidity 2019–21 [Internet]. 2023. www.npeu.ox.ac.uk/mbrrace-uk/reports.

M'Balilara K., Swendsen J. et al. Baby blues: Characterisation and influence of psycho-social factors. *L'Encephale* 2005, 31(3):331–6.

Moyo G., Djoda N. Relationship between the baby blues and postpartum depression: A study among Cameroonian women. *Am. J. Psychiatry Neurosci.* 2020, 8(1):26–9.

NICE. Antenatal and Postnatal Mental Health: Clinical Management and Service Guidance [Internet]. 2020. www.nice.org.uk/guidance/cg192/resources/antenatal-and-postnatal-mental-health-clinical-management-and-service-guidance-pdf-35109869806789.

Poeira A., Zngao M. Construct of the association between sleep quality and perinatal depression: A literature review. *Healthcare (Basel)* [Internet] 2022, 10(7):1156. www.ncbi.nlm.nih.gov/pmc/articles/PMC9319957/.

Qiaomeng L., Xiao X. The risk factors of postnatal urinary retention after vaginal delivery: A systematic review. *Int. J. Nurs. Sci.* 2020, 7(4):484–92.

UNFPA. Obstetric Fistula [Internet]. 2022. www.unfpa.org/obstetric-fistula.

WHO. WHO Recommendations on Maternal and Newborn Care for a Positive Postnatal Experience [Internet]. 2022. www.who.int/publications/i/item/9789240045989.

Whooley M., Avins A. et al. Case-finding instruments for depression: Two questions are as good as many. *J. Gen. Int. Med.* 1997, 12(7):439–45.

The transition from fetal to neonatal life

Sarah Fleming and Kirsten Baker

LEARNING OUTCOMES

- ▶ Understand and explain the fetal circulatory system, and the changes it undergoes at birth
- ▶ Describe how to assess circulatory changes after birth
- ▶ Describe the metabolic, thermal and respiratory adaptations of the newborn, including counter-regulatory mechanisms
- ▶ Understand the relationship between hypothermia, hypoxia and hypoglycaemia (the energy triangle)
- ▶ Identify elements of care around birth which support the transition to neonatal life
- ▶ Explain the aetiology of physiological jaundice, understand the difference between physiological and pathological jaundice, and apply this knowledge to practice
- ▶ Describe key newborn checks and screening tests and relate these to relevant neonatal anatomy and physiology

At birth, a fetus transitions from an environment where all its needs are met by its mother, to a world in which they must meet many of their needs independently. The physiological transitions undergone at this time are complex and finely tuned, and yet many rely on relatively simple science, such as pressure and concentration gradients. This chapter charts the amazing transformation of the water-dwelling

DOI: 10.4324/9781003227571-30

fetus to the air-breathing, independently functioning neonate.

Neonatal transitions at birth

In order to live independently, a neonate needs to take control of its own oxygenation, blood glucose regulation, temperature stabilisation and protection from infection.

Oxygenation

The fetal circulatory system

There are five unique features of fetal circulation: the **placenta** and **umbilical cord** containing the umbilical vein and arteries, the **ductus venosus**, the **foramen ovale** and the **ductus arteriosus** (see Figure 5.2.1). These features are all designed to get oxygenated blood in, and deoxygenated blood out, of the fetus *without* them using their lungs. The process of fetal circulation is outlined below and summarised in Figure 5.2.2.

- ▶ Oxygenated blood enters the fetus through the **placenta**, via the **umbilical vein**.
- ▶ Approximately half this blood travels to the liver and then to the heart, and the other half travels directly to the heart via the **ductus venosus**. The ductus venosus is a blood vessel which acts as a 'shunt', allowing oxygenated blood in the umbilical vein to bypass the liver and travel directly to the **right atrium** of the heart via the inferior vena cava. When the lungs take over after birth, oxygenated blood will be deposited in the **left atrium**.
- ▶ Once in the heart, most of the blood moves directly from the right atrium to the left atrium through a small flap-like opening called the **foramen ovale**. It does this because, in fetal life, the pressure in the right atrium is greater

than the pressure in the left atrium. This mechanism allows the blood to bypass the pulmonary circulation; the lungs have no role in gas exchange during fetal life.

- ▶ From the left atrium, the blood moves into the left ventricle then travels to the trunk of the body and the brain via the ascending aorta, exactly as it will after birth.
- ▶ The small amount of blood which was left in the right atrium (see third bullet above) moves into the right ventricle.
- ▶ From the right ventricle, this small proportion of blood travels to the pulmonary artery and towards the lungs. Most of it does not reach the lungs, however, but instead passes through another shunt – the **ductus arteriosus**. The ductus arteriosus links the pulmonary artery directly to the aorta, where the blood mixes with the oxygenated blood that passed through the foramen ovale and travels on with it around the lower body and limbs. The very small proportion of blood that does reach the lungs is enough to keep the lung tissue alive, and it returns to the heart via the pulmonary veins.
- ▶ Deoxygenated blood returns to the **placenta** via the **umbilical arteries**, encouraged by the low resistance to blood flow in the placenta. This low resistance facilitates optimum gaseous exchange within the placental blood vessels.

INTERRUPTER

Fill in the blanks in the 'fetal circulation' exercise in your workbook to help embed your knowledge.

There are further factors in the fetal circulatory system which promote optimal

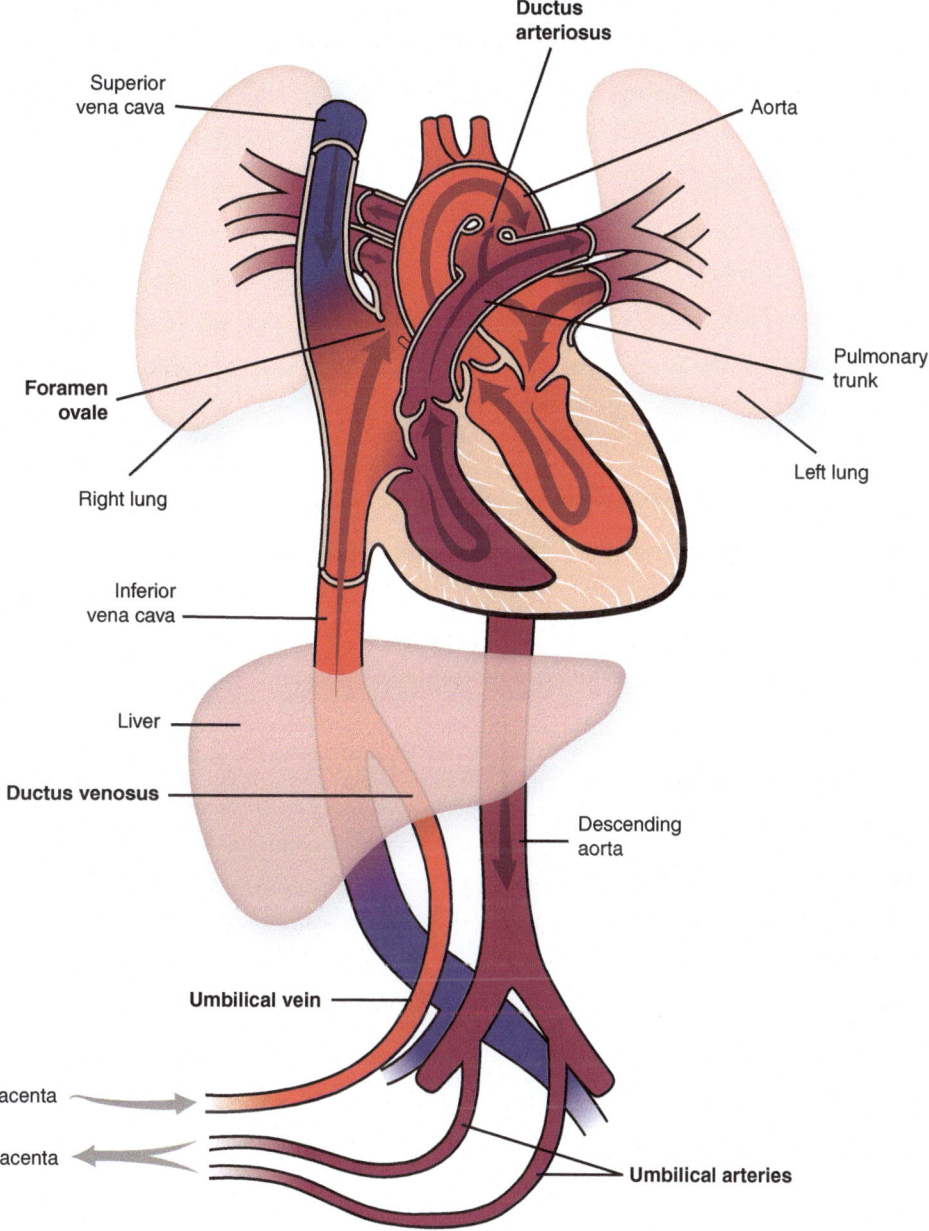

Figure 5.2.1 Fetal circulation

5.2

blood flow, growth and development. **Prostaglandins** produced by the placenta facilitate the patency of the ductus arteriosus during fetal life. The **fetal lungs** are filled with **fluid** and not air, maintaining **hypoxic vasoconstriction** – the arterioles in the lungs constrict (vasoconstriction) in response to the low level of available oxygen (hypoxia). This results in a **high resistance to blood flow** which, in turn, encourages the blood to flow through the foramen ovale and ductus arteriosus instead of through the lungs.

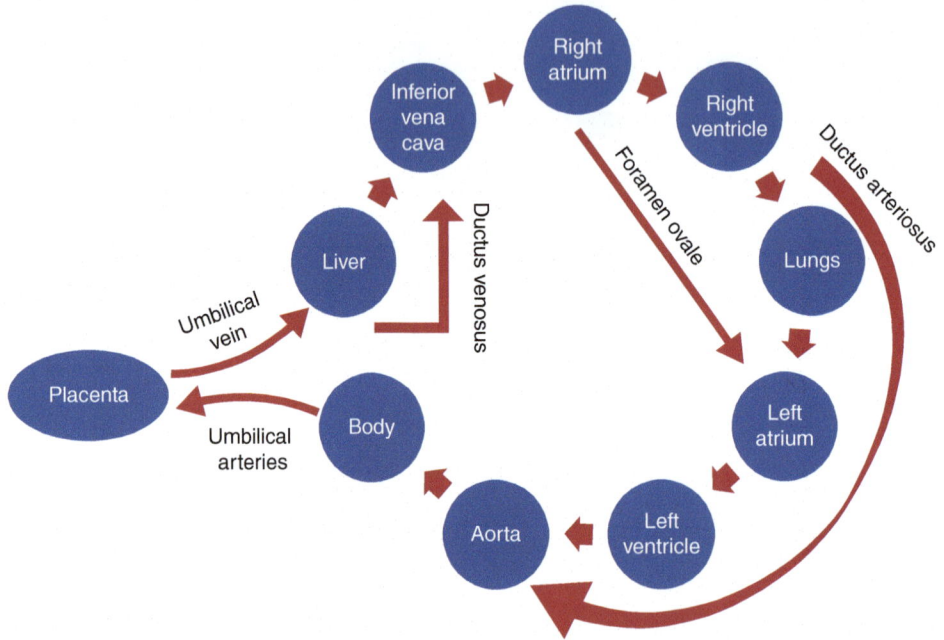

Figure 5.2.2 Flow diagram of fetal circulation

Fetal lung fluid supports the development and maintenance of optimal lung shape. Towards the end of a term pregnancy, the fetal lungs begin to absorb the fluid contained in them. The increase in adrenaline levels during labour is also believed to contribute to the absorption of fetal lung fluid. A baby born at term therefore has little residual fluid left in the lungs. This increases the chance of effective ventilation of the lungs with respiratory efforts, which in turn promotes effective gaseous exchange. Impaired lung fluid reabsorption can lead to an increased risk of the newborn developing respiratory distress symptoms.

The fetus has a high concentration of **haemoglobin**, the oxygen-carrying component of red blood cells. In addition, fetal haemoglobin has a stronger affinity for oxygen, which enables maternal haemoglobin to transfer its oxygen to the fetus. These differences optimise fetal oxygen levels.

From fetal to neonatal circulation

Following birth, fetal circulation rapidly adapts in response to:

▶ The **termination of the blood supply from the placenta**, either due to placental separation, the clamping of the umbilical cord or the constriction of the umbilical vein and arteries (the Wharton's jelly which surrounds them expands in the colder air). If the cord is left unclamped, some oxygenated blood will continue to enter the baby's circulation while it establishes respiration. This is helpful for the lungs, which require an influx of blood to start working.

▶ An onslaught of **sensory stimulation** as the baby enters a world of light, sound, touch and a cooler temperature triggers a release of stress hormones including cortisol and catecholamines. This directly stimulates the taking of the first breaths, which push fluid out of the lungs, replacing it with air.

These two relatively immediate changes initiate other changes within the newborn's body:

1. When the blood flow in the **umbilical vein** stops, the **ductus venosus** gradually closes and blood flow is redirected for hepatic circulation.

2. The presence of oxygen stimulates the **dilation of the blood vessels** in the lungs which had previously been subjected to hypoxic vasoconstriction. The lungs then change from being an area of **high resistance** to being an area of **low resistance** which encourages blood flow to them rather than away from them, as occurred *in utero*.

3. The decreased resistance within the lungs has the effect of **reducing the pressure** within the **right atrium** of the heart. This decreased pressure, together with the **increased pressure** in the **left atrium** (a result of the increased amount of blood now flowing back into the heart from the lungs), causes the **foramen ovale** to close (as the foramen ovale only opens from right – left, so the pressure in the left atrium is now pushing it shut).

4. The decreased resistance within the lungs also has the effect of reducing the flow of blood through the **ductus arteriosus** which gradually closes. A lower level of circulating prostaglandins following the birth of the placenta further supports the closure of the **ductus arteriosus**, as does the general increase in oxygen levels in the newborn compared with the fetus.

Assessing the transition from fetal to newborn circulation

Although the majority of babies make the transition to newborn life independently, ongoing assessment at this time is essential. This can normally take place while the baby is in skin-to-skin contact with the mother, and the cord is intact:

Tone: Muscle tone is the degree of tension, or resistance to movement, in the voluntary muscles. A newborn should have flexed rather than floppy, limp muscles. Newborns should respond to stimulation such as being moved or picked up by moving and flexing their limbs. A very floppy baby is likely to need help with establishing, and possibly maintaining, normal breathing.

Breathing: A newborn should begin breathing within the first minute of life. The first breaths, often associated with loud crying, are designed to push the remaining fluid out of the lungs and into the pulmonary lymphatic system then replace it with air. A baby who does not cry shortly after birth needs careful assessment. Gasping breaths are not normal especially if they occur alongside sternal recession and/or nasal flaring. A gasping baby may require help to open their airway and establish normal breathing. Although breathing can be irregular at first, by the time a baby is approximately 30 minutes old, the respiratory rate should fall between 30 and 60 breaths per minute.

Heart rate: By the time a healthy baby is two minutes of age, the heart rate should be more than 100 beats per minute.

Colour: The baby's trunk, lips and tongue should be well perfused as respirations become established. Regardless of colour, the skin should take on more red tones, and the mucous membranes inside the mouth and the tongue should appear pink. A grey or bluish appearance of the trunk and/or mucous membranes can indicate central cyanosis – this results from a lack of

5.2

oxygen and may mean that the baby requires some assistance to establish effective respirations. However, initial central cyanosis in a baby who is breathing regularly and has a fast heart rate will usually resolve spontaneously. Cyanosis of the extremities is termed acrocyanosis and is normal in newborns as priority for oxygenated blood is given to the heart, brain and other vital organs and there is a slower blood flow through the peripheral areas.

Apgar scoring: This scoring system, widely used since its development in the 1950s, is a method of assessing a newborn's transition at birth. Scores of 0, 1 or 2 are given for each of the following five areas: **heart rate**, **response to stimulation**, **muscle tone**, **respiratory effort** and **colour**. A score is then calculated out of a possible maximum of ten and the process repeated at one, five and ten minutes after birth. Colour is regarded as the least objective and least satisfactory element of the Apgar score as it varies so widely between individuals. Perfusion is perhaps better judged by reference to the mucous membranes rather than the newborn's trunk. Table 5.2.1 shows how the scoring is completed.

Maintaining glucose levels – Metabolism

During fetal life, nutrition as well as oxygenation was provided via the placenta. Following birth, the initial nutritional need is for **carbohydrate** in the form of **glucose**; this provides the instant energy necessary to sustain the newborn so it can take its first breaths and recover from the birth process. Although a newborn's blood glucose level is approximately 70–80% of the birth mothers at first, this falls quickly within the first hour or so of life. Healthy,

term babies develop the ability to raise their own blood sugar levels by around four hours of age, through a process known as **counter-regulation**:

▶ Circulating catecholamines **suppress insulin** which ensures that glucose stays in the bloodstream rather than moving out into the cells.

▶ **Glycogenolysis** – catecholamines also stimulate enzymes in the liver to promote the conversion of stored glycogen to glucose.

▶ **Glucogenolysis** – glucose is produced by the liver and kidneys from substrates such as fatty acids and amino acids.

▶ **Alternative fuel sources** such as **ketones**, which are processed from fat stores, are utilised to protect the brain until more glucose is available.

Maintenance of a normal blood sugar level is most effectively achieved through feeding as glycogen stores are quickly depleted. Human milk contains a relatively high proportion of carbohydrate, and babies are 'programmed' to want to feed within an hour of birth.

Hypoglycaemia occurs when the demand for glucose is higher than the newborn's ability to produce it, or when too much insulin is produced which moves glucose out of the blood and into the body's tissues. Some babies will be less able to maintain their blood sugar levels:

▶ Newborns who have reduced glycogen and fat stores, such as **preterm**, **small for gestational age** and **growth restricted babies**. These babies are reliant on immediately available glucose as they are less able to counter-regulate.

▶ **Babies of diabetic mothers** can experience fetal hyperglycaemia *in utero* if their mother has elevated blood sugar levels during pregnancy. This hyperglycaemia results in increased

Table 5.2.1 Apgar scoring system

	Score 0 if:	Score 1 if:	Score 2 if:
Heart rate	Absent	Below 100 bpm	Above 100 bpm
Respiratory effort	Absent	Gasping or irregular	Regular or crying
Muscle tone	Limp	Some flexion	Active, good tone
Response to stimulation	Nil	Grimace	Cry or cough
Colour	No evidence of perfusion – skin/mucous membranes pale/grey pallor	Body appears partially perfused, blue tones in skin and/or white/blue mucous membranes	Appears well perfused all over – red tones in skin/mucous membranes and extremities (palms and soles of feet)

5.2

insulin production as the fetus attempts to control their blood sugar level. The increased insulin production continues after birth, resulting in the newborn having unusually high glucose requirements. Compounding this situation, babies of diabetic mothers can also struggle to mobilise their glycogen stores.

▶ Newborns who have experienced **fetal distress** during labour, have become **hypothermic**, have developed **sepsis** or who have **congenital heart disease** have increased energy requirements as the body tries to cope with their condition. This means that their energy requirement is likely to exceed what is available even considering glycogen and fat stores.

▶ Babies who are **cold**, **compromised** (due to birth asphyxia or illness) or whose mothers have taken **beta blockers** antenatally may also struggle to maintain their blood glucose levels.

Midwives and other health professionals will need to work alongside parents to provide additional support to these infants, to ensure that they are kept warm and well fed. Breastmilk will stabilise blood sugar levels more effectively than formula milk, and if challenges are foreseen, such as in the case of mothers with diabetes, breastmilk can be expressed antenatally to help meet the baby's demands in the early days after birth.

Temperature stabilisation – Thermoregulation

In utero, a fetus' temperature is maintained at approximately 0.5°C, higher than the maternal body temperature. Following birth, the baby is exposed to a much cooler environment and has to begin the process of controlling and maintaining their own body temperature between approximately 36.5°C and 37.5°C. Given that neonates have a high surface area to body weight ratio and are wet at birth, it is easy for rapid heat loss to occur. There are four methods of heat loss: **radiation**, **convection**, **conduction** and **evaporation**. These are explained in Figure 5.2.3 and Table 5.2.2.

Healthy term newborns are able to generate some heat via increased **muscle activity** and a process called '**non-shivering thermogenesis**', both of which require oxygen and glucose. Non-shivering thermogenesis occurs when the cooler environmental temperature to which the baby is exposed immediately following birth stimulates the release of noradrenaline which activates brown

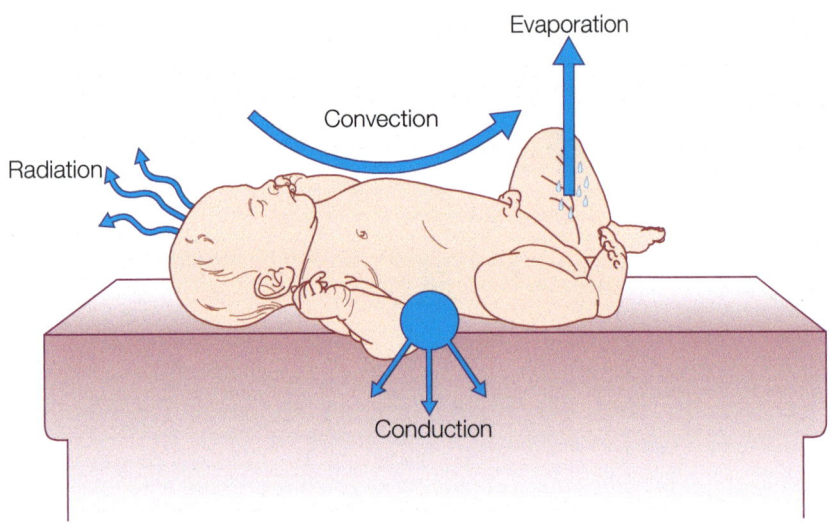

Figure 5.2.3 Heat loss mechanisms
Source: Figure 8.1, p.91, Lumsden and Holmes (2010)

Table 5.2.2 Heat loss mechanisms explained

Criterion/ method of heat loss	Radiation	Convection	Conduction	Evaporation
Definition	Transfer of heat from the baby's body to a cooler surface or object placed near the baby	Transfer of heat from the baby's body to cooler, moving air near the baby	Transfer of heat from the baby's body to a cooler object or surface which is touching the baby	Transfer of heat away from the baby's body through the conversion of liquid to vapour
Example(s)	Plastic cot sides Sides of weighing scales Walls of the room	Gusts of air from an open window Gusts of air caused by the opening and closing of doors Electric fan	Weighing scales Changing mat Plastic-coated cot mattress Cold, wet towels/bedding/ clothes	Wet baby exposed to the air Wet nappy/ clothing/towels/ bedding
How to prevent	Ensure that surfaces and objects placed in close proximity to the baby are warm For example, a warmed sheet or towel can be placed on weighing scales The mother's body provides an ideal, warm environment for the newborn	When birth is approaching, turn off any electric fans, shut doors and windows, and keep peoples' entries and exits to and from the room to a minimum	Surfaces on which a baby is going to lie can be made warm beforehand For example, a warmed towel can be placed on weighing scales and in the cot The mother's chest and abdomen provide an ideal, warm surface for the newborn Check clothing, bedding and nappies regularly and change them quickly if wet	Dry babies as soon as possible after birth, and consider placing a hat on the baby Check clothing, bedding and nappies regularly and change them quickly if wet

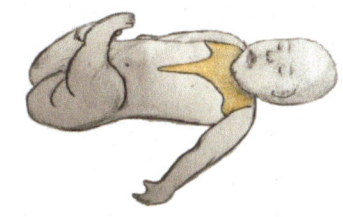

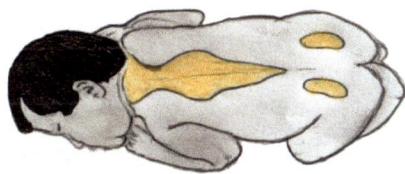

Figure 5.2.4 Locations of neonatal brown adipose tissue (BAT)

adipose tissue (BAT) metabolism (Figure 5.2.4). Brown fat contains many mitochondria, and triglycerides within these mitochondria are broken down into glycerol and fatty acids. The oxidation of these fatty acids produces energy which is released in the form of heat.

Some babies are more at risk than others of not being able to regulate their own body temperature:

▶ **Preterm and growth restricted babies** do not have as much BAT, and preterm babies are less able to generate heat through muscle activity.

▶ **Babies who have required resuscitation after birth** may have used their readily available glucose and glycogen stores, and will also have experienced a degree of hypoxia; both these issues make them less able to generate heat through non-shivering thermogenesis and increased muscle activity.

▶ **Sepsis** is likely to affect a baby's ability to metabolise BAT efficiently.

These babies will require additional temperature monitoring and will particularly appreciate heat transferred during

skin-to-skin contact (see below), or from a heat lamp.

> **INTERRUPTER**
>
> Using the table in the fetal circulation section of your workbook, list and explain in your own words the ways in which a newborn can counter-regulate.
>
> Given that healthy, term newborns can mobilise alternative fuel supplies, is blood glucose measurement an absolute measure of well-being?

5.2

The relationship between hypoglycaemia, hypoxia and hypothermia

Hypoglycaemia, hypoxia and hypothermia are interlinked, as illustrated in the '**energy triangle**' in Figure 5.2.5.

Hypoglycaemia: If a newborn is experiencing hypoxia and/or hypothermia, then hypoglycaemia is more likely. Breathing will be harder work during hypoxia, requiring additional energy, and in hypothermia additional energy is required to produce heat. The generation of heat uses glucose.

Hypoxia: This occurs when there is a lack of an adequate supply of oxygen which, in turn, leads to a deficiency in the tissues of the body. Hypoglycaemic babies are more likely to have difficulties with breathing, which can then result in respiratory distress and subsequently hypoxia. A hypothermic baby will have an increased need for oxygen in order to produce heat, which makes hypoxia more likely as demand outstrips supply. A hypothermic baby may also have periods of apnoea (cessation of breathing), which causes a reduction in oxygen which can then further contribute to hypoxia.

317

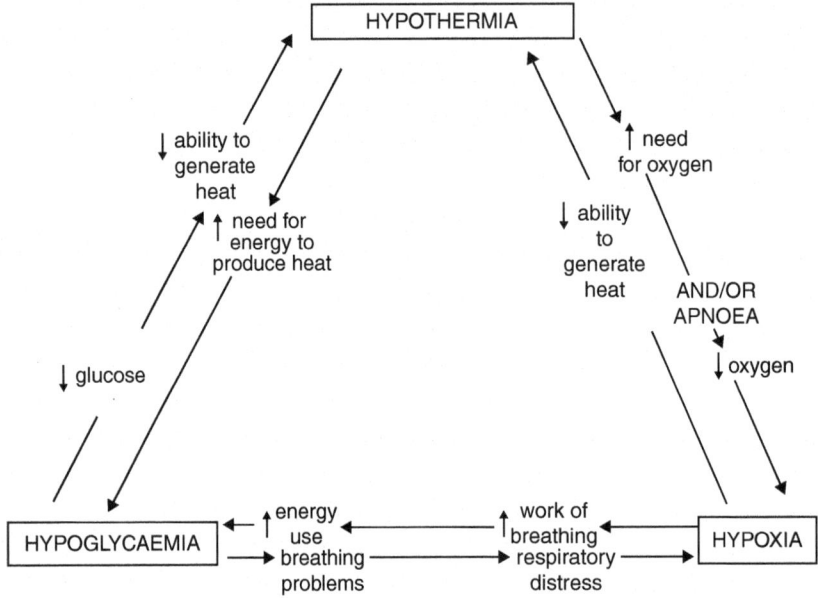

Figure 5.2.5 The energy triangle

Hypothermia: This occurs when the body temperature falls below a normal range (36.5–37.5 °C for a newborn). Hypothermia can negatively impact on growth and development, and is a contributing factor to neonatal morbidity. As oxygen and glucose are both required to produce heat through non-shivering thermogenesis and increased muscle activity, hypoglycaemic and hypoxic babies are less able to maintain their temperatures.

> ## INTERRUPTER
>
> Annotate the neonatal energy triangle in your workbook to embed this knowledge.

Protection from infection – Microbial colonisation

As the fetus travels along the birth canal, its oral cavity and gut become colonised with microbes from the mother which start to lay down the foundations of a **microbiome**.

A microbiome is the collection of microorganisms in a particular environment. These microorganisms have a vested interest in keeping their host (the neonate) alive and form an important part of the human immune system. Over 400 species of bacteria enter the gut during vaginal birth and the early days of breastfeeding. They work symbiotically with the neonate to form an ongoing immune defence (see Chapter 6.1 for more information on the constituents of breastmilk). The gut bacteria influence barrier function, mucin and IgA secretion, inflammation, and cell proliferation and apoptosis. Although the precise mechanisms of this influence are as yet poorly understood, it is thought that microbes have an epigenetic effect, directly influencing gene expression.

Supporting the physiological transition to life

Vaginal birth, breastfeeding, delayed cord clamping and skin-to-skin contact all support neonatal transition to extrauterine life.

Vaginal birth

Compression of the chest during vaginal birth

Compression of the chest as the baby passes through the vagina in the second stage of labour creates negative pressure. This facilitates the sucking of air into the lungs as the chest expands immediately following birth. The compression of the chest also helps to squeeze out the residual fluid within the lungs.

Microbial colonisation

If an infant gut is exposed to insufficient bacteria or different bacteria during and in the early days after birth, the immune system will develop differently, leaving the individual more vulnerable to autoimmune disorders, obesity and other conditions. The increased risk of immune and metabolic conditions in babies born by Caesarean section has been associated with their different gut microbiota. Attempts have been made to provide the maternal microbes lacking in a Caesarean-born baby by swabbing them with vaginal fluids shortly after birth, but the safety and effectiveness of this procedure has yet to be tested in large-scale randomised controlled trials. See Section 6 for further information on microbes present in breastmilk.

Delayed cord clamping

The baby's pulmonary circulation needs additional blood volume in order to effectively take over from the placenta as the site of gaseous exchange. This blood is drawn into the baby's system from the placenta, provided the cord is left unclamped for at least the first one to three minutes after birth. In addition, this extra volume of blood from the placenta has the effect of increasing the newborn's iron stores for up to three to six months after birth.

Skin-to-skin contact

Skin-to-skin contact is derived from placing an unclothed newborn directly on their mother's bare chest, with their head between or just below her breasts. Mother and baby can be covered with a dry towel to keep them warm. Benefits of this practice include:

- ▶ Calm, relaxed mother and baby
- ▶ Facilitates regulation of the baby's heart rate
- ▶ Facilitates regulation of the baby's breathing
- ▶ Ensures that the baby's skin is colonised with the commensal bacteria on their mother's skin. These bacteria will support skin health and barrier function
- ▶ Keeps the baby warm (oxytocin stimulates blood flow to the mothers' breasts)
- ▶ Initiates a series of neonatal behaviours which culminate in them moving to and feeding from the breast (see Chapter 6.3, The Breast Crawl)
- ▶ Facilitates maternal and neonatal oxytocin release and promotes bonding and attachment

Unless they require medical attention, babies should be placed in skin-to-skin contact with their mother for at least an hour after birth. If this is not possible, skin-to-skin contact can be undertaken by a second parent or carer.

Red blood cell changes and neonatal jaundice

In utero, oxygen crosses the placenta via passive diffusion. This requires fetal red blood cells to have a higher affinity for oxygen than maternal red blood cells, as outlined above. After birth, fetal red blood cells are broken down and replaced with neonatal red blood cells, which are smaller, less numerous and have a lower haemoglobin content. The fetal red blood cells are then broken down and their components are either reused or expelled. The **haemoglobin** component breaks down into **haem**, and **globin**. **Globin**, a protein, is broken down further into **amino acids** which are recycled. **Haem** is converted first to **biliverdin**, and then further to **bilirubin** by enzymes in the liver, spleen and lymph nodes. Bilirubin is a waste product that needs to be excreted from the body.

Metabolism of bilirubin

Bilirubin is fat soluble. In order to be excreted, it must first be converted to a water-soluble form through **conjugation** with glucuronic acid. This takes place in the **liver**:

▶ Bilirubin needs to bind with **albumin** to be transported to the liver.
▶ In the liver, bilirubin becomes **conjugated** with **glucuronic acid** in the presence of the enzyme gluceronyl transferase.
▶ Conjugated bilirubin is water soluble and is transported to the neonatal gut, where it is worked on by gut bacteria and

excreted in the form of **urobilinogen** (in urine) and **stercobilinogen** (in faeces). It is bilirubin that causes these to be yellow in colour.

▶ However, the neonatal gut contains a substance called **beta gluceronidase** which *un*conjugates conjugated bilirubin. The relatively high levels of beta gluceronidase in the neonatal gut suggests that some level of **unconjugated bilirubin** may be beneficial to the neonate, possibly as an evolutionary safeguard against sepsis (Hansen et al., 2018). However, as with all finely balanced physiological processes, any disruption has consequences. If, for any reason, gut motility is slow (such as inadequate milk intake), there is a higher risk of bilirubin becoming unconjugated as it has more exposure to beta glucuronidase.
▶ Once unconjugated, bilirubin needs to return to the liver to begin the process of conjugation again. This occurs via the enterohepatic circulation. A schematic of bilirubin metabolism is shown in Figure 5.2.6.

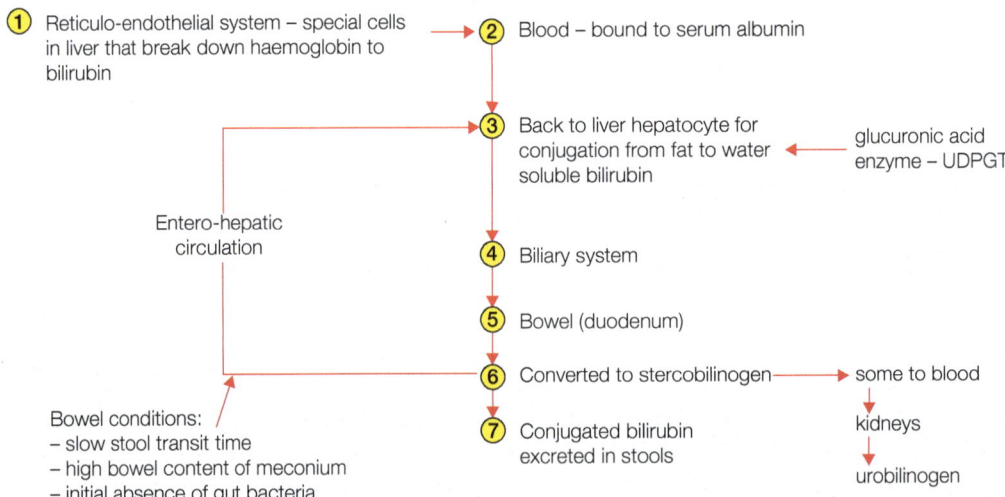

Figure 5.2.6 Schematic of bilirubin metabolism
Source: Figure 9.1, p.102, Lumsden and Holmes (2010)

Jaundice results when the amount of bilirubin present in the body exceeds the baby's capacity to process or metabolise it. This means that excess unconjugated bilirubin is circulating within its system. Jaundice can be **physiological** (meaning that it presents no compromise to the neonate) or **pathological** (high levels of bilirubin can cause cerebral palsy, hearing loss, learning difficulties and problems with vision and teeth). Physiological jaundice is relatively common: about 60% of neonates experience this, with a slightly higher incidence amongst boys. Jaundice causes discoloration of the baby's skin, sclera (the white outer area of the eyeball) and lunula (nail beds) which take on a yellowish hue. The extent to which skin discoloration is discernible depends, of course, on skin tone. Jaundice is over-diagnosed in babies of East Asian heritage, while midwives can fail to spot dangerously high levels of bilirubin in babies of African heritage if they rely on skin colour alone to rule out the condition.

It is important to note that the process of breaking down fetal red blood cells begins soon after birth, but the build up of bilirubin does not manifest until 24 hours of age. Therefore, if jaundice is apparent in the neonate *within* the first 24 hours, it is not physiological but pathological. Physiological jaundice can last several weeks, decreasing over time as the number of senescent red blood cells declines.

INTERRUPTER

Now, using the space indicated in the jaundice section of your workbook, use your own way (an image, a story, text notes – whatever makes sense to you!) to describe the process of bilirubin metabolism. Make sure you include all of the key stages and words in the process.

Challenges to bilirubin metabolism

For a healthy neonate who is feeding well, the process of conjugating and excreting bilirubin is unproblematic, and the presence of some unconjugated bilirubin is likely to have some benefits. However, if levels of unbound or unconjugated bilirubin exceed the neonate's capacity to metabolise it, a vicious circle ensues. Once fat soluble bilirubin crosses the blood brain barrier it causes lethargy which makes a baby difficult to rouse. This in turn makes feeding difficult, which means calorific intake is insufficient to conjugate the high levels of bilirubin. Therefore, any conjugated bilirubin will potentially sit for longer in the gut, where it might become unconjugated once more. At very high levels, bilirubin can cause neurological damage and in extreme cases, death. This condition is known as **hyperbilirubinaemia** or **kernicterus** (meaning 'yellow kern', as brain cells acquire a yellow discoloration). In low- and middle-income countries, where treatment options are limited and can be difficult to access, hyperbilirubinaemia is a leading cause of neurological impairment such as cerebral palsy, deafness and intestinal problems.

The neonate's metabolic capacity (and therefore, risk of hyperbilirubinaemia) may be challenged by a number of factors including:

- ▶ **Prematurity** – levels of gluceronyl transferase are too low in a premature neonate's liver to allow sufficient quantities of bilirubin to be conjugated.
- ▶ **Hypoxia** – bilirubin metabolism requires oxygen.
- ▶ **Hypothermia** – energy available for bilirubin metabolism is depleted as the neonate uses energy for thermogenesis (see above).

5.2

- **Polycythaemia** (a high number of red blood cells, for example as a result of twin-to-twin transfusion or maternal diabetes). This means there is additional bilirubin to conjugate.
- **Rhesus incompatibility** – neonatal red blood cells are destroyed by maternal antibodies, creating more bilirubin.
- **Bruising** – for example as a result of an instrumental delivery – resulting in high levels of red blood cell breakdown.

Diagnosis and care

Identifying the threshold between physiological and pathological jaundice is a key component of early neonatal care. NICE (2016) recommendations are to use a transcutaneous bilirubinometer for babies of over 35 weeks gestational age, and who are >24 hours old, following this up with a serum bilirubin measurement. As shown in Figure 5.2.7, the safe threshold changes over time.

APPLICATION TO PRACTICE

Elevated bilirubin levels can be managed and treated by:

- **Frequent feeding**: A good milk intake will increase gut transit times, meaning that conjugated bilirubin is not reabsorbed.
- **Exposure to weak sunlight**: Although this must be carefully managed to avoid sun damage and over- or under-heating, evidence suggests that exposing skin to sunlight will help decrease bilirubin levels (Horn et al., 2021). Ultraviolet (UV) light disrupts bilirubin molecules, rendering them excretable.
- **Prebiotics**: A very small amount of evidence (Armanian et al., 2019) suggests that these may boost populations of beneficial bacteria in the colon, helping to process bilirubin in bile.
- **Phototherapy**: This is recommended if bilirubin levels exceed the treatment threshold, and is based on the action of

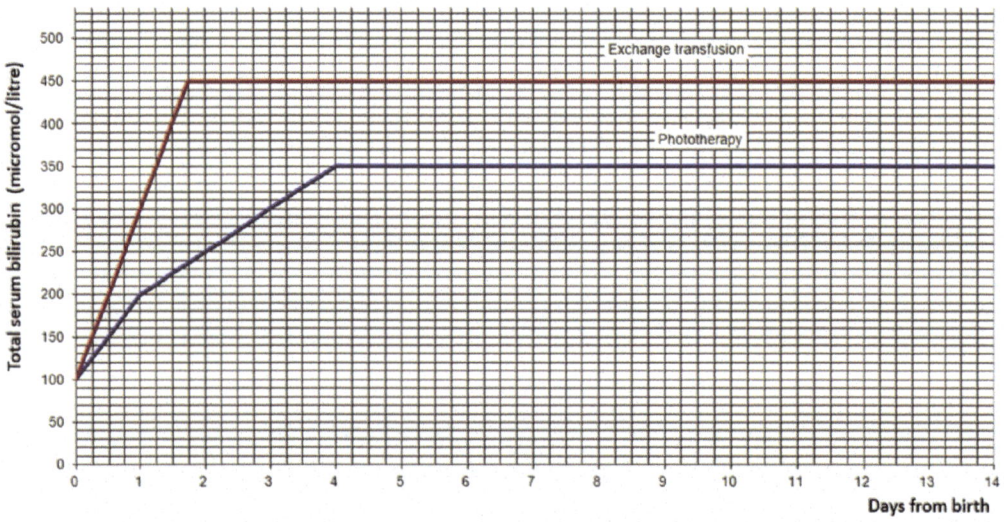

Figure 5.2.7 Bilirubin thresholds for intervention for babies born at or over 38 weeks' gestation

UV light on bilirubin, similar to sunlight. Phototherapy can be administered by placing the baby under UV lights, or by wrapping them in a 'bili blanket': a portable phototherapy device which uses a fibre optic pad to swathe the neonate's body in light.

▶ **Exchange transfusion**: This may be necessary if the degree of unbound, unconjugated bilirubin is very high relative to the neonate's age. This procedure removes the bilirubin-ridden blood and replaces it with donor blood.

Newborn physical checks and examinations

Initial neonatal check

The Apgar score (see Table 5.2.1) is used to assess the newborn's airway, breathing and circulation immediately after birth. Further checks are usually carried out after a period of uninterrupted skin-to-skin contact to assess physical health. The temperature of the newborn will be checked to ensure they are able establishing thermoregulation (see above). The **birth weight** is usually established, although this need not be immediate (and should not be prioritised over skin-to-skin contact and the first breastfeed). The average term newborn weighs approximately 3500 g, although this can vary substantially. Babies who have a **low birth weight** (less than 2500 g) may be at greater risk of having low oxygen levels at birth, difficulties establishing effective breathing, difficulties maintaining a normal body temperature, developing infections and having poor feeding. Links have also been made between low birthweight and an increased risk of infant mortality, childhood developmental problems and poor health as an adult. Babies who have a **high birth weight** (more than 4000 g) may have increased

risk of birth trauma such as brachial plexus injury and may be at increased risk of initial hypoglycaemia after birth.

A newborn's **head circumference** is about half its body length plus 10 cm. Therefore, if the average newborn's body length is 50 cm, the average head circumference will be 35 cm. Anything from 32 to 38 cm is considered normal. An unusually **small head circumference** at birth may indicate **microcephaly**, a rare condition affecting brain growth which, in turn, can affect normal growth and development. An unusually **large head circumference** may indicate a condition such as **hydrocephalus**, where there is excess cerebrospinal fluid within the ventricles of the brain. Hydrocephalus at birth can arise due to congenital conditions such as spina bifida or can be the result of certain maternal infections during pregnancy. Hydrocephalus can lead to seizures and/or developmental delays.

Top to toe baby check

Using a systematic top to toe approach to check a newborn baby in the first days of life helps to ensure that no anomalies or symptoms of underlying conditions that may affect the baby's well-being are overlooked. Conducting this examination with the baby's parents can help them get to know their newborn and provide reassurance regarding any benign physical quirks or irregularities. The elements of a systematic examination of a newborn are outlined in Figure 5.2.8.

Systematic examination of the newborn

A second physical examination within 72 hours of birth provides a further opportunity to check for certain abnormalities and confirm that the newborn is adapting effectively to extrauterine life. In England, this forms the first part of the **Newborn and Infant**

5.2

General
- Skin - colour, integrity, bruises, abrasions, rashes, birth marks, blue spots, presence of vernix (common in pre-term babies) orany dryness (common in post-term babies)
- Oedema - pitting (check albumin levels) or non-pitting (a sign of Turner's syndrome in female infants)
- Alertness and muscle tone
- Weight

Head and neck
- Head - circumference and shape, fontanelles (normal, sunken (a sign of dehydration), bulging), caput, moulding, cephalhaematoma
- Neck - length (normal, short, long), evidence of lumps or swellings

Face
- Eyes - size and shape, spacing (wide or narrow set?), conjunctivitis, discharge, burst or bleeding vessels, evidence of squint
- Nose and ears - symmetry, position (normal, low set), apparent patency, nasal flaring
- Mouth - intact lips and palate, tongue, jaw size, colour of mucous membrane
- Milia - white spots on the nose, chin or cheeks - caused by sebaceous glands and resolve after two-three weeks

Arms and hands
- Arms - length and symmetry, tone, movement, evidence of birth injury (such as Erb's palsy)
- Hands - number of digits, shape (straight, inward curving), webbing, presence of palmer creases (one (can indicate Downs Syndrome), multiple)

Chest and abdomen
- Size, shape, symmetry, breast tissue (palpable breast tissue is normal in males and females), nipples
- Breath sounds, bowel sounds
- Umbilicus - smell, discharge, hernia
- Palpate abdomen gently for organs, masses or herniaae

Genitourinary
- Genitalia - female: labia majora and minora, clitoris (enlarged?)
- Genitalia - male: penis, foreskin, testes (see below)
- Anus - position/patency
- Urine and stools

Hips, legs and feet
- Hips - any obvious dislocation (see below)
- Legs - length, symmetry, movement
- Feet - number of digits, webbing, evidence of talipes

Back and spine
- Spine - intact, shape (any evidence of defects or curvature)
- Scapulae and buttocks - symmetry
- Dimples, hair tufts (can be sign of occult spina bifida if on spine)

Neurological
- Tone, sleepiness, rousability, cry
- Reflexes - Moro, rooting, suck, grasp, stepping

Key:
Can be checked shortly after birth and at 72 hours
Check at around 72 hours

Figure 5.2.8 Top to toe baby check

Physical Examination (NIPE) which aims to reduce infant morbidity and mortality by:

► Identifying detectable congenital abnormalities of the **eyes**, **heart**, **hips** and **(in males) testes**, and referring affected infants for treatment

► Identifying abnormalities that may become detectable and require referral by the time of the 6–8 week infant physical examination

Other countries have similar versions of this check (such as the Routine Examination of the Newborn in Scotland). The systematic examination of the newborn may include aspects of the top to toe check if these have not already been completed.

The eye

The examination of the eye enables the newborn to be screened for the presence of **congenital cataracts**; the most treatable cause of sight loss during childhood. Approximately 2–3 per 10000 babies in the UK are born with cataracts and, for more than half of these babies, both eyes will be affected (Public Health England, 2021).

Pathophysiology of cataracts

The lens of the eye is an ellipsoid structure which refracts (bends) light onto the retina. It is the processing of this light, initiated in the retina, which enables us to both see and understand the objects in our surroundings. Congenital cataracts occur when proteins within the lens of the eye change, and form dense, cloudy areas on the otherwise transparent lens. This affects how light enters the eye, and subsequently the quality of vision. If the cataracts are severe, then surgery is generally required to remove the affected lens; this is then replaced with an artificial lens or contact lens.

5.2

Newborns at increased risk

Babies with a first degree relative who had congenital cataracts are considered to be at particular risk.

Testing for cataracts

Sometimes, the presence of a cataract can be detected simply by observing the baby's eyes, but use of the '**red reflex**' examination is advised. The 'red reflex' is the reflection of light from the retina which causes the baby's entire pupil to appear orange, pink or red when the light from an ophthalmoscope is shone into the eye.

If congenital cataracts are present, the 'red reflex' will either be partially obscured, in which case it will appear as a ring rather than circle, or completely obscured, in which case the pupil will appear blue or white (see Table 5.2.3). An

Table 5.2.3 Normal and abnormal red reflexes

Appearance of iris and pupil	Description	Diagnosis
a.	a. Entire pupil appears orange, pink or red (exact colour varies with genetic heritage)	Normal. No cataract present
b.	b. Orange, red or pink ring around pupil	Abnormal. Partially obscured. Cataract present
c.	c. Pupil appears blue or white	Abnormal. Obscured. Cataract present

abnormal 'red reflex' should result in an urgent referral to ophthalmology services.

The heart

The aim of the examination of the cardiovascular system is early detection of **congenital heart disease (CHD)**. The incidence of CHD is approximately 8 per 1000 live births (Public Health England, 2021). Critical congenital heart defects can be life threatening and require intervention within the first 28 days of life. These types of defect account for between 15% and 25% of babies with CHD.

Pathophysiology of CHD

The main forms of CHD are summarised in Table 5.2.4. They may be diagnosed before the newborn examination, either via an antenatal ultrasound scan or following circulatory difficulties after birth.

Newborns at increased risk of CHD

- Babies with a first degree relative with CHD
- Babies with trisomy 21 or another trisomy
- Babies with a cardiac abnormality suspected on ultrasound scan during pregnancy
- Babies of mothers who had a virus such as rubella during early pregnancy
- Babies of birth mothers with conditions such as diabetes, epilepsy and lupus
- Babies whose birth mothers took certain teratogenic medications during pregnancy (for example, diazepam, and also isotretinoin and topical retinoids which are used for treating acne)

Testing for CHD

There are several elements of the examination of the cardiovascular system, and a baby is considered to be at high risk of having a form of CHD if any of the following are present:

Difficulties with breathing

Breathing should be assessed by both watching and listening. The number of breaths per minute should also be counted.

- **Tachypnoea** (unusually fast breathing; the normal rate is approximately 40–60 breaths per minute) can occur in babies with CHD due to too much blood flowing to the lungs, or blood not flowing correctly out of the lungs – resulting either from an obstruction in the heart or major blood vessels or to the heart pumping ineffectively.
- **Periods of apnoea** (no breathing) lasting longer than 20 seconds or associated with cyanosis can occur in babies with CHD due to a lack of adequate blood flow to the brain. This can result in the failure of the respiratory centre to be normally stimulated.
- **Sternal recession** (drawing in of the centre of the chest) occurs because babies have soft, pliable rib cages; increased work of breathing can cause indrawing of the sternum and rib cage. This is especially evident when accessory muscles in the neck, ribcage or abdomen have to be used in order to inflate the lungs.
- **Nasal flaring** is a compensatory mechanism which increases the diameter of the upper airways which assists with the work of breathing.
- **Breathlessness associated with feeding** can occur in babies with CHD as the necessary coordination of 'suck, breathe, swallow' can be very tiring for them.

Colour and behaviour

Central cyanosis (blue tones discernible in the face, especially the lips and mucous membranes in the mouth, and the trunk of the body) either all the time or just when the baby is at rest and/or feeding, limp muscle tone or lethargy.

Examination of the heart

The examination of the heart includes feeling the heartbeat through the baby's chest wall, auscultating the heart using a stethoscope and palpating the femoral pulses (these are the pulses in the groin midway between the pubic bone and the iliac crest). Signs of concern are:

▶ 'heaves and thrills' (a 'heave' is a palpable, forceful, contraction of the heart and a 'thrill' is a palpable heart murmur that feels like a vibration when a hand is placed over the chest)

▶ absent or weak femoral pulses (Figure 5.2.9) and/or

▶ audible heart murmurs (extra or unusual heart sounds) on auscultation of each area of the chest (Figure 5.2.10), including the coarctation area, which is between the scapulae on the baby's back

It is important to remember that some heart murmurs in very young newborns can be completely benign, and are associated with the normal changes occurring within the cardiovascular system after birth. It is equally important to remember that not all forms of CHD present with a heart murmur.

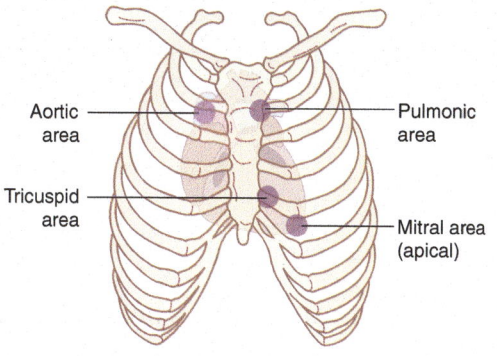

Figure 5.2.10 Auscultation of the heart
Source: Figure 4.5, p.47, Lumsden and Holmes (2010)

5.2

Referral following identification of risk factors will depend on the clinical condition of the baby but will involve an assessment by a neonatologist and subsequent referral to a cardiologist if appropriate.

INTERRUPTER

During a newborn examination, an extra heart sound is heard on auscultation and the baby's respiratory rate is 70 per minute. It is also evident that the baby's lips are slightly cyanosed. What might be the problem? What action(s) would you take?

You can give your answer to this, and other questions about the newborn examination, in your workbook.

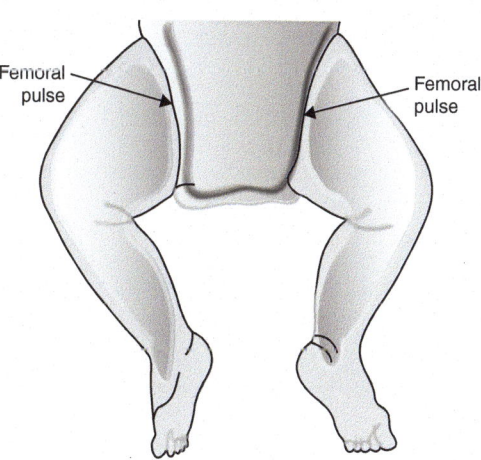

Figure 5.2.9 Location of femoral pulses

The hips

The aim of the examination of the hips is detection of **developmental dysplasia of the hips (DDH)**. DDH is a general term for a shallow acetabulum (hip socket), unstable hips or dislocated hips. Between 3–5 babies per 1000 live births (Public Health England, 2021) may require treatment with a Pavlik's harness to stabilise the hip joint (Figure 5.2.11).

327

Table 5.2.4 Presentations of CHD

Type of CHD	Description	Diagnosis (made in partnership with the multidisciplinary team)
Aortic stenosis	Narrowing of the aortic valve Affects the oxygen rich blood supply from the heart to the aorta and therefore, the baby's body Can lead to increased work for the left ventricle which can, in turn, lead to a thickening of the muscle of the ventricle The muscle thickening results in reduced efficiency of the pumping action of the heart	Severe cases sometimes diagnosed via ultrasound scan during pregnancy Most cases diagnosed after birth via detection of a heart murmur and subsequent echocardiogram (an ultrasound scan of the heart) Femoral pulses may be weak or absent
Coarctation of the aorta	Narrowing of the aorta which prevents blood circulating to the lower parts of the body Blood can flow to the lower parts of the body *in utero* via the ductus arteriosus If this duct is allowed to naturally close, it is not possible for blood to reach the lower body	Some cases are suspected during pregnancy, via an ultrasound scan Affected newborns can be pale and breathless, and they may also have difficulties feeding A heart murmur may be heard on auscultation, particularly between the scapulae, and femoral pulses may be weak or absent
Hypoplastic left heart syndrome (HLHS)	There are several features of HLHS, a form of critical CHD: Narrowing of the mitral valve and/or aortic valve Small and under-developed left ventricle and aorta Atrial-septal defect (ASD); a hole between the right and left atria These defects result in an abnormal flow of blood through the left side of the heart: blood passes from the lungs into the left atrium and then straight into the right atrium through the ASD, rather than to the left ventricle and then around the body Blood then travels from the right atrium back to the lungs The only way for blood to reach the aorta and then the body of newborns with HLHS is via the ductus arteriosus	Usually diagnosed via an ultrasound scan in pregnancy, but in some cases it is not diagnosed until after birth Babies with HLHS can become breathless and unwell soon after birth Femoral pulses may be weak or absent, and a heart murmur may be audible Initial treatment of HLHS is through administration of prostaglandins which keep the ductus arteriosus patent
Pulmonary atresia with intact ventricular septum	There are two abnormalities associated with this critical form of CHD: Blockage of the pulmonary valve – this prevents blood flowing from the heart to the lungs Abnormally developed right ventricle In newborns with this condition, blood has to flow through the ductus arteriosus in order to travel from the heart to the lungs	The low blood oxygen levels in newborns with this condition means that they can have cyanosis Femoral pulses may be weak or absent and a heart murmur may be audible Diagnosis is usually after birth, following an echocardiogram Initial treatment is the administration of prostaglandins which keep the ductus arteriosus patent Surgery is usually required within the first weeks of life

(*Continued*)

Table 5.2.4 (Continued)

Type of CHD	Description	Diagnosis (made in partnership with the multidisciplinary team)
Pulmonary atresia with ventricular septal defect	There are two abnormalities associated with this critical form of CHD: Blockage of the pulmonary valve which prevents blood flow from the heart to the lungs A hole between the left and right ventricles (ventricular septal defect – VSD) In newborns, blood has to flow through the ductus arteriosus in order to travel from the heart to the lungs The VSD allows blood to move across from the left to the right ventricle This results in the mixing of oxygenated and deoxygenated blood and, subsequently, a reduced level of oxygen flowing to the body A large VSD also results in a greatly increased flow of blood to the lungs – the usual amount from the right ventricle plus blood from the left ventricle which has passed through the VSD	The low blood oxygen levels caused by pulmonary atresia and VSD in newborns means that they can have cyanosis Femoral pulses may be weak or absent and a heart murmur may be heard If the VSD is large, the increased blood flow to the lungs can cause breathlessness Diagnosis is usually after birth, following an echocardiogram Initial treatment is the administration of prostaglandins which keep the ductus arteriosus patent
Pulmonary stenosis	Narrowing of the pulmonary valve The narrowing means that the right ventricle has to work harder to force the blood into the pulmonary artery which, in turn, can cause thickening of the ventricular muscle tissue Severe pulmonary stenosis can lead to low blood oxygen levels due to the reduction in the amount of blood flowing to the lungs	Newborns do not usually have symptoms although a heart murmur may be audible Pulmonary stenosis is not usually diagnosed prior to birth unless it is particularly severe: newborns with severe pulmonary stenosis are likely to be cyanotic
Tetralogy of Fallot	There are four main abnormalities associated with this critical form of CHD: Pulmonary stenosis VSD Overriding aorta – this is when the aorta is positioned above both ventricles rather than just the left one Enlarged, muscular right ventricle The two abnormalities which cause the main problems associated with this condition are pulmonary stenosis and VSD (refer to pulmonary stenosis and pulmonary atresia with VSD for a full explanation)	The pulmonary stenosis and VSD, both leading to a generally reduced blood oxygen level in the body, can lead to cyanosis The cyanosis may be evident all the time, or may only be evident when the baby cries There may be weak or absent femoral pulses A heart murmur may be audible Hypercyanotic attacks can occur; this is when a baby becomes suddenly cyanosed and may even collapse Tetralogy of Fallot is not usually diagnosed during pregnancy

5.2

(Continued)

Table 5.2.4 (Continued)

Type of CHD	Description	Diagnosis (made in partnership with the multidisciplinary team)
Transposition of the great arteries (TGA)	With this condition, a form of critical CHD, the pulmonary artery connects to the left ventricle rather than the right, and the aorta connects to the right ventricle rather than the left As a result of this transposition, blood flows to the lungs and becomes oxygenated, but then flows back to the lungs again rather than around the body Blood flowing around the body is unable to travel to the lungs for oxygenation In newborns with TGA, the patent ductus arteriosus allows some oxygenated blood to reach the body	Babies with TGA are usually cyanosed This cyanosis can worsen, or in some cases only be apparent, when the baby cries There may be weak or absent femoral pulses, and a heart murmur may be audible In many cases, TGA is diagnosed prior to a baby's birth via ultrasound scan A treatment plan can then be made in advance, which usually includes initial treatment with prostaglandins to keep the ductus arteriosus patent

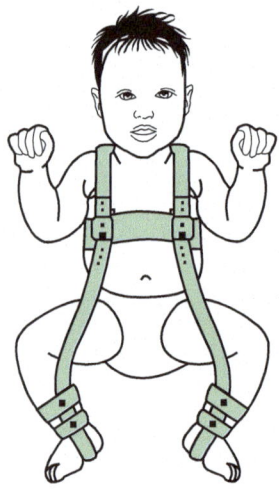 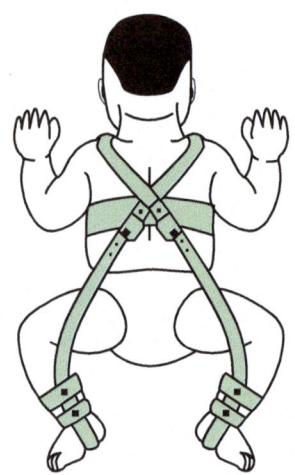

Figure 5.2.11 A Pavlik harness

Between 1 and 2 babies per 1000 live births may require surgery in order to resolve DDH. Early diagnosis and treatment of DDH helps to prevent lifelong difficulties with pain and mobility, including osteoarthritis.

Pathophysiology of DDH

It is, theoretically, comparatively easy for a fetal or newborn femoral head and acetabulum to become misaligned due the acetabulum being shallower than a child's or adults, and the joint being formed predominantly of soft, flexible cartilage rather than hard bone. In addition to these factors, the maternal pregnancy hormones relaxin and progesterone can also affect the fetus and newborn, causing ligament laxity and subsequent instability of the hip joint. However, the majority of babies' hips

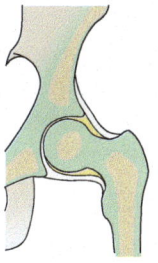 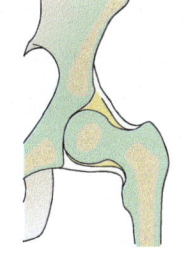 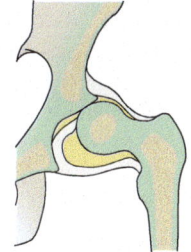

Normal   Acetabular dysplasia   Subluxation

Figure 5.2.12 Types of hip dysplasia

develop normally. There are different forms of DDH (Figure 5.2.12).

Acetabular dysplasia – the femoral head is located in the acetabulum, but the acetabulum is abnormally shallow or malformed and cannot always hold it securely in place. As a result, the femoral head is at risk of migrating out of the acetabulum – dislocating.

Subluxatable/dislocatable – the femoral head is able to move – completely or partially – in and out of the acetabulum.

Dislocated – the femoral head rests completely outside the acetabulum and may or may not be able to be replaced into the acetabulum.

Neonates at increased risk

▶ Infants with a first degree relative who had DDH
▶ Breech presentation at or after 36 weeks of pregnancy
▶ Babies born in a breech position after 28 weeks of pregnancy

The breech position in later pregnancy and during birth can put pressure on the hip and thigh muscles in such a way that instability of the hip joint is more likely. It

has also been suggested that the breech presentation does not allow for the range of movement necessary to naturally develop and deepen the acetabulum.

Testing for DDH

Examination of the hips involves checking that both legs are of equal length, that the knees are at the same level when each leg is bent with the feet placed flat on a flat surface, and that each hip is easily abductable. A lack of parity in leg length or knee height suggests that the hip is dislocated. Failure of the hip to abduct normally is indicative of DDH.

The **Barlow** and **Ortolani** manoeuvres should also be performed. Ortolani's manoeuvre (Figure 5.2.13a) assesses whether or not a hip is dislocated. A dislocated hip will be felt 'clunking' back into place within the acetabulum. Barlow's manoeuvre (Figure 5.2.13b) assesses whether or not a hip is dislocatable. A dislocatable hip will be felt sliding out of the posterior aspect of the acetabulum. If a newborn is assessed as being in a 'high risk' category for DDH, or has a positive hip screen, a referral for a hip ultrasound and further assessment should be made within six weeks of birth.

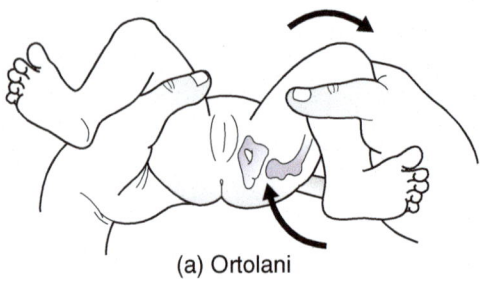

(a) Ortolani

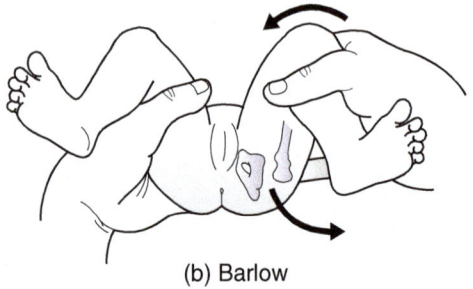

(b) Barlow

Figure 5.2.13 a) Ortolani and b) Barlow manoeuvres

Source: Figure 4.3, p.43, Lumsden and Holmes (2010)

The testes

The absence of one (unilateral) or both (bilateral) of the testes in the scrotum is known as **cryptorchidism**, or undescended teste(s). Between 2–6% of term baby boys are born with cryptorchidism and approximately 1% of these babies will require surgery to correct the issue. Uncorrected cryptorchidism can result in an increased risk of testicular cancer and impaired fertility.

Pathophysiology of cryptorchidism

Little is known about the causes of cryptorchidism, although in preterm babies, the normal process of descent of the testes may have yet to be completed by the time of their birth.

Both male and female embryos have two small ducts called the Wolffian and Mullerian ducts and two gonads in the abdomen which have the potential to become either male or female reproductive systems. The first stage of sex differentiation is controlled by chromosomes. The SRY gene on a male embryo's Y chromosome produces testis determining factor (TDF) which initiates the development of the male sex organs. From their initial position in the abdomen, the testes need to descend into the scrotum, which occurs from about 28 weeks gestation and is usually complete by full term (Figure 5.2.14).

Neonates at increased risk of cryptorchidism

▶ Babies who have a first degree relative who had/has cryptorchidism
▶ Preterm babies
▶ Small for gestational age babies

Testing for cryptorchidism

The scrotum should be gently palpated to assess for the presence of two testes. If not present in the scrotum, the palpation should extend to the inguinal canals and perineum. A teste/testes located anywhere other than in the scrotum should be treated as 'undescended' and a 'screen positive'. A unilateral undescended teste can be reviewed at 6–8 weeks, by which time it is likely to have descended spontaneously. Bilateral undescended testes warrant an urgent medical review to rule out Androgen Insensitivity Syndrome and Congenital Adrenal Hyperplasia.

Androgen insensitivity syndrome (AIS) occurs in males who are insensitive to testosterone. This can result in the development of a blind-ended vagina and intra-abdominal testes. The external genitalia often look ambiguous or more feminine than masculine.

Congenital adrenal hyperplasia (CAH) can occur in males or females and affects the adrenal glands and their production of cortisol and aldosterone (producing too little) and sometimes androgens, including testosterone, as well (producing too much). Too little cortisol can affect the physiological response to stresses such as injury, and

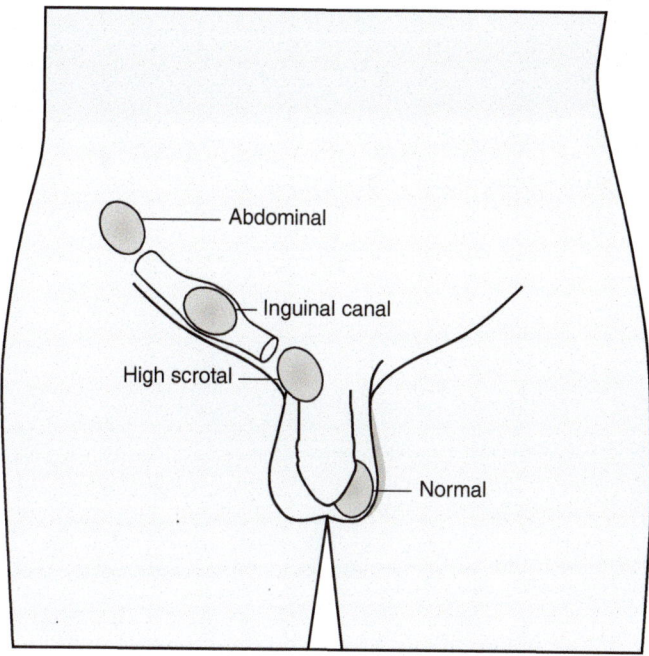

Figure 5.2.14 Descent of testes

also the regulation of blood pressure, blood sugar, heart function and the immune system. Too little aldosterone affects the levels of salts such as sodium and potassium in the blood which can result in early onset dehydration in newborns.

Overproduction of androgens can lead to ambiguous genitalia in baby girls, or genitalia which are more masculine than feminine. However, the internal sexual organs are generally unaffected.

References

Armanian A.M., Jahanfar S. et al. Prebiotics for the prevention of hyperbilirubinaemia in neonates. *Cochrane Database Syst. Rev.* [Internet] 2019. www.cochranelibrary.com/cdsr/doi/10.1002/14651858.CD012731.pub2/full.

Hansen R., Gibson S. et al. Adaptive response of neonatal sepsis-derived Group B Streptococcus to bilirubin. *Sci. Rep.* [Internet] 2018, 8:6470. doi:10.1038/s41598-018-24811-3.

Horn D., Ehret D. et al. Sunlight for the prevention and treatment of hyperbilirubinemia in term and late preterm neonates. *Cochrane Database Syst. Rev* [Internet] 2021. www.cochranelibrary.com/cdsr/doi/10.1002/14651858.CD013277.pub2/full.

NICE. Jaundice in Babies under 28 Days [Internet]. 2016. www.nice.org.uk/guidance/cg98/chapter/Recommendations#information-for-parents-or-carers.

Public Health England. Newborn and Infant Physical Examination Screening Standards [Internet]. 2021. www.gov.uk/government/publications/newborn-and-infant-physical-examination-screening-standards/newborn-and-infant-physical-examination-screening-standards-valid-for-data-collected-from-1-april-2021.

Lactation

Louise Hunter

Developments in ultrasound technology and microbial science have transformed our understanding of the anatomy and physiology of lactation and highlighted the key role of breastfeeding in child health and survival. A recent Lancet Series drew attention to the extent to which industrialised societies have been hoodwinked into believing that this vital, free resource can be replaced with financially and environmentally expensive commercial milk formula (Rollins et al., 2023). This section draws on the latest research to demonstrate the fundamental importance of breastmilk and breastfeeding in resource-rich and poorer societies, and outlines the anatomical and physiological knowledge base necessary to enable midwives to support women to breastfeed.

DOI: 10.4324/9781003227571-31

The constituents of breastmilk

Louise Hunter

LEARNING OUTCOMES

▶ Understand and explain the importance of human milk and breastfeeding to the health and development of babies

▶ Appreciate the physiological interactions underpinning the key role of exclusive breastfeeding up to six months, and the ongoing importance of breastmilk as part of a healthy diet beyond that point

Breastmilk supports three key factors necessary to ensure a newborn survives and thrives outside the womb: protection against disease, adequate nutrition and a highly developed brain. Breastmilk cannot be replicated – replacing it with other substances leads to increased mortality and morbidity in both high- and lower-income settings.

An evolving, changing fluid

Breastmilk changes over time, over the course of a day and during a single feed, responding to a baby's needs as it grows and develops. At the time of her baby's birth, a mother's breasts will contain **colostrum**, a thick, viscous, yellow fluid that is particularly high in antibacterial and antiviral properties (it contains more white blood cells and around ten times more secretory immunoglobulin A (sIgA) than later milks). Colostrum is only present in small amounts, so that it does not overwhelm the newborn's kidneys, and making it easier to learn to coordinate suckling and breathing. It has a laxative effect, helping the passage of meconium, and contains relatively high concentrations of pancreatic secretory trypsin inhibitor, which protects the gut from damage by digestive enzymes, protecting and preparing the intestines for the processing of food.

DOI: 10.4324/9781003227571-32

As maternal progesterone levels fall following the birth of the placenta, colostrum is replaced with **transitional milk** around four days after birth, and then **mature milk** by around day 13. Mature milk is more plentiful and tends to leave the breast in two stages as a baby feeds. Initially, the milk leaving the breast is high in protein, lactose and water. As the feed progresses, the fat level gradually increases but volume decreases (see Figure 6.1.1). This is because water flows more readily than fat, so it leaves the breast first. Think about dipping a sponge into a bowl of oil and water and lifting it up – the water will immediately drip back into the bowl, but most of the oil will need to be squeezed out. For this reason, it is important that infants can feed from a breast until they release it spontaneously, enabling them to access as much fat-rich milk (represented in dark purple in the image below) as they need. A baby's suckling behaviour will change over a feed depending on milk flow and consistency.

Breastmilk contains approximately 750 calories per litre, and is made up of over 200 components, the roles of some of which are as yet unclear. It is not only species specific (for example, it contains less protein than cow's milk as human babies mature more slowly than calves, and more carbohydrates than most mammalian milks to support brain growth and development) but is also tailored to particular individuals. The milk of a mother who gives birth to a premature baby will be different to that of a mother giving birth at term, including containing over twice as many macrophages and lymphocytes to ward off pathogens. In addition to its natural fluctuations, the constituents of expressed breastmilk are also impacted by microwaving (which destroys IgA) and pasteurisation (which reduces the effectiveness of defence factors including IgA and B and T cells).

A crucial immune defence and immune system trigger

Up until birth, an infant is protected from disease by its mother's immune system. They are therefore particularly vulnerable to pathogens when separated from this at birth. Neonates have no acquired immunity, as they have not been directly exposed to any pathogens, and many of their innate immune defences are underdeveloped. Phagocyte function and responses are immature, antibody production is limited and slow (it takes up to 30 days postpartum

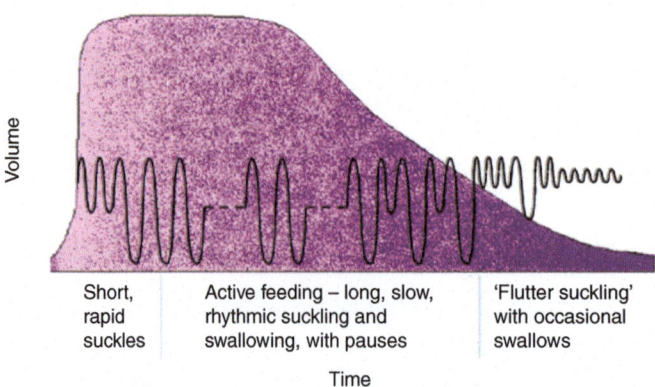

Short, rapid suckles | Active feeding – long, slow, rhythmic suckling and swallowing, with pauses | 'Flutter suckling' with occasional swallows

Time

Figure 6.1.1 The whale of milk. Copyright © UNICEF UK Baby Friendly Initiative
Source: © UNICEF UK Baby Friendly Initiative

for the neonatal gut to produce high enough levels of sIgA for protection), and the newborn infant lacks the capacity to produce a contained inflammatory response, tending instead to over-react and cause cell damage. On top of all this, the newborn gut, which forms the largest internal interface with external organisms, is functionally immature – the tight junctions in the gut mucosa, which maintain the intestinal barrier and regulate permeability, take weeks to mature and prevent the passage of whole proteins and pathogens into the bloodstream. The newborn is both vulnerable to attack and unable to defend itself.

Breastmilk provides **passive immunity** and **stimulates and directs the development of the newborn immune system**. It is beyond the scope of this book to list all the ways in which it does this, and indeed new immunologic properties are still being discovered, but some key functions are discussed below.

Passive immunity

A number of agents in breastmilk protect the baby while its own immune system matures. These are generally found in higher quantities in colostrum and in the milk of the mothers of premature babies, offering protection at particularly vulnerable times. Mediators of passive immunity include:

▶ **White blood cells** (leukocytes). These contain phagocytes and lymphocytes which engulf and destroy pathogens. About 80% of the cells present in colostrum are leukocytes.

▶ **Antibodies** (immunoglobulins). Breastmilk contains IgA, IgG, IgM and IgD. IgA (known as sIgA in its secretory form) coats the newborn gut, preventing the entry of bacteria and viruses, including E. coli, salmonellae, streptococci, staphylococci, pneumococci, poliovirus and the

rotaviruses. IgG antibodies can make pathogenic bacteria more susceptible to phagocytosis, IgM antibodies are made as an initial response to infection and IgD functions as an antigen receptor on activated B cells. Immunoglobulins are antigen specific. If a lactating mother ingests, inhales or otherwise comes into contact with pathogens, she will synthesise specific antibodies to target them. These are transferred into breastmilk and protect the baby (IgA is even made and stored in the breast). It is therefore essential that mothers and their babies stay close to one another, so that they are exposed to the same pathogens. Babies will also transmit small amounts of saliva into their mothers' breasts while feeding, and a mother will then make antibodies to any pathogens found in this, transmitting them back into the baby as early as the next feed.

▶ **Lactoferrin**. Like antibodies, lactoferrin is a protein. It is present in its highest levels in colostrum immediately after birth, and then decreases significantly over the first three days. Lactoferrin binds iron, making it easier to absorb and removing it as a food source for pathogenic bacteria in the intestine. It also alters the properties of bacterial cell membranes, making them more susceptible to degradation by the enzyme lysozyme (see below), and has antiviral properties, including against the human immunodeficiency virus (HIV), cytomegalovirus and hepatitis B and C.

▶ **Alpha-lactalbumin**. Alpha-lactalbumin is a principal protein in human milk. When mixed with acid found in milk and in the infant's stomach, it produces a compound called human alpha-lactalbumin made lethal to tumour cells (HAMLET), which causes cell suicide in over 40 types of cancer.

6.1

▶ **Enzymes**. There are multiple enzymes in breastmilk that assist in the destruction of pathogens. They include lysozyme, which degrades the outer wall of gram-positive bacteria and is active against HIV, and platelet-activating factor acetylhydrolase which helps prevent necrotising enterocolitis (NEC).

▶ **Oligosaccharides**. These important non-digestible sugars have a number of functions, including acting as decoy receptors for pathogens. The pathogens attach to the oligosaccharides, rather than the gut wall, and are then carried through the baby's system.

▶ **Fats**. Milk lipids attack bacteria and damage the outer surface of some viruses, leaving them unable to replicate.

Anti-inflammatory mechanisms

These prevent the immature newborn immune system going into overdrive, protecting neonates from conditions such as NEC, which mostly affects premature babies, where intestinal tissue becomes inflamed and dies, causing perforations in the intestine. The passive immunity features described above also prevent the neonate initiating an inflammatory response as they remove pathogens before they are recognised by the neonatal immune system. Other anti-inflammatory mechanisms include:

▶ **Vitamins A, C, E**. These antioxidants neutralise free radicals – unstable molecules produced during normal cell metabolism which can cause cell damage and inflammation.

▶ **Lactoferrin**. Decreases pro-inflammatory cytokine expression.

▶ **Cytokines**. The presence of cytokines in breastmilk further discourages the neonate from producing its own inflammatory response. Cytokines also combine with dietary antigens to induce tolerance to dietary and microflora antigens (further preventing inflammation).

Promotion of immune defences

There are several components in breastmilk which actively promote and direct the development of immune defences, which will protect the neonate throughout their life. These include:

▶ **Growth factors**. These promote growth and development of the immature gut. Foremost is epidermal growth factor, a peptide which is also found in amniotic fluid and supports cell growth and differentiation in the gut lining. It supports the development of a functional barrier, protecting the neonate from pathogens while allowing the transport of nutrients. Epidermal growth factor is more abundant in the milk of mothers who have preterm babies and is linked to a reduced risk of NEC.

▶ **Lactoferrin**. This also promotes growth of the gut lining, inducing cell proliferation at high concentrations (in the first 3 days of life) and cell differentiation at low concentrations (day 3 onwards).

▶ **Cytokines**. Cytokines orchestrate the development and functioning of the immune system. For example, IL-7 promotes development of the thymus, where T cells, a crucial part of the body's acquired immune response, mature and differentiate. It is known that the concentration of IL-7 in breastmilk is positively correlated to the size of the infant's thymus and the number of T cells it is able to release (Hossny et al., 2020). The size of the thymus in a breastfed baby is up to twice that of an infant who has not been breastfed. IL-7 also has an important role in promoting the production of B cells, which produce antibodies.

- **Viral fragments**. These stimulate an acquired immune response, making a neonate better able to respond to later assaults. Breastfed babies respond much better to vaccines than infants who are not breastfed.
- **Vitamin A**. Levels of this vitamin are twice as high in colostrum than in mature milk. It supports cell growth and promotes the growth and development of T cells.
- **Commensal bacteria**. These are bacteria that act on the infant's immune system to induce protective responses and are essential for appropriate seeding of the gut microbiome (see Chapter 5.2 for more information about the microbiome).
- **Oligosaccharides**. Over 200 different oligosaccharides have been identified, and they constitute the third largest solid component of human milk. Oligosaccharides pass through the small intestine to the colon, where they produce short-chain fatty acids through fermentation, creating a favourable acidic environment for growth of probiotic, anti-inflammatory bacteria such as bifidobacteria and lactobacilli.
- **Lactose and lactoferrin**. Promote the growth of commensal bacteria in the gut.

INTERRUPTER

How would you explain breastmilk's role in immune protection to parents? Use the space in your workbook to detail this. Try to include all of the key functions above, and some examples of how each works.

A complete source of nutrition for healthy growth and development

The constituents of breastmilk change as a baby develops, providing a complete source of nutrition until six months of age. Until this point, an infant is unlikely to have the motor and oral skills needed to cope with solid foods. After this point, the World Health Organization (2023) recommends that breastmilk remains a principal source of nutrition until around a year, and an important supplementary food source until two years and beyond. It can provide half or more of a child's energy needs between the ages of 6–12 months, and one-third of energy needs between 12 and 24 months. The nutritional components of breastmilk are outlined below.

Water

Breastmilk is around 87.5% water, meaning that babies do not need supplements of other drinks, even on hot days.

Carbohydrates

Around 7% of breastmilk is made up of carbohydrates, with lactose making up the largest proportion of this. Lactose contains galactocerebrosides for brain development and enhances calcium and iron absorption. It is easily broken down into glucose for energy. Around 40% of breastmilk's calorific value is made up of carbohydrates.

Fats

Fats make up around 4% of breastmilk. They are a major energy source, constituting about 50% of milk's calorific value, and are essential for the absorption of the fat-soluble vitamins A, D, E and K. Breastmilk fat is made up of globules of triglycerides, which are easy to digest, and includes long chain polyunsaturated fatty acids (LCPs), which support the development of the brain, eyes and nervous and vascular systems. It also

6.1

contains cholesterol, which is an essential part of all membranes and a vital ingredient of the myelin sheath involved in nerve conduction in the brain.

Protein

Protein is essential for muscle and tissue growth. Its low concentration in breastmilk (around 1% of breastmilk is protein) reflects the fact that human young have evolved to grow and mature slowly. Breastmilk protein is whey based – the whey:casein ratio is around 60:40 – making it easy to digest and use. The proportion of casein, which takes longer to digest, rises over the course of the lactation. Proteins also assist with the absorption of calcium and phosphate. For comparison, cow's milk is 3.5% protein, 80% of which is casein. This makes cow's milk formula challenging for human babies to digest.

Vitamins

Breasts cannot synthesise vitamins – these are taken directly from the maternal diet and are mostly present in breastmilk in roughly the same levels as in maternal serum. It is therefore important to ensure that breastfeeding mothers eat healthily and that 'hard to acquire' vitamins such as B12 in plant-based diets, are accounted for. The fat-soluble vitamins A, E and K, and vitamin C, are present in higher levels in colostrum than in maternal serum, suggesting that active transport mechanisms transfer these important nutrients into milk. Vitamin K is important for blood clotting and levels in breastmilk are considered insufficient to protect newborns from vitamin K deficiency bleeding. Although this is a rare condition, vitamin K administration to newborns is common practice in many parts of the world. After a few days, this vitamin will be produced by the neonate's intestinal flora. Levels of vitamin D in breastmilk have recently come under scrutiny due to a reported rise in cases of rickets in young children in developed countries. This probably reflects a move to

lifestyles where more time is spent indoors and in polluted, urban environments, as well as increased use of sunscreen. Supplements of vitamin D are now routinely offered to babies in many settings.

Minerals

The concentration of minerals such as iron in breastmilk is highest in colostrum. Although the iron level in breastmilk is considered to be low, it is far more bioavailable than iron in other food sources, thanks to the presence of lactoferrin. Furthermore, an excess of iron would promote the growth of pathogens. Term infants have sufficient physiological stores of iron to supplement what they ingest from breastmilk for the first six months of life.

Trace elements

Trace elements such as growth and transfer factors maximise the utilisation and absorption of nutrients. Breastmilk also contains nucleotides, which help with cell repair; taurine, which is required for the conjugation of bile salts; hormones which support the infant's immature endocrine system; and stem cells which can migrate from the gut to other areas of the body and differentiate into specialised cells. There is some evidence that breastmilk stem cells remain in the baby's system long after breastfeeding has stopped.

References

Hossny E.M., El-Ghoneimy D.H. et al. Breast milk interleukin-7 and thymic gland development in infancy. *Eur. J. Nutr.* 2020, 59(1):111–18.

Rollins N., Piwoz E. et al. Marketing of commercial milk formula: A system to capture parents, communities, science, and policy. *Lancet* 2023, 401 (10375):486–502.

World Health Organization. Breastfeeding [Internet]. 2023. www.who.int/health-topics/breastfeeding#tab=tab_1.

The anatomy of the breast and the physiology of lactation

Louise Hunter

LEARNING OUTCOMES

▶ Understand and explain the anatomy of the breast and the physiology of lactation

▶ Apply your knowledge of the anatomy and physiology of lactation to support mothers to successfully establish and maintain breastfeeding

The anatomy of the female breast

Adult female breasts are separate, glandular structures specialised for milk synthesis and removal. They are commonly classified as part of the integumentary system – an organ system which also includes skin, hair, nails and sweat and sebaceous glands. However, aside from a common glandular origin they do not work in tandem with these structures and, as a collection of tissues which work together to form a particular function, they are perhaps better viewed as organs in their own right.

Situation

Breasts are situated on either side of the sternum, on top of the pectoralis major muscle, and extend vertically from

DOI: 10.4324/9781003227571-33

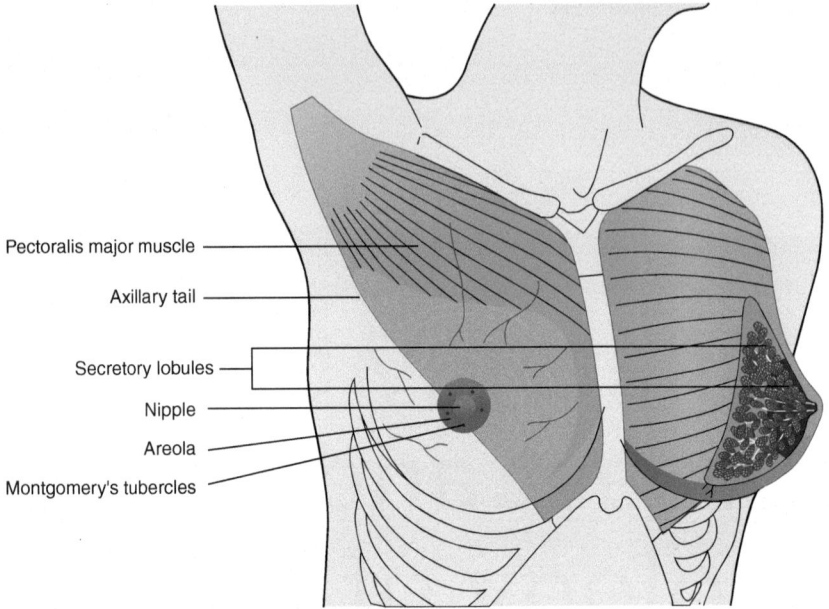

Pectoralis major muscle

Axillary tail

Secretory lobules

Nipple

Areola

Montgomery's tubercles

Figure 6.2.1 Anatomy of the breast

around the second to the sixth rib (see Figure 6.2.1). Suspensory ligaments known as **Cooper's ligaments** anchor the breast to the underlying muscle. Cooper's ligaments are slightly lax, allowing breasts a degree of movement while maintaining structural integrity.

External appearance and anatomy

Breasts are roughly hemispherical in shape, but can also appear conical, pear-shaped or flat, and have an **axillary tail** extending towards the axilla (armpit). A woman's breasts are rarely the same size and shape, and breast appearance varies greatly between women, with genetics, race, diet, age, parity and menopausal status all influencing breast size and shape. The size of a breast is not indicative of how much milk it can produce.

A circular, pigmented area known as the **areola**, measuring around 3–4 cm in

diameter, sits in the centre of the breast. Small, pimple-like sebaceous glands called **Montgomery's tubercles** open onto the areola and secrete an oily liquid which is thought to be protective during feeding and emit an odour which attracts the baby towards the centre of the breast to feed after birth (it is said to smell like amniotic fluid).

In the centre of the areola is the **nipple**, a sensitive erectile structure made up of smooth muscle, collagen and elastic connective tissue. The nipple contains between 4–18 (usually between 5 and 9) openings from which breastmilk flows during suckling. Nipples can protrude, be relatively or completely flat against the areola, or even inverted. They usually become erect when stimulated but can also retract. The shape and size of the nipple does not generally impact on feeding, as babies breast, rather than nipple, feed. Some women may have additional, accessory nipples which may even secrete milk – these are usually found along a 'milk line' that stretches on each side of the body from the armpit, through the breast and down to the inner thigh. Humans are relatively unusual in only having two functioning breasts – many other mammals have several along two milk lines. Accessory breast tissue or nipples may look like moles or be more developed.

The areola and nipple together form the **nipple-areola complex**. The size and colour of the nipple-areola complex is again dependent on genetics, race and parity. It can vary in colour from pink to black, but due to an increased density of melanocytes it is generally a shade or two darker than the surrounding skin. It is sometimes stated that the darkened appearance of the areola helps the baby to locate it after birth so

that they can feed, but given that sight is quite underdeveloped in neonates, and that in many women there is in fact very little difference in colour between the skin and the areola, this seems unlikely.

Blood supply and lymphatic drainage

Breasts are **highly vascular** (milk is synthesised principally from blood, so a good supply is essential), receiving blood from branches of the internal thoracic artery, lateral thoracic artery and thoracoacromial artery (see Figure 6.2.2). Accompanying the blood vessels is a relatively dense network of **sensory and autonomic nerves**, enabling the breasts to respond to touch and other stimuli to produce

6.2

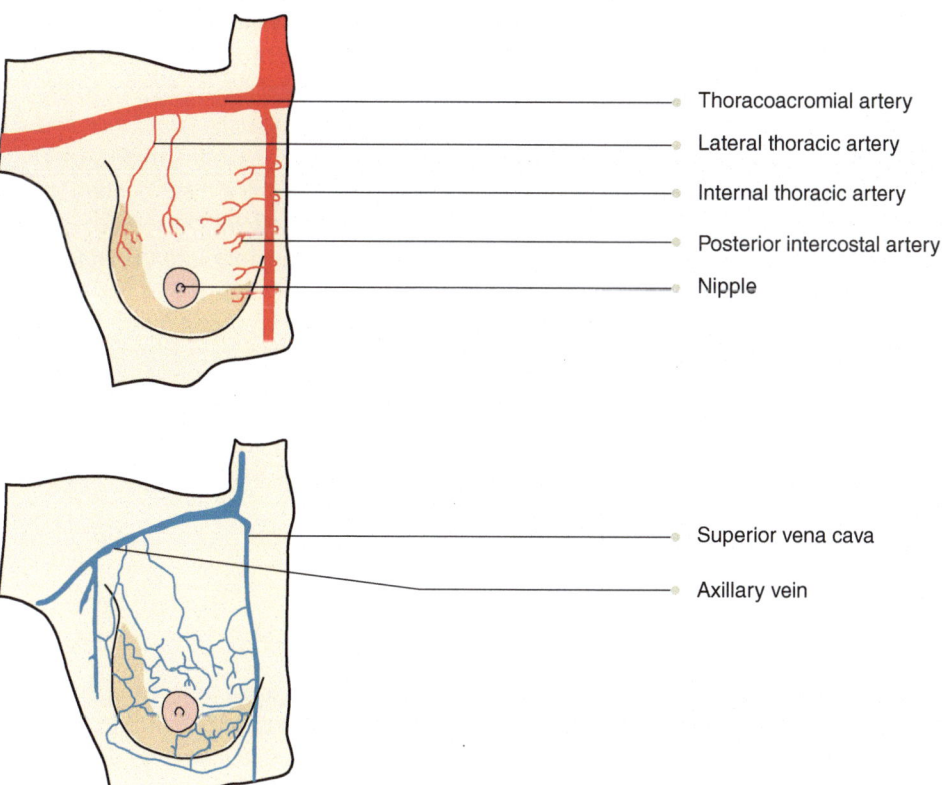

Thoracoacromial artery

Lateral thoracic artery

Internal thoracic artery

Posterior intercostal artery

Nipple

Superior vena cava

Axillary vein

Figure 6.2.2 Blood supply to, and venous drainage from, the breast

345

and release milk. A further network of **lymphatic vessels and nodes**, extending into the armpit and neck, drains inactivated bacteria and other cell parts, and any excess fluid that seeps into the breast tissue. The nodes protect the breast by producing and storing **lymphocytes** and other pathogenic entities. It is highly likely that these entities are transferred from the lymph nodes into breastmilk – it is known that the nodes can become swollen as they react to pathogens transferred from the baby into the mother during suckling.

Internal structures

Behind the nipple openings are small **lactiferous ducts**, approximately 2 mm in diameter. There can be between 4 and 18 (mean 9) ducts in an individual breast. They are superficial and easily compressible. It is possible for there to be more nipple openings than ducts, as some openings can be superficial, and also for there to be more ducts than openings, as some ducts can join together very close to the nipple. About 5–8 mm back from the nipple, the ducts start to acquire branches, or **ductules**, which terminate in clusters of **alveoli** known as **lobules**. Each duct will house between 20 and 40 lobules, and each lobule will consist of 10–100 alveoli (see Figure 6.2.3). Each complex of duct, ductules and lobules is known as a **lobe**. It is sometimes helpful to think of lobes as resembling bunches of grapes (the ducts are the stems) or a head of broccoli. Lobes are intertwined in the breast, rather than being sited evenly or radially around the nipple. More are actually located in the upper outer quadrant (up towards the armpit – this is one of the reasons why breast cancer is more commonly found here). Lobes are glandular tissue – lobules and alveoli are sometimes referred to as **mammary glands**. They are supported by fibrous connective tissue and embedded in fatty tissue. The proportion of glandular:fatty tissue in a lactating breast is around 2:1, although this varies between individuals, and it is the fatty tissue that largely determines breast size. There is minimal fatty tissue immediately under the areola, but it gradually builds towards the back of the breast. Sixty-five per cent of the glandular tissue is located within a 30 mm radius from the base of the nipple.

Milk synthesis

Milk synthesis occurs in the **alveoli**. Each alveolus has a rich vascular supply and is lined with a single layer of milk producing cells called **lactocytes**, giving the lactocytes ready access to blood for milk synthesis. The lactocytes are connected by tight junctions and have **prolactin receptor sites** on their outer surfaces which, when activated, allow **prolactin** to message the cells to make milk. The lactocytes take in blood from the capillaries adjacent to their outer surface, synthesise it into milk and eject it into the lumen in the middle of the alveoli. The alveoli are surrounded by **myoepithelial (muscle) cells** which, when they contract, expel milk into the lactiferous ducts (see Figure 6.2.3).

INTERRUPTER

Label the diagrams of breast anatomy in your workbook to embed this knowledge.

Breast changes in puberty and beyond

Breast budding is often one of the first signs of adolescence in girls. Up to this point, the breast contains some lactiferous ducts but no alveoli. As puberty arrives, hormones of the reproductive system such as oestrogen and growth hormone

6.2

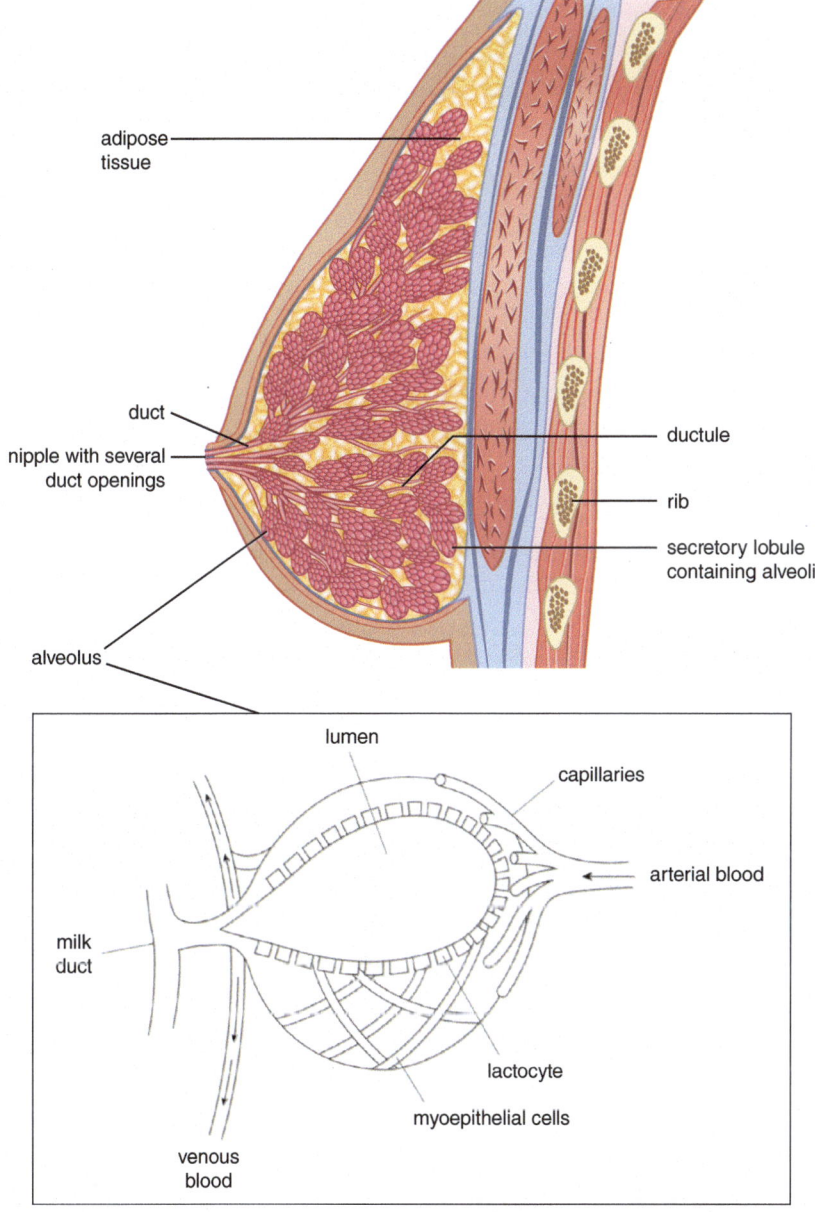

Figure 6.2.3 Internal anatomy of the breast, with magnified cross section of an alveolus

stimulate development of the ductal system. Lobular development commences under the influence of progesterone. Hormonal fluctuations in each menstrual cycle facilitate a little more mammary development, up to around the age of

35. The areola enlarges and darkens, and breasts increase to adult size, initially mostly due to adipose tissue.

The loss of oestrogen and progesterone during the menopause causes the glandular tissue in the breast to atrophy. It is replaced with adipose tissue. The connective tissue in the breast also becomes less cellular and the amount of collagen decreases, causing the breast to shrink and droop.

Breast changes in pregnancy

Breast development is accelerated from early pregnancy as high levels of **oestrogen** and **progesterone** are maintained initially by the corpus luteum and then by the placenta. A cocktail of other hormones assists this process, including human placental lactogen, produced by the placenta, and prolactin. Levels of both these hormones rise throughout pregnancy and further support progesterone with lobular and alveolar development. Prolactin also supports oestrogen to stimulate the growth of lactiferous ducts and helps differentiate alveolar cells into lactocytes. It is thought that the intense cell differentiation in the breast throughout pregnancy has a role in protecting women from breast cancer. It also makes breast changes one of the first visible signs of pregnancy, with many women experiencing tingling sensations, sensitivity, growth and heaviness of their breasts.

The blood supply to the breasts doubles in the first 24 weeks of pregnancy, giving some breasts a marbled appearance as veins become visible on the surface. By 12 weeks there is greater pigmentation to the areola and nipples, causing them to darken. They may also increase in size, and some women develop a 'secondary areola' around the areola at around 24 weeks. Montgomery's tubercles become more prominent and start to excrete small amounts of their oily lubricant. By around 16 weeks gestation, the breasts are capable of secreting colostrum. Further milk synthesis is prevented by progesterone and human placental lactogen until after the birth of the placenta.

The physiology of lactation

Lactogenesis

Lactogenesis (the production of milk) is generally divided into three phases. Lactogenesis I and II are hormonally driven and occur whether or not breastfeeding takes place, whereas lactogenesis III only occurs in the presence of breastfeeding:

▶ **Lactogenesis I** covers breast changes and colostrum production in pregnancy, discussed above.

▶ **Lactogenesis II** is the onset of **milk production** after the birth of the placenta and membranes. After the birth of the placenta, circulating levels of progesterone, oestrogen and human placental lactogen fall, allowing **prolactin** to 'dock' on the prolactin receptor sites on the **lactocytes** and instruct the cell to make milk. Insulin and cortisol also have a part to play in milk synthesis. Furthermore, the **tight junctions** between the lactocytes are initially open, allowing immunoglobulins, lymphocytes and macrophages, so important for early immunity against pathogens, to travel into the colostrum. After 2–3 days, the tight junctions close, enabling the lactocytes to work together and increasing milk production. While there is around 5 ml of colostrum available to the baby at birth, by the end of the first week an individual's breasts can be producing up to 868 ml of milk a day.

▶ **Lactogenesis III** is the regulation of ongoing milk production. Although partially under hormonal control, this is also dependent on the regular removal of milk from the breasts. Milk removal stimulates milk production, so the more milk that is removed, the more will be produced. There are two mechanisms that prevent over-production:

▶ A whey protein in the milk itself called the **feedback inhibitor of lactation (FIL)**; when the breasts are full, and levels of FIL are consequently high, it signals the lactocytes to stop making milk. When the milk is removed, the signal is removed along with it.

▶ Lactocytes are cuboidal in shape when they are full, and columnar if they are empty. This changes the shape of the prolactin receptor sites on their surface, so that prolactin finds it more difficult to 'dock' when the cells are full.

Each breast works independently to control milk synthesis, so milk needs to be removed from each breast to ensure continued milk production from that breast. It is not unusual for one breast (usually the right one) to produce more milk than the other.

The role of prolactin

Prolactin is produced in and secreted by the **anterior pituitary gland**; a small pea-sized gland located at the base of the brain below the **hypothalamus**. The hypothalamus regulates the secretion of prolactin. It travels through the bloodstream to the breasts, where it lands on the prolactin receptor sites on the lactocytes and instructs them to make milk.

The earlier and more frequently the receptor sites are put to work, the greater the milk producing capacity of the breast becomes for that lactation cycle (until the next time the mother gives birth). Unused receptor sites will close after a period of time, limiting milk production in a lactocyte. Prolactin receptor sites can also be found in other locations such as the ovaries and central nervous system. It is thought that this may facilitate this hormone's role in promoting protective and loving behaviour towards the baby.

Prolactin levels increase throughout pregnancy. Further temporary rises occur in response to touch and stimulation of the breast, areola and nipple. Babies therefore actively stimulate prolactin production in their mothers by bringing their hands to the breast, nuzzling and licking breast tissue prior to and during feeding, and prolactin levels can double at this time. They reach a peak around 30–45 minutes after a baby starts to feed, ensuring that the milk the baby removes is replaced, and/or that further milk production is triggered. Prolactin concentration in plasma follows a circadian rhythm and is highest during rapid eye movement (REM) sleep, when the brain is more active. Suckling at night can therefore elevate prolactin levels more effectively and is important for ongoing milk production. Prolactin levels increase less with suckling over time, as the lactocytes become more sensitive to its effects. It is inhibited by stress, making good support for breastfeeding people essential.

Milk transfer

The transfer of milk from the mother to the baby during suckling relies on a complex interplay of hormonal and mechanical factors, in which both mother and baby play an active role.

The role of oxytocin

The maternal contribution to the process of milk transfer is largely mediated by oxytocin. Oxytocin causes the **myoepithelial (muscle) cells** surrounding the alveoli to contract, forcing milk into the milk ducts and down towards the nipple. As the milk is pushed into the **lactiferous ducts** they widen and shorten in response to the increased pressure. Oxytocin also increases blood circulation to the breast, warming a feeding baby and ensuring the ingredients

6.2

349

for further milk synthesis are present, and releases stored nutrients into milk.

Oxytocin is synthesised in the **hypothalamus** and released by the **posterior pituitary gland** in pulsatile bursts lasting 3–4 seconds and occurring every 5–15 minutes. The first of these bursts (also referred to as '**milk ejection reflexes**' or 'MER's') in each feed is the strongest, and experienced by the woman shortly after the feed commences as a 'let down reflex', involving sensations of tingling and tightening in the breast, and sometimes thirst, warm flushes or even sleepiness. With each subsequent oxytocin burst, smaller amounts of increasingly fat rich milk are released into the milk ducts, meaning that over the course of a feed the 'whale of milk' depicted in Figure 6.1.1 (Chapter 6.1) becomes a series of increasingly smaller and denser humps. MER's can cause milk to be ejected from the breast even if the baby is not feeding.

Oxytocin is particularly responsive to nipple stimulation and closeness to the baby. It works best in a warm, calm environment, and its release can be delayed by stress. Over time, the milk ejection reflex becomes conditioned to other stimuli, such as particular sights or smells associated with feeding, or hearing other babies cry.

Oxytocin's contractile effects are not limited to the breasts – it will also cause the **smooth muscle cells** around the uterus to contract, helping to minimise bleeding postnatally. Multiparous women in particular may experience these contractions as 'afterpains' during the early days of feeding. It also produces analgesic effects and reduces cortisol levels, leading to reduced stress, anxiety and blood pressure. Oxytocin works with prolactin to induce feelings of calmness, love and protection, helping to ensure that the baby's needs for closeness and security are met. As described in Chapter 3.4, the way that prolactin and oxytocin work to produce and transfer milk, as described here, is an example of a positive feedback loop.

INTERRUPTER

Using Figure 6.2.3, summarise the anatomy and physiology of lactation in a way that will make sense to parents. Space is given for this in the lactation section of your workbook.

The mechanisms of suckling

Babies are programmed to feed – they have a rooting reflex compelling them to turn their heads towards anything that strokes their cheeks, and a suckling reflex compelling them to suckle on anything placed in their mouths.

When a baby latches on to the breast, they use their tongue to bring breast tissue into the mouth, shaping it into a teat with the nipple at the far end. The tongue, lips and jaw form a seal around this teat. Milk is then drawn into the baby's mouth by negative pressure as the tongue presses up against the breast and then moves down with the lower jaw, expanding the space in the oral cavity and reducing the pressure, so that milk flows from the high pressure environment in the lactiferous ducts into the lower pressure environment in the baby's mouth. As the baby's tongue moves back up, the pressure equalises and milk flow stops. Simultaneously, the soft palate rises and seals off the nasal cavity, the epiglottis seals off the airway and the milk that has flowed into the mouth is channelled in a bolus towards the baby's throat, triggering swallowing (see Figure 6.2.4). A suckling baby will begin a feed with a short series of quick suckles, thought to stimulate oxytocin release, and then settle into periods of deeper suckling and swallowing. The ratio of suckles to swallows can be 1:1 at the start of a feed, and then settle to 2:1 and even 3:1 towards the end of the feed. Rests during feeds are thought to correspond to pauses between milk ejections.

A baby's tongue is uniquely adapted to suckling, being relatively large and having an ability to curl laterally and create a channel along which milk can flow; this is lost over time. The cheeks and palate also contribute to successful suckling. A term baby's cheeks contain fatty pads (buccinators), which prevent the cheeks from imploding in response to the negative pressure created by the tongue. These diminish over time and are replaced with cheek muscles. The hard palate stabilises the breast, and the soft palate protects the baby's upper airway.

The swallowing reflex in newborns is reasonably well developed, as they routinely ingest amniotic fluid in the womb. In order to feed effectively, however, an infant needs to coordinate suckling, swallowing and breathing. This can take a while to perfect, and 1–3-day old infants show interruptions in breathing movements when they swallow. By about four days, breathing continues unhindered through feeding with swallows occurring at the boundary between inspiration and expiration.

Further reading

Walker M. *Breastfeeding management for the clinician* (2nd edition). Sudbury, MA: Jones and Bartlett, 2011.

6.2

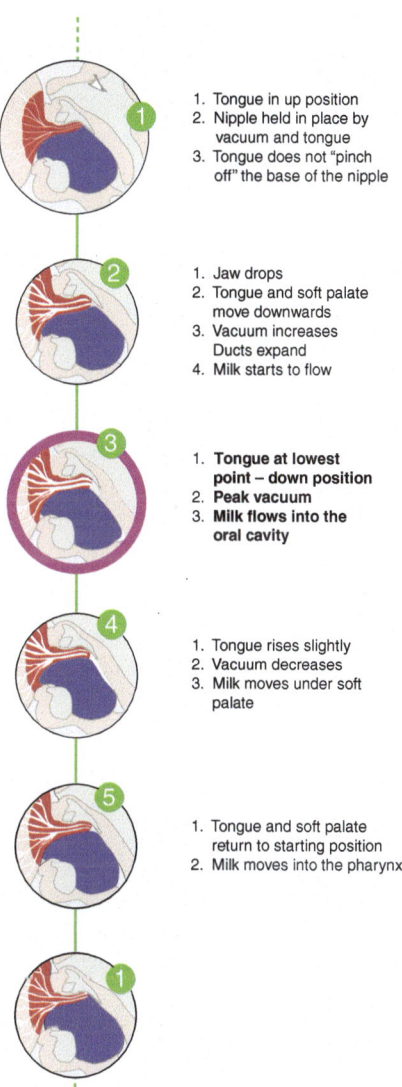

1. Tongue in up position
2. Nipple held in place by vacuum and tongue
3. Tongue does not "pinch off" the base of the nipple

1. Jaw drops
2. Tongue and soft palate move downwards
3. Vacuum increases Ducts expand
4. Milk starts to flow

1. **Tongue at lowest point – down position**
2. **Peak vacuum**
3. **Milk flows into the oral cavity**

1. Tongue rises slightly
2. Vacuum decreases
3. Milk moves under soft palate

1. Tongue and soft palate return to starting position
2. Milk moves into the pharynx

Figure 6.2.4 Suckling

Supporting and maintaining breastfeeding

Louise Hunter

Positioning and attachment

Positioning refers to the way in which a baby is held and/or supported in order to feed. **Attachment** is the way a baby latches onto the breast to feed. Good positioning supports effective attachment, and both are essential to optimise milk transfer, stimulate ongoing milk production and prevent pain and damage to the breast.

Positioning

There are a plethora of different positions in which a baby could feed effectively (see Figure 6.3.1 for some examples), but there

DOI: 10.4324/9781003227571-34

are a number of key principles that need to be in play. The UNICEF Baby Friendly Initiative (BFI) recommends using the acronym 'CHINS' to remember and teach these:

▶ **Close** – the baby needs to be close to the breast in order to take sufficient breast tissue into their mouth.
▶ **Head free** – A baby needs to be able to tilt their head back when latching and approach the breast with their chin leading. Feeding with an extended head helps maintain the baby's airway. It also enables the baby to open their mouth wide enough to latch on properly (the jaw cannot drop sufficiently if the head is flexed).
▶ **In line** – A baby's head and body should be in alignment – twisting the neck in order to latch would make breathing, feeding and swallowing challenging. The baby should be positioned so that they are facing the nipple and can latch without the breast being moved.
▶ **Nose opposite nipple** – if a baby's nose is opposite their mother's nipple before they start to latch, when they tip their head back and gape to come onto the breast, they will be able to fill their mouth with the underlying breast tissue, and the nipple will be perfectly positioned to slip under the baby's top gum and rest at the back of their mouth (see Figure 6.3.2A).
▶ **Sustainable** – both mother and baby should be relaxed and comfortable.

Attachment

Unless they are being supported in a position that enables self-attachment, an infant should be brought to the breast when they gape. It is important that pressure is put on their upper back and not on their head or neck, so that the head is able to extend. A **wide gape** (which can be elicited by gently brushing the nipple along the infant's upper lip), with the tongue at the base of the mouth, is essential for effective attachment and suckling (see Figure 6.3.2B). As infants tend to raise their tongues when they cry, it is therefore important that they are calm when coming to the breast. An infant should approach the breast with their **chin leading** and with their **lower lip as far away from the nipple as possible**, so they have to stretch their mouth to allow the nipple to slip under the top gum (see Figure 6.3.2C). This will ensure that they take **a large mouthful of breast tissue**, triggering suckling and milk release (see Figure 6.3.2D).

APPLICATION TO PRACTICE

Key indications of effective attachment are:

▶ An **asymmetrical orientation** on the breast. If any of the areola is visible, more of it should be showing above the baby's top lip than below their bottom lip. An asymmetrical latch enables the tongue to compress the breast tissue underlying the nipple, forcing the nipple up into the space under the soft palate where it will not be damaged by tongue movements.
▶ The **chin** should be **indenting the breast**, indicating that the tongue is close enough to the breast tissue to apply negative pressure, and the nostrils should be free, so that the baby can breathe. If the nostrils appear to be compressed against the breast, the mother can apply a little extra pressure on the baby's shoulders to encourage further head extension.
▶ The baby's **mouth** should be **wide open**, with the lower lip turned outward and the upper lip appearing stretched. A flanged upper lip is indicative of an insufficiently wide gape.
▶ The baby's **cheeks** should appear **rounded**. Dimpled cheeks are

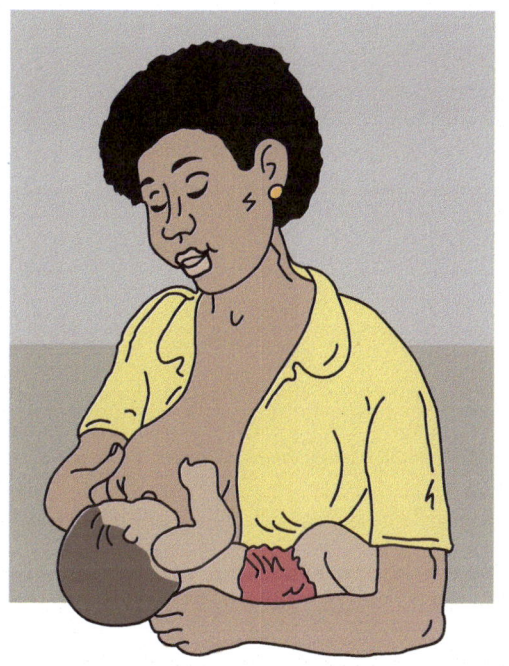

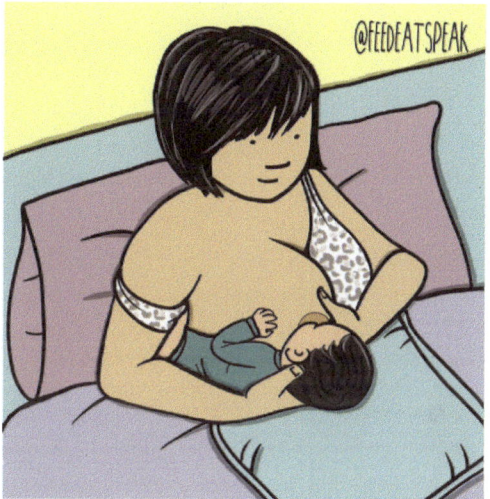

6.3

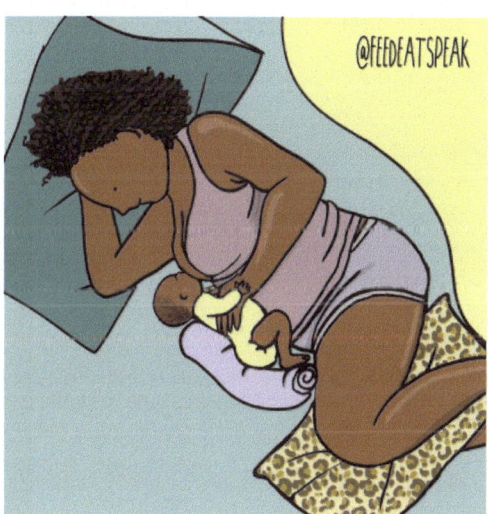

Figure 6.3.1 Examples of breastfeeding positions. Images 2 and 3 copyright Stacey Zimmels, IBCLC, feeding and swallowing specialist SLT. www.feedeatspeak.co.uk, @feedeatspeak

indicative of insufficient breast tissue in the mouth. If the cheeks are pulled inwards while the infant is suckling, this could suggest an absence of sufficient fat pads to support effective feeding.

▶ The feed should **not be painful** for the mother.
▶ At the end of a feed, the **nipple** should **not** appear **squashed**, **squeezed** or **damaged**.

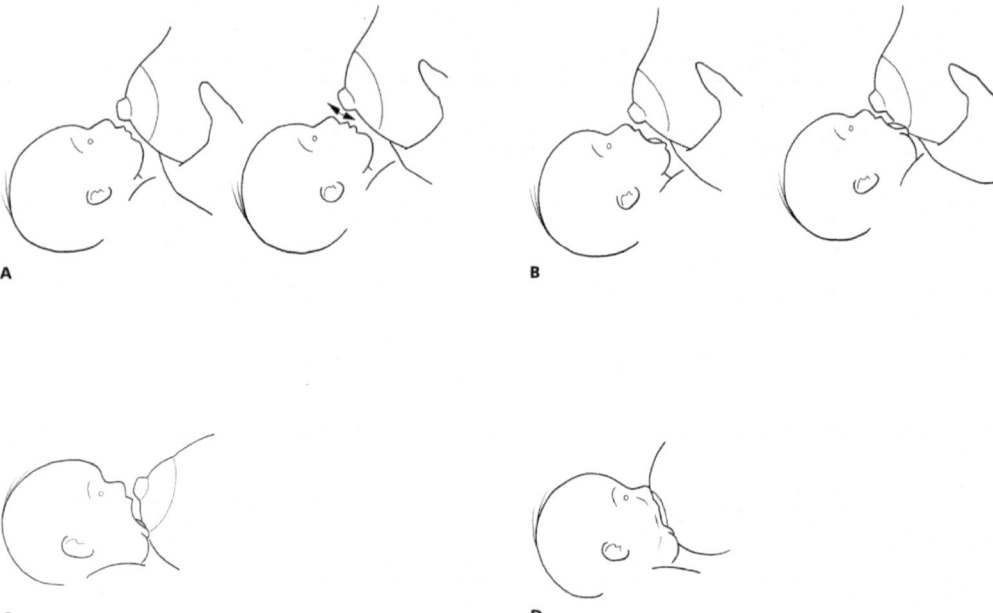

Figure 6.3.2 Latching.
Source: © UNICEF UK Baby Friendly Initiative

A baby may engage in **pre-latching behaviour** such as head bobbing, licking the areola and nipple, and/or massaging the breast with their hands before latching and suckling. Fighting these behaviours, for example by swaddling the baby, is unlikely to promote successful feeding. Massaging movements are designed to promote oxytocin release, and are not a sign that the baby is pushing the breast away and not wanting to feed. In her seminal research into **biological nurturing**, Suzanne Colson noted that holding a baby close and upright, with their head between their mother's breasts and their mother reclining slightly, appears to promote the expression of maternal and neonatal reflexes that support feeding. A baby in this position is better able to bob their head, and any massaging movements are less likely to be interpreted as pushing away the breast. Holding her baby in this position encourages a mother to make a nest around the baby with one arm, stroke her baby's feet (this appears to

relax the lips and tongue ready for latching), and guide her baby to the breast, where they will self-latch (Colson et al., 2008). Positions that encourage self-latching are shown in Figure 6.3.3

APPLICATION TO PRACTICE

It is said that a picture is equivalent to 1000 words. Sharing pictures of positioning and attachment with families that are physiologically accurate is therefore hugely important.

Take a closer look at the images used in this chapter, and at the other resources provided by **UNICEF BFI** and **FeedEatSpeak**. Compare them to other images that are widely available online and think about how images showing suboptimal positioning or attachment might undermine breastfeeding. Put together a list of reliable sources to signpost people to.

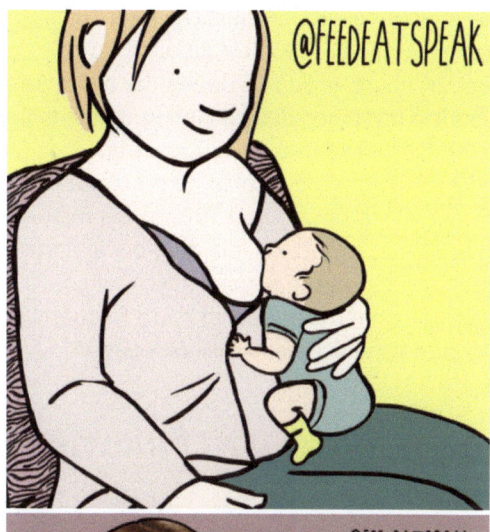

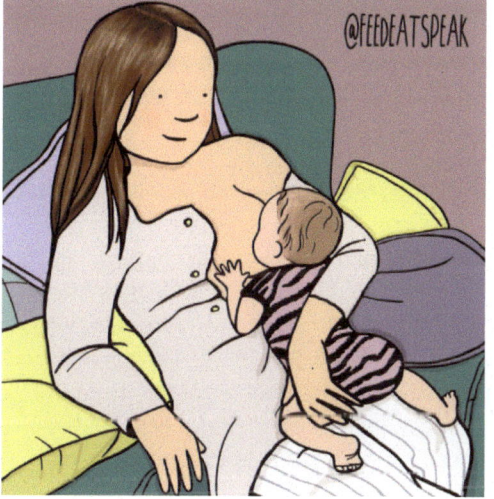

Figure 6.3.3 Positions enabling self-latching. Copyright Stacey Zimmels, IBCLC, feeding and swallowing specialist SLT. www. feedeatspeak.co.uk, @feedeatspeak

Effective milk transfer

Good positioning and attachment will almost always result in effective and sufficient milk transfer, unless there are issues with the baby's suckling ability or milk production and release. Reassuring signs include:

▶ **Suckling pattern** – A baby will begin a feed with a series of fast suckles, designed to trigger the release of oxytocin and a milk ejection. They will

then settle into deeper, rhythmic suckles with swallowing in a ratio of one-two suckles to each swallow. As the milk volume reduces, the baby's suckling rate will slow down and their jaw movements will be less pronounced, resulting in **flutter suckling** rather than active feeding. Flutter suckles may stimulate a further milk ejection, in which case the baby may revert to deeper rhythmic suckles and swallows. The baby should come off the breast spontaneously, indicating that they are full or would like a break or to move to the other side. A full baby will often appear drowsy and satiated.

6.3

▶ **Behaviour** – A baby should appear calm and relaxed at the breast, with periods of active feeding interspersed with short breaks.

▶ **Urine output** – From day 1–6 after birth, the number of wet nappies produced by the baby should at least correlate to their age in days. From day 6, the number should level off but the volume of urine may increase.

▶ **Stooling pattern** – Well fed babies will usually produce a minimum of two soft yellow stools, around the size of a £2 coin, per day after day four and until around six weeks of age. Before day four, stools will consist of black, tarry meconium followed by green sludgy stools. From six weeks, the number of stools can vary from multiple times a day to as few as one every ten days.

▶ **Weight** – Any loss greater than 7% is an indication of possible insufficient milk intake. However, weight loss and gain are late indicators of intake – urine and stool output are more immediate signs.

Ineffective milk transfer can result in the baby wanting to feed more frequently, becoming frustrated at the breast, and developing jaundice and hypernatraemia (dehydration, causing levels of salt in the blood to rise).

Feeding frequency and volume

Babies feed for a number of different reasons, including hunger, thirst and a need to feel comforted and secure. They may feed very efficiently for a short time, or have a long feed interspersed with many breaks. Unless they are vulnerable or unwell, there is no need for babies to be fed to any externally imposed schedule. Such schedules can in fact limit the number of times a baby feeds.

Frequent feeding and/or nuzzling at the breast in the early days after birth increases the sensitivity of prolactin receptors, increasing the breast's capacity for milk synthesis. Early and frequent feeding also helps to stabilise a newborn's blood sugars and promotes the removal of meconium from the baby's gut, preventing the reabsorption of any bilirubin it contains.

A newborn will only ingest small amounts of colostrum, and their gastric tone will gradually relax to accommodate increased volumes of milk. It is not unusual for newborns to be sleepy and feed infrequently in the first 2–3 days. This is not an issue for healthy, term babies, who rapidly develop the ability to **counter-regulate** (see Chapter 5.2) and **produce ketones** as an alternative fuel source in response to low blood sugar. However, if a baby does not feed frequently initially, it is important to protect the mothers' milk supply by encouraging her to hand express.

Human milk is digested easily and quickly. It has a mean gastric half emptying time (the time required by the stomach to empty 50% of an ingested meal) of 47 minutes. Infants are therefore predisposed to feed frequently, and milk is synthesised to accommodate this. It is not unusual for a newborn to feed every 2–3 hours, or to have periods of frequent feeding followed by a longer sleep. Overall, an infant should be expected to feed at least eight times per 24 hours, including during the night. As feeding becomes established, mothers will produce between 500–1200 ml of milk a day. On average over a 24-hour period, an infant will remove about 76% of the milk available at a feed. As infants grow and their demand for milk increases, they will go through periods of feeding more frequently to stimulate increased milk production.

APPLICATION TO PRACTICE

Hand expression

Hand expression can enable mothers to maintain their milk supply when their baby is unable to latch, and produce milk to feed their baby at times when they are unable to offer the breast. It is a skill that fosters mothers' confidence in their body's ability to produce milk, and knowledge of their breast anatomy. Hand expression, as opposed to using a breast pump, is particularly useful for removing colostrum, which is thick, viscous and only present in small amounts, from the breast. Investigations have also shown that mothers are able to remove up to 50% more milk from their breasts if they hand express after pumping, rather than just using a pump alone (Morton, 2017). Increasingly, women are learning to hand express antenatally, collecting colostrum from 37 weeks' gestation, giving them time to practise this important skill before their baby arrives. Expressed colostrum can be kept at room temperature for 24 hours as it is so rich in antibodies. Mature milk can be kept at room temperature for six hours, and both milks can be kept in a fridge at 4°C for five days and in a freezer for six months.

The instructions below can be given to women, lactating people or whoever, with their consent, is undertaking the expression:

▶ **Wash your hands** to prevent any contamination of the milk and **have a clean container or syringe to hand** in which to collect it. This receptacle does not need to be sterile as breastmilk is a living fluid packed with antibodies and other antibacterial and antiviral ingredients.

▶ **Encourage oxytocin to flow**. Good oxytocin release is essential as unlike suckling, hand expression does not include the benefit of negative pressure created by the lowering of the baby's tongue. Oxytocin release can be stimulated by warmth, being close to the baby (or having a picture or item of their clothing to hand if that is not possible), comfort, privacy and **breast massage**. Massage is likely to be most effective if performed by the mother themselves or someone very close to them. Techniques include gentle stroking from the back of the breast (including under the axilla) towards the nipple and making a fist and rocking the knuckles over the breast. Massaging should include stimulation of the areola and nipple, which have a rich nerve supply.

▶ After around 5 minutes of breast massage, **make a 'C' shape with your thumb and index finger and place this on the breast**, with the thumb uppermost, about **2–3 cm back from the base of the nipple**. The thumb and index finger should be on opposite sides of the nipple, and over some of the lobules in the breast.

▶ Without pulling the breast tissue forwards, or sliding the thumb or forefinger over the breast, **gently bring your thumb and finger closer together**, applying pressure on the underlying breast tissue. **Hold the pressure for 2–3 seconds before releasing it**, keeping the thumb and finger in the same position on the breast. This process should be repeated in a rhythmic fashion. Droplets of milk should start to appear after a short time. If this does not happen, move your thumb and forefinger a little further back or forwards on the breast and try again, until you find a position that works for you. Some people find expressing works better if they push their thumb and forefinger towards the chest wall before squeezing them together.

▶ **Continue pressing and releasing until milk stops flowing, then rotate your thumb and forefinger to a different position around the nipple** (it might help to think of them as hands moving round a clock face). This should bring them above a different set of lobules to milk.

▶ After expressing from different points in a circle around 2–3 cm back from the nipple, you can **repeat the process on the other breast**.

Supporting innate and relational feeding behaviours

Humans are social creatures, and in many societies, bonds are forged and friendship and love are expressed through the giving and sharing of food. The intertwining of food and relationship building starts from birth, with maternal and neonatal oxytocin surges that support feeding, bonding and attachment. These behaviours are best enabled by keeping a mother and baby close together, preferably by placing a neonate in skin-to-skin contact on their mother's chest. Neonates are particularly responsive to smell and touch after birth – holding a baby close to their mother will help them feel secure and encourage them to gravitate towards the smell of the fluid secreted by the Montgomery's tubercles on the areola.

Skin-to-skin contact

Skin-to-skin contact (see Chapter 5.2) can be practised at any time, but when it is undertaken immediately after birth, a healthy term infant will initiate a sequence of innate behaviours that culminate in their finding and feeding from the breast, usually within an hour. These behaviours are designed to promote the survival of both the mother and baby, and must be allowed to happen without external interruption. It is thought that the high levels of adrenaline present in the neonate in the first 1–2 hours after birth facilitate feeding behaviour. The behaviours expressed by babies in skin-to-skin contact (often referred to as the 'breast crawl') are shown in Box 6.3.1. As the neonate works through them, the mother will begin to smell, stroke and greet her baby.

BOX 6.3.1 Behaviours expressed by newborn infants in skin-to-skin contact: the breast crawl

▶ A brief, distinctive '**birth cry**', possibly designed to promote respiration.
▶ A short period of **rest and recovery**.
▶ A period of **awakening**, where the baby opens their eyes, is alert, and can stretch, make hand to mouth movements (triggering gaping and suckling), and start to salivate.
▶ A period of **movement**, where the baby moves their head, arms and shoulders, and then draws up their knees and kicks down with their feet to move towards a breast. The kicking down movements help to stimulate maternal contractions and expel the placenta.
▶ A possible further short period of **rest** once they arrive at the breast.
▶ A period of **familiarisation** with the breast. The baby may nuzzle, smell and lick around the areola and nipple, and massage the breast with their hands. As well as familiarising the baby with the breast, this behaviour encourages maternal oxytocin and prolactin release, ensuring a readily available supply of milk when the baby latches and for subsequent feeds.
▶ A period of **suckling**. Usually after a series of head bobs, the baby will latch and start to feed. Their mother will instinctively cradle them in their arms as they do so.
▶ A period of **sleep**. The baby will release the breast and fall asleep.

APPLICATION TO PRACTICE

Next time you are at a birth, try and take a step back and look at the environment. What are the factors that are facilitating feeding, bonding and attachment, and what factors are inhibiting this? How could the environment be improved?

Take time to observe the baby in skin-to-skin contact and watch physiology in action as they move to the breast to feed.

Responsive feeding and brain development

Feeding necessitates that mothers and infants spend time together, and the relationship forged as they interact with each other during this time has a long-lasting impact on the development of the neonatal brain. The neonatal period is a time of intense brain growth, during which **connections in neural pathways** can be forged at the rate of more than a million a second. Although the blueprint for this process is imprinted in the baby's genes, it is **epigenetics** – the interaction with their environment – that dictates how many, and how strongly, connections are built. When neurons are stimulated through events such as communication and interaction with others (verbally or otherwise), pathways are built in the brain. The more these pathways are used, the stronger they become. During early life, an infant lays down pathways which will determine their emotional capacity, behavioural control, motor skills, language and memory. An infant that is exposed to repeated, predictable, episodes of interaction and love will develop a strong and healthy network of connections from which more complex pathways can develop. This process is fuelled by **oxytocin** and can be damaged by prolonged exposure to **cortisol** (for example in conditions of chronic stress such as repeated episodes of prolonged crying), when pathways will be actively pruned back. **Insecure attachment** not only leads to reduced brain growth, but also directly impacts health throughout life. It is associated with a higher risk of strokes, heart attacks, high blood pressure and suffering pain, for example from headaches or arthritis.

Responding to a baby's **feeding cues**, which include rooting, suckling, hand to mouth and rapid eye movements, 'chattering' noises and restlessness, lays the foundations for their future emotional well-being. Cultural beliefs involving ignoring infants and imposing strict schedules on them are misinformed. **Responsive feeding** is also associated with reduced neonatal weight loss, a lower incidence of engorgement,

blocked ducts and mastitis, reduced bilirubin levels in the infant and an increased overall duration of breastfeeding.

Responsive feeding includes **reciprocity** – a mother may sometimes want to offer her baby a feed in order to feel close to them, or in order to accommodate feeding around other aspects of her or her family's life. In this way, a baby is assimilated into a family and wider social network. Building **strong bonds** with her baby through feeding also promotes a mothers' mental well-being. Receiving positive affirmations from her baby (such as eye contact, and their being soothed by her presence) will increase her confidence, and the oxytocin-rich environment of feeding is associated with reduced anxiety, stress and obsessiveness, lowering the risk of psychiatric and cardiovascular disorders.

Potential challenges to the physiological mechanisms of lactation

Thanks to a better understanding of breastfeeding physiology, the routine separation of mothers and babies in the early days after birth is no longer common practice in many birth settings. There are, however, still many conditions and routine cultural and professional practices, often working in tandem, which have the potential to disrupt breastfeeding physiology. Challenges can arise from pre-existing maternal conditions and behaviours, intrapartum events and care, the condition and gestational age of the baby at birth, and postpartum breast damage and pathology.

Pre-existing maternal conditions and behaviours

Hypothyroidism, **diabetes insipidus** and **polycystic ovary syndrome** can all affect **prolactin** secretion, potentially impacting milk synthesis. Women with

insulin-dependent (type I) diabetes may have lower serum prolactin levels, and their milk production will be further affected by a lack of readily available insulin (insulin is required to initiate milk production). Prolactin levels are also impacted by certain **medications** and oral contraceptives, particularly those containing oestrogen.

Smoking decreases the fat content of a mother's milk, potentially making it less able to meet an infant's needs. **Alcohol**, **stress** and **pain** can all have an effect on oxytocin release and hence, on the availability of synthesised milk to an infant.

It is suggested that **obesity** is associated with delayed lactogenesis II due to fat soluble progesterone levels decreasing more slowly postpartum, inhibiting the effect of prolactin. However, there is an ongoing debate as to whether obesity in and of itself leads to breastfeeding challenges, or whether it is the conditions and treatment that accompany plus sized women that are the problem. Larger women are more likely to have or develop diabetes in pregnancy, to develop pre-eclampsia, give birth by Caesarean section and sustain a postpartum haemorrhage. They are also less likely to be given the support to help them breastfeed due to prejudice and stigma surrounding their weight (Chang et al., 2020).

Breastfeeding can be successful after **breast surgery**, depending on the extent of tissue removal. It will probably require intense support. Breast surgery is a common cosmetic surgery in the UK and US. There have been reports of inadequate milk supply following breast augmentation, and the removal and reattachment of the areola and nipple complex during some breast reduction procedures can make breastfeeding incredibly problematic.

Intrapartum events and care

Any **medications** given to a woman in labour will cross the placenta. Newborns may be sleepy, lethargic, lack the energy to reach the breast themselves, and be unwilling to feed if their mothers have been given narcotic drugs. These may also inhibit the mother's ability to respond to her infant, and morphine in particular can lower the maternal oxytocin response to neonatal suckling. There is conflicting evidence around epidural use and breastfeeding, but not receiving any pain medication in labour is positively associated with continuing to breastfeed beyond six weeks (Dekker, 2018).

Neonates may also be unwilling to feed after birth if their mothers have been given large amounts of **intravenous fluid** in labour. These can also inflate the baby's birth weight, leading to excessive weight loss and subsequent concerns over milk supply in the early days after birth. Administration of synthetic oxytocin to women in labour can also inhibit the release of endogenous oxytocin, impacting milk release.

Caesarean birth can result in the delayed onset of lactogenesis II, probably due to a delayed rise in prolactin levels. Mothers will also experience fewer oxytocin pulses after a Caesarean. Lactogenesis II can also be delayed in women who experience significant **stress** in labour, and in the presence of **retained placental fragments**, which may prevent progesterone levels from decreasing. A severe **postpartum haemorrhage** and subsequent **reduced haemoglobin level** can result in fewer raw ingredients being available for milk synthesis, and also cause vascular injury to the pituitary gland.

Neonatal conditions

The **gestational age** of the baby at birth can affect its ability to suckle effectively. An infant born before 34 weeks gestation is unlikely to be able to draw enough breast tissue into their mouth to feed effectively, although they will root for, lick and nuzzle at the breast, stimulating milk supply. An infant born between 34–36 weeks may not initially be able to maintain their airway in some breastfeeding positions, and they are likely to tire quickly, lack tone in their cheeks to support negative pressure and have at least some episodes of uncoordinated suckling – the ability to suckle, swallow and breathe should emerge at some point over this period. Term infants of mothers with insulin-dependent diabetes can also display poor suckling patterns and may be less neurologically mature.

Gestational age also potentially impacts a mother's ability to produce milk. Breast development is ongoing in pregnancy, and there may not be sufficient lobular development before 28 weeks to support lactation. However, although this may result in a delay in lactogenesis II, lobular development can continue post pregnancy to meet an infant's need.

Some babies cannot **counter-regulate** effectively and so are at risk of hypoglycaemia if they do not feed frequently (see Chapter 5.2).

If a mother and/or baby experience **stress or trauma** around feeding (for example if the baby is pushed onto the breast by a clinician, or the mother is extremely tense), a baby may 'refuse' the breast and become agitated and upset when offered a breastfeed. Breast refusal can also be a reaction to the smell of a particular washing powder or soap. The removal of the stressor and a warm, calm environment including skin-to-skin contact can help resolve this situation.

Postpartum care, breast damage and pathology

The introduction of **breastmilk substitutes** has been shown to negatively impact breastfeeding by diminishing breastmilk synthesis (as the baby removes less milk from the breast); have a significant adverse effect on gut flora, potentially leading to conditions such as necrotising enterocolitis (NEC); promote sensitivity to cow's milk protein; and trigger the development of diabetes in babies from susceptible families. Any **separation of mother and baby**, or **delay in initial skin-to-skin contact or feeding**, also has the potential to adversely affect breastfeeding and harm the baby. A systematic review found that the risk of mortality was reduced by 33% in neonates initiating breastfeeding within an hour of birth, compared to those initiating breastfeeding between 2–23 hours. Infants initiating breastfeeding 24 hours after birth had an 85% greater risk of mortality (Smith et al., 2017). **Pacifier use** may also impact breastmilk supply and delay lactogenesis II, as babies are likely to be brought to the breast less often. **Ineffective** and/or **infrequent suckling**, and not bringing the baby to the breast each time they indicate a wish to feed, will have the same effect.

The aetiology and management of some common **lactation pathologies** is outlined in Table 6.3.1.

Contraindications to breastfeeding

There are very few situations in which breastfeeding or giving infants breastmilk is contraindicated. Infants with **galactosemia** (a metabolic condition where infants cannot convert breastmilk sugars into glucose) cannot tolerate breastmilk. In most developed countries, breastfeeding is not advised if a mother is **HIV positive**. However, in countries where morbidity

6.3

and mortality due to diarrhoea, pneumonia and malnutrition are high, the risks of not breastfeeding are considered higher than the risk of contracting HIV through breastmilk. Caution is required for **viral infections** such as herpes and hepatitis B and C, and **bacterial infections** such as tuberculosis. Individual circumstances should be considered in these cases, but breastfeeding is usually possible.

Medications taken by the mother will inevitably transfer to her milk. Breastfeeding is not usually recommended if a mother is receiving **radiation** or **chemotherapy**. Again, the risks and benefits need to be considered on a case-by-case basis. Antibiotics in breastmilk may cause a baby to become unsettled and produce foamy green stools. They will also destroy the baby's gut flora. It can be difficult for clinicians to access information about the effects of medications in breastmilk, as many drug companies will routinely label their products as unsuitable for breastfeeding mothers. The use of **specialist lactation resources** such as the UK Drugs in Lactation Advisory Service (UKDILAS) (www.midlandsmedicines. nhs.uk) or the Spanish service E-lactancia (www.e-lactancia.org) is advised.

APPLICATION TO PRACTICE

Use your usual source of medication knowledge (such as the British National Formulary (BNF)) to look up the anti-depressant drug sertraline. What does it say about prescribing this drug to breastfeeding mothers?

Now look up the same drug on the UKDILAS site, or on E-lactancia. If a mother in your care was requiring medication, which resource is more useful?

The physiological implications of not breastfeeding

Breastmilk and breastfeeding have evolved over centuries to optimise the survival and well-being of humankind. Infants who are fed breastmilk substitutes are at greater risk of **necrotising enterocolitis, gastroenteritis, severe respiratory illness, ear, chest** and **urinary tract infections**. Their guts will develop differently, and their microbiome will be less able to protect them from certain conditions in later life, making them more likely to be **obese** and suffer from **hypertension, cardiovascular disease, diabetes** and **other autoimmune disorders such as Crohn's**. The brain architecture of formula fed infants is also compromised, with reduced mental and psychomotor development leading to **lower IQ scores**.

Supporting exclusive breastfeeding for the first six months of life is therefore a health priority. Formula milk is an inert fluid that contains none of the live protective factors in breastmilk. The introduction of any formula substitutes will potentially **sensitise** the baby, leading to future **allergic reactions**, and will **alter the acidic environment in the gut**. It will take 2–4 weeks of exclusive breastfeeding following formula ingestion to correct this. That being said, many midwives work in settings where formula milk is heavily promoted and considered a desirable alternative to breastmilk. If a mother chooses to introduce supplementary feeds, gently supporting her to maximise her baby's breastmilk intake alongside this will be less damaging to the baby's long-term health than not being fed any breastmilk at all. Mothers can also be shown how to offer formula feeds responsively, in order to capture some of the relational benefits of breastfeeding. The UNICEF BFI website contains information about responsive bottle feeding that can be shared with mothers.

Not breastfeeding also has a physiological impact on **mothers**. The oxytocin released through breastfeeding immediately after birth stimulates further contraction of the uterus, assisting placental separation and reducing **blood loss**. Lactation also promotes calcium uptake in the maternal duodenum, leading to increased **bone mass** in the lumbar spine and protecting mothers from **osteoporosis** and **hip problems** in later life. Women who breastfeed for longer than thirteen months are less likely to suffer from **arthritis**. Breastfeeding is further known to be protective against **ovarian** and **breast cancer** and **type II diabetes**, and breastfeeding mothers are better able to space their conceptions.

6.3

Table 6.3.1 Common lactation pathology

Symptoms	Likely cause	Suggested management	Possible alternative diagnosis
Painful, damaged nipples Nipples can be sore (inflamed and painful), and/or cracked (the skin is broken and there is a wound)	Poor positioning and attachment	Observe a feed Gentle support with positioning and attachment If the nipple is sore, correct positioning and attachment should result in pain-free feeding (although until the soreness has resolved there may be some initial discomfort when the baby latches) A Cochrane review (Dennis et al., 2014) which did not differentiate between sore or cracked nipples, found that applying nothing or expressed breastmilk may improve pain symptoms in the short term more effectively than the application of ointment If the nipple is cracked and wounded, most authorities concur that moist wound healing should be encouraged: apply petroleum jelly or purified lanolin after a feed to keep the wound moist and prevent a scab forming (which would be damaged and removed as the baby fed) Support the mother to find a comfortable feeding position while the wound heals Feeding is likely to be less painful than expressing Temporarily resting the breast is a last resort Offer analgesics for pain management	1. Tongue tie – refer to lactation specialist for diagnosis and treatment if correct positioning and attachment does not resolve symptoms 2. Thrush (see below)

(Continued)

Table 6.3.1 (Continued)

Symptoms	Likely cause	Suggested management	Possible alternative diagnosis
Painful, possibly damaged nipple and/or breast Usually sudden in onset, present in both breasts, and experienced as a severe pain extending deep into the breast and persisting after each feed	Thrush	Swab mother's nipples and baby's mouth to confirm (it is likely that both will be infected, and both should be treated) Observe a feed to rule out problems with latch If diagnosis confirmed, miconazole cream is recommended for the nipples, and miconazole oral gel for the baby To help prevent reinfection, strict hand hygiene should be observed, and family members should use separate towels	1. Poor positioning and attachment (see above) 2. Allergic reaction to breast pad, bra or creams 3. Bacterial infection
Warm, firm, tender, heavy breasts	Breast fullness – this is normal and not problematic unless the mother has a fever, the baby cannot latch and/or milk does not flow readily	Hand express a little milk prior to offering feed in order to soften the breast to help the baby to latch	
'Pin-point' pain radiating from a white spot/blister on the nipple	The white spot usually indicates a blockage at the tip of a duct, and the pain is caused by milk building up behind it	The white spot can be opened up by being gently rubbed with a clean cloth, or using a sterile needle	
Hot, hard, tight, shiny, painful breast Possible localised areas of soreness/inflammation and or palpable lump/abscess Possible maternal fever	Mastitis: includes a spectrum of symptoms from engorgement to a severe infection and/or inflammatory response Symptoms can result from poor feeding technique, restricted feeding or anything that causes a restriction of milk flow (e.g. a tight or underwired bra or a finger pressed into the breast during a feed)	Continue to feed/express according to baby's needs Do not remove more milk than necessary as this could make the inflammation worse Engorgement results in oedematous tissue, so milk ducts will be narrowed and it will be harder for milk to flow Warm flannels or a warm shower can encourage milk flow (but use these judiciously, as they can exacerbate inflammation) Hand expression will help soften the breast so that the baby can latch (if the breast is hard, the baby will not be able to mould it to stabilise it in their mouth)	1.Sepsis. Symptoms of mastitis are extremely similar to the symptoms of sepsis; therefore, although there is no physiological basis for treating non-infective mastitis with antibiotics, antibiotics are now recommended as a first line treatment If a woman is deteriorating rapidly, and/ or does not respond to initial management measures, refer for urgent medical attention

(Continued)

Table 6.3.1 (Continued)

Symptoms	Likely cause	Suggested management	Possible alternative diagnosis
	Mastitis can be non-infective as the body mounts a systemic response to milk leaking into the surrounding tissue as it is prevented from flowing freely through the ducts, or infective as the same response is mounted to a foreign pathogen, usually entering the breast through a damaged nipple	Cold compresses after feeding/expressing can help reduce inflammation Check positioning and attachment to ensure that the baby is draining the breast effectively Position the baby so that they latch with their chin adjacent to any hot, hard and/or inflamed areas of breast tissue, to facilitate drainage of these areas Secure a course of antibiotics; these will treat infective mastitis and lessen any inflammation associated with non-infective mastitis Offer further analgesics and anti-inflammatories to ease symptoms of pain, fever and inflammation If an abscess is present, surgical removal may be necessary	2. Breast cancer: any unusual breast swellings or lumps that do not respond to antibiotics should be urgently referred to rule out cancer

6.3

CHAPTER CHALLENGE

The latest research on breastfeeding and a number of maternal health issues can be found on the UNICEF BFI website: www.unicef.org.uk/babyfriendly/news-and-research/baby-friendly-research/maternal-health-research/

Have a look at the research in one of the areas listed and answer the following questions:

In what ways does the condition impact physiologically on breastfeeding?

How would breastfeeding benefit the babies of mothers with the condition?

How can midwives better support these particular women to breastfeed?

In your opinion, to what extent is the research free from bias, and what further research is required?

References

Chang Y.S., Glaria A.A. et al. Breastfeeding experiences and support for women who are overweight or obese: A mixed-methods systematic review. *Matern. Child Nutr.* [Internet] 2020, 16(1). https://pubmed.ncbi.nlm.nih.gov/31240826/.

Colson S., Meek J. et al. Optimal positions for the release of primitive neonatal reflexes stimulating breastfeeding. *Early Hum. Dev.* [Internet] 2008, 84(7):441–9. www.sciencedirect.com/science/article/pii/S0378378207002423.

Dekker R. Effect of epidurals on breastfeeding. Evidence Based Birth [Internet]. 2018. https://evidencebasedbirth.com/effect-of-epidurals-on-breastfeeding/.

Dennis C.-L., Jackson K. et al. Interventions for treating painful nipples among breastfeeding women. *Cochrane Database Syst. Rev.* 2014. doi:10.1002/14651858.CD007366.pub2.

Morton J. How to Use Your Hands When You Pump [Video]. 2017. https://med.stanford.edu/newborns/professional-education/breastfeeding/maximizing-milk-production.html.

Smith E.R., Hurt L. et al. Delayed breastfeeding initiation and infant survival: A systematic review and meta-analysis. *PLoS ONE* [Internet] 2017, 12(7). https://journals.plos.org/plosone/article?id=10.1371/journal.pone.0180722.

Further reading

Wambach K., Riordan J. *Breastfeeding and human lactation* (5th edition). Burlington, MA: Jones and Bartlett Learning, 2016.

Index

Note: Page numbers in *italics* indicate figures, and those in **bold** indicate tables.